The Dizzy Patient

Editors

MAJA SVRAKIC
MEREDITH E. ADAMS

OTOLARYNGOLOGIC CLINICS OF NORTH AMERICA

www.oto.theclinics.com

Consulting Editor
SUJANA S. CHANDRASEKHAR

October 2021 • Volume 54 • Number 5

ELSEVIER

1600 John F. Kennedy Boulevard • Suite 1800 • Philadelphia, Pennsylvania, 19103-2899

http://www.oto.theclinics.com

OTOLARYNGOLOGIC CLINICS OF NORTH AMERICA Volume 54, Number 5
October 2021 ISSN 0030-6665, ISBN-13: 978-0-323-89674-0

Editor: Stacy Eastman
Developmental Editor: Diana Ang

Otolaryngologic Clinics of North America (ISSN 0030-6665) is published bimonthly by Elsevier, Inc., 360 Park Avenue South, New York, NY 10010-1710. Months of issue are February, April, June, August, October, and December. Business and Editorial Offices: 1600 John F. Kennedy Blvd., Suite 1800, Philadelphia, PA 19103-2899. Customer Service Office: 6277 Sea Harbor Drive, Orlando, FL 32887-4800. Periodicals postage paid at New York, NY and additional mailing offices. Subscription prices are $437.00 per year (US individuals), $1278.00 per year (US institutions), $100.00 per year (US & Canadian student/resident), $559.00 per year (Canadian individuals), $1348.00 per year (Canadian institutions), $610.00 per year (international individuals), $1348.00 per year (international institutions), $270.00 per year (international student/resident). Foreign air speed delivery is included in all *Clinics*' subscription prices. All prices are subject to change without notice. **POSTMASTER:** Send address changes to *Otolaryngologic Clinics of North America*, Elsevier Health Sciences Division, Subscription Customer Service, 3251 Riverport Lane, Maryland Heights, MO 63043. **Telephone: 1-800-654-2452 (U.S. and Canada); 314-447-8871 (outside U.S. and Canada). Fax: 314-447-8029. E-mail: journalscustomerservice-usa@elsevier.com (for print support); journalsonlinesupport-usa@elsevier.com (for online support).**

Reprints. For copies of 100 or more of articles in this publication, please contact the Commercial Reprints Department, Elsevier Inc., 360 Park Avenue South, New York, NY 10010-1710. Tel.: 212-633-3874; Fax: 212-633-3820; E-mail: reprints@elsevier.com.

Otolaryngologic Clinics of North America is also published in Spanish by McGraw-Hill Interamericana Editores S.A., P.O. Box 5-237, 06500 Mexico D.F., Mexico.

Otolaryngologic Clinics of North America is covered in *MEDLINE/PubMed (Index Medicus), Current Contents/Clinical Medicine, Excerpta Medica, BIOSIS, Science Citation Index,* and *ISI/BIOMED.*

Contributors

CONSULTING EDITOR

SUJANA S. CHANDRASEKHAR, MD, FACS, FAAOHNS
Past President, American Academy of Otolaryngology–Head and Neck Surgery, Secretary-Treasurer, American Otological Society, Partner, ENT & Allergy Associates, LLP, Clinical Professor, Department of Otolaryngology–Head and Neck Surgery, Donald and Barbara Zucker School of Medicine at Hofstra/Northwell, Hempstead, New York; Clinical Associate Professor, Department of Otolaryngology–Head and Neck Surgery, Icahn School of Medicine at Mount Sinai, New York, New York

EDITORS

MAJA SVRAKIC, MD, MSEd
Associate Professor, Department of Otolaryngology, Donald and Barbara Zucker School of Medicine at Hofstra/Northwell, Northwell Health, New Hyde Park, New York

MEREDITH E. ADAMS, MD, MS
Associate Professor, Department of Otolaryngology–Head and Neck Surgery, University of Minnesota, Minneapolis, Minnesota

AUTHORS

MEREDITH E. ADAMS, MD, MS
Associate Professor, Department of Otolaryngology–Head and Neck Surgery, University of Minnesota, Minneapolis, Minnesota

YURI AGRAWAL, MD, MPH
Professor, Department of Otolaryngology–Head and Neck Surgery, Professor, Johns Hopkins University, Baltimore, Maryland

JENNIFER ALYONO, MD, MS, FACS
Clinical Assistant Professor, Department of Otolaryngology–Head and Neck Surgery, Stanford University School of Medicine, Stanford, California

RICHARD BARON, MD
Adult Neurology Resident, Department of Neurology and Neurological Sciences, Stanford University School of Medicine, Stanford, California

SHIN C. BEH, MD
Assistant Professor of Neurology, Director, Vestibular and Neuro-Visual Disorders Clinic, The University of Texas Southwestern Medical Center, Dallas, Texas

WENDY J. CARENDER, PT, MPT
Department of Otolaryngology–Head and Neck Surgery, Michigan Medicine, University of Michigan, Michigan Balance Vestibular Testing and Rehabilitation, Ann Arbor, Michigan

DIVYA A. CHARI, MD
Clinical Fellow in Otology, Neurotology, and Skull Base Surgery, Department of Otolaryngology–Head and Neck Surgery, Massachusetts Eye and Ear, Department of Otolaryngology–Head and Neck Surgery, Harvard Medical School, Boston, Massachusetts

LAURA CHRISTOPHER, MD
Jackson Ear Clinic, Flowood, Mississippi

MAURA K. COSETTI, MD
Department of Otolaryngology–Head and Neck Surgery, Icahn School of Medicine at Mount Sinai, Ear Institute, New York Eye and Ear Infirmary of Mount Sinai, New York, New York

M. JENNIFER DEREBERY, MD, FACS
House Ear Clinic and Institute, Los Angeles, California

DANIEL R. GOLD, DO
Department of Neurology, Johns Hopkins School of Medicine, Baltimore, Maryland

MELISSA GRZESIAK, PT, DPT
Department of Otolaryngology–Head and Neck Surgery, Michigan Medicine, University of Michigan, Michigan Balance Vestibular Testing and Rehabilitation, Ann Arbor, Michigan

MARI HAGIWARA, MD
Associate Professor, Department of Radiology, NYU Langone Health, New York, New York

ERIN ISANHART, PT, DPT, NCS
Angular Momentum Physical Therapy, San Jose, California

KRISTEN L. JANKY, AuD, PhD
Department of Audiology, Boys Town National Research Hospital, Omaha, Nebraska

NICOLE T. JIAM, MD
Department of Otolaryngology–Head and Neck Surgery, University of California San Francisco School of Medicine, San Francisco, California

ELIZABETH A. KELLY, MD
Department of Otolaryngology, Boys Town National Research Hospital, Omaha, Nebraska

JENNIFER KELLY, DPT
Ear Institute, New York Eye and Ear Infirmary of Mount Sinai, New York, New York

CHRISTINE LITTLE, BA
Department of Otolaryngology–Head and Neck Surgery, Icahn School of Medicine at Mount Sinai, New York, New York

YUAN F. LIU, MD
Assistant Professor, Department of Otolaryngology–Head and Neck Surgery, Loma Linda University Health, Loma Linda, California

WASSIM MALAK, MD
Neuroradiology Fellow, Department of Radiology, NYU Langone Health, New York, New York

EMMA MARTIN, MD
Department of Otolaryngology–Head and Neck Surgery, Otolaryngology Resident, University of Illinois at Chicago, Chicago, Illinois

BIBHUTI MISHRA, MD
Director of Neurology, LIJ Forest Hills Hospital, New York; Professor of Surgery, George Washington University, Washington, DC

ASHKAN MONFARED, MD
Professor of Surgery and Neurosurgery, Division of Otolaryngology, The GW Medical Faculty Associates, Washington, DC

OLWEN C. MURPHY, MBBCh, MRCPI
Department of Neurology, Johns Hopkins School of Medicine, Baltimore, Maryland

VINH NGUYEN, MD
Clinical Associate Professor, Department of Radiology, NYU Langone Health, New York, New York

JESSIE N. PATTERSON, AuD, PhD
Department of Audiology, Boys Town National Research Hospital, Omaha, Nebraska

STEVEN D. RAUCH, MD
Professor, Department of Otolaryngology–Head and Neck Surgery, Massachusetts Eye and Ear, Department of Otolaryngology–Head and Neck Surgery, Harvard Medical School, Boston, Massachusetts

MALLORY J. RAYMOND, MD
Department of Otolaryngology–Head and Neck Surgery, Medical University of South Carolina, Charleston, South Carolina

HABIB G. RIZK, MD, MSCR
Associate Professor, Chair Clinical and Translational Research Ethics, Department of Otolaryngology–Head and Neck Surgery, Charleston, South Carolina

DESI P. SCHOO, MD
Department of Otolaryngology–Head and Neck Surgery, Johns Hopkins School of Medicine, Baltimore, Maryland

JEFFREY D. SHARON, MD
Department of Otolaryngology–Head and Neck Surgery, University of California San Francisco School of Medicine, San Francisco, California

NEERAJ SINGH, MD
Assistant Professor of Neurology, Zucker School of Medicine at Hofstra/Northwell, Director of Epilepsy and EEG, LIJ Forest Hills Hospital, Northwell Health, New York

DONG-IN SINN, MD
Department of Neurology and Neurological Sciences, Stanford University School of Medicine, Palo Alto, California

KRISTEN K. STEENERSON, MD
Clinical Assistant Professor, Departments of Neurology and Neurological Sciences, and Otolaryngology–Head and Neck Surgery, Stanford University School of Medicine, Palo Alto, California

MAJA SVRAKIC, MD, MSEd
Associate Professor, Department of Otolaryngology, Donald and Barbara Zucker School
of Medicine at Hofstra/Northwell, Northwell Health, New Hyde Park, New York

STEVEN A. TELIAN, MD
John L. Kemink Professor of Neurotology, Department of Otolaryngology–Head and Neck
Surgery, University of Michigan, Ann Arbor, Michigan

ESTHER X. VIVAS, MD
Associate Professor, Department of Otolaryngology–Head and Neck Surgery, Emory
University School of Medicine, Atlanta, Georgia

BRYAN K. WARD, MD
Department of Otolaryngology–Head and Neck Surgery, Johns Hopkins School of
Medicine, Baltimore, Maryland

HEATHER M. WEINREICH, MD, MPH
Assistant Professor, Department of Otolaryngology–Head and Neck Surgery, Assistant
Professor, University of Illinois at Chicago, Chicago, Illinois

ILANA YELLIN, MD
Resident Physician, Department of Otolaryngology, Donald and Barbara Zucker School of
Medicine at Hofstra/Northwell, New Hyde Park, New York

ASHLEY ZALESKI-KING, AuD, PhD
Assistant Research Professor, Otolaryngology, The GW Medical Faculty Associates,
Washington, DC

STEVEN A. ZUNIGA, MD
Neurotology Fellow, Department of Otolaryngology—Head and Neck Surgery, University
of Minnesota, Minneapolis, Minnesota

Contents

The evaluation of dizziness as a chief complaint can be exceptionally challenging to otolaryngologists. The critical piece in evaluating dizzy patients is to have a plan for how to screen and schedule, how to gather data, and to develop a workflow for testing that allows clinical efficiency. This article provides an overview of evidence-based practices on how to screen dizzy patients before being scheduled, how to efficiently move patients through the otolaryngologist's clinic, and strategies for managing a dizzy practice.

When interviewing a patient presenting with dizziness, it is imperative to both diagnosis and treatment for the clinician to identify the impact dizziness has on the patient's productivity, general function level and cognition. and cognition. Psychiatric comorbidities and concurrent sleep disturbances are common in this patient population and identification of these additional factors is important in implementing a holistic, multidisciplinary treatment plan and ultimately improves the patient's outcome.

Dizziness is a common complaint in otolaryngology clinics and can present a diagnostic challenge. A thorough history including onset, duration, and exacerbating and alleviating factors, along with physician persistence, can help differentiate between otologic and nonotologic forms of dizziness. An otologic and neurotologic physical examination, including vestibulo-ocular reflex and cranial nerve function evaluation and postural examination, can shed further light on symptom etiology. Otologic forms of dizziness often result in vertigo and may be associated with unilateral symptoms of hearing loss, aural fullness, or tinnitus. Primary causes of dizziness are more often constant and insidious in onset.

Central vestibulopathies involve disorders of the central nervous system that lead to problems with balance, often manifested as dizziness, vertigo, and gait difficulty. Central vestibulopathies can be distinguished from peripheral vestibulopathies with the use of certain tests, including nystagmography and posturography. The neuroanatomy of individuals with central vestibulopathies may reveal structural abnormalities in the posterior cerebrum or cerebellum. Various medications may be used to manage central vestibulopathies, including vestibular migraine.

Vestibular migraine (VM) is one of the most common neurologic causes of vertigo. Symptoms and International Classification of Headache Disorders criteria are used to diagnose VM because no objective tests, imaging or audiologic, have been shown to reliably diagnose this condition. Central auditory, peripheral, and central vestibular pathway involvement has been associated with VM. Although the interaction between migraine and other vestibular disorders can be a challenging scenario for diagnosis and treatment, there are data to show that vestibular rehabilitation and a variety of pharmacologic agents improve reported symptoms and vertigo frequency.

 Video content accompanies this article at http://www.pmr.theclinics. com.

Initial diagnosis of peripheral vestibulopathy requires a detailed history, physical examination, and, in some cases, audiovestibular testing, radiographic imaging, or serology. Differentiation of a peripheral vestibulopathy as progressive or degenerative is often nuanced and influenced by a characterization of a patient's symptoms or natural history over time. A diverse group of vestibular pathology may fit into this category, including Ménière's disease, autoimmune conditions, congenital pathologies, ototoxic medications, radiation therapy, and perilymphatic fistula. Differentiation among these entities may be guided by initial or subsequent symptomatology, with various combinations of audiovestibular testing, serology, and imaging. Treatment options are disparate and disease-specific, ranging from observation to medical management or surgical intervention, underscoring the need for astute investigation and diagnosis.

Dizziness occurs in children with an estimated prevalence of 0.45% to 15.0%. Vestibular disorders in the pediatric population can impact gross motor function development, visual acuity, and contribute to psychological distress. Appropriate case history and focused direct examination can be helpful when determining the etiology of dizziness. Vestibular testing can be completed in children and guide management of suspected vestibular dysfunction. Vestibular dysfunction is commonly seen in patients with sensorineural hearing loss. Migraine disorders are the most common cause of dizziness in childhood. Etiologies of dizziness in children differ from those commonly seen in adults.

There is a reciprocal relationship between vestibular and neuropsychological disorders. People with vertigo and dizziness are at higher risk of various psychiatric disorders, particularly anxiety, depression, and panic disorder. On the other hand, people with mood disorders are at higher risk of experiencing vertigo and dizziness. Vestibular information plays a crucial role in cognitive processes, especially visuo-spatial abilities. Consequently, vestibular disorders (both peripheral and central) often result in visuo-spatial deficits. In addition, lesions of the cortical and subcortical components of the vestibular system result in disorders of higher vestibular function, such as hemispatial neglect, pusher syndrome, and topographagnosia.

 Video content accompanies this article at http://www.pmr.theclinics. com.

Dizziness is a common chief complaint with an extensive differential diagnosis that ranges from peripheral, central, to nonvestibular conditions. An understanding of nonvestibular conditions will aid accurate diagnosis and initiation of appropriate management. Thus, the objective of this article is to present an overview of nonvestibular etiologies that may plague a dizzy patient and the recommended treatment options.

 Video content accompanies this article at http://www.pmr.theclinics. com.

Vestibular physical therapy (VPT) is a specialized form of evidence-based therapy designed to alleviate primary (vertigo, dizziness, imbalance, gait instability, falls) and secondary (deconditioning, cervical muscle tension, anxiety, poor quality of life, fear of falling/fear avoidance behavior) symptoms related to vestibular disorders. This article provides an overview of VPT, highlighting various exercise modalities used to treat a variety of vestibular disorders. Patient safety and fall prevention are paramount; therefore, fall risk assessment and treatment are also addressed.

Medical therapies for dizziness are aimed at vertigo reduction, secondary symptom management, or the root cause of the pathologic process. Acute peripheral vertigo pharmacotherapies include antihistamines, calcium channel blockers, and benzodiazepines. Prophylactic pharmacotherapies vary between causes. For Meniere disease, betahistine and diuretics remain initial first-line oral options, whereas intratympanic steroids and intratympanic gentamicin are reserved for uncontrolled symptoms. For cerebellar dizziness and oculomotor disorders, 4-aminopyridine may provide benefit. For vestibular migraine, persistent postural perceptual dizziness and mal de débarquement, treatment options overlap and include selective serotonin reuptake inhibitors, serotonin-norepinephrine reuptake inhibitors, tricyclic antidepressants and calcium channel blockers.

Allergic reactions may result in central symptoms of dizziness, including nonspecific chronic imbalance, Meniere's disease, and autoimmune inner ear disease. Excepting first-generation antihistamines, and short-term use of steroids, most pharmacotherapies used to treat allergic rhinitis have limited benefit in treating allergically induced or related dizziness. Allergy immunotherapy and/or an elimination diet for diagnosed food allergies have been found to be effective treatments. Individuals diagnosed with autoimmune inner ear disease remain challenging to treat and may require high-dose, long-term steroid treatment, biologics, or immunomodulators for symptom control.

Despite progress in vestibular research in the last 20 years, much remains poorly understood about vestibular pathophysiology and its management. A shared language is a critical first step in understanding vestibular disorders and is under development. Telehealth will continue for patients with dizziness, and ambulatory monitoring of nystagmus will become a diagnostic tool. In the next 2 decades, it is anticipated that vestibular perceptual threshold testing will become common in tertiary centers, imaging with improved spatial resolution will yield better understanding of vestibular pathophysiology, and that vestibular implants will become a part of clinical practice.

OTOLARYNGOLOGIC CLINICS
OF NORTH AMERICA

SERIES OF RELATED INTEREST

Facial Plastic Surgery Clinics
Available at: https://www.facialplastic.theclinics.com/

THE CLINICS ARE AVAILABLE ONLINE!
Access your subscription at:
www.theclinics.com

Foreword

"Doctor, I'm Dizzy": Approaching the Dizzy Patient Comprehensively and Compassionately

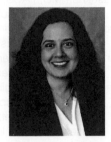

Sujana S. Chandrasekhar, MD, FACS, FAAOHNS
Consulting Editor

Trying to help patients who are dizzy can be most frustrating and challenging, but if one takes time, patience, and effort, their care can be the most rewarding as well.

Dizziness is a broadly encompassing symptom that affects 15% to 20% of the population annually, with one-quarter of the cases being classified as vestibular vertigo.[1] The lifetime prevalence estimates of significant dizziness range between 17% and 30%, and for vertigo range between 3% and 10%.[2] Dizziness accounts for 5% of walk-in clinic and 4% of emergency department (ED) visits. In the ED, patients with this complaint are evaluated for longer times, imaged more, and admitted more often than those with other complaints. One-third of patients in the ED receive an otologic/vestibular diagnosis; half are given a medical diagnosis; 11% receive a neurologic diagnosis; 7% are given a psychiatric diagnosis, and nearly one-quarter leave with the symptom of dizziness or vertigo as their "diagnosis." Medical diagnoses found in the ED include cardiovascular, respiratory, metabolic, injury/poisoning, digestive, genitourinary, and infectious.[3] Likewise, dizziness accounts for 5% of primary care office visits, where the importance of history distinguishing between vertigo, disequilibrium, presyncope, and lightheadedness is emphasized, but with 20% again not receiving a diagnosis.[4] Most of these patients are referred on to the otolaryngologist or neurologist.

"Doctor, I'm dizzy" is such a nonspecific statement that the importance of obtaining a focused yet comprehensive history including defining the patient's actual symptoms cannot be overemphasized. Only then can the assessment proceed in a logical fashion, streamlining the workup and facilitating the arrival at a diagnosis as often as possible, so that appropriate treatment can be instituted.

Otolaryngol Clin N Am 54 (2021) xiii–xiv
https://doi.org/10.1016/j.otc.2021.06.008
0030-6665/21/© 2021 Published by Elsevier Inc.

oto.theclinics.com

Drs Maja Svrakic and Meredith Adams, the Guest Editors of this comprehensive issue of *Otolaryngologic Clinics of North America* on The Dizzy Patient, have ensured that the reader has access to the most up-to-date knowledge on vestibular dizziness. The reader is encouraged to savor the attention to historical detail, quality of life, targeted testing, and thoughtful treatment that is covered in this issue and share some of the "out of the box" thinking with their colleagues in other specialties. The next time a patient comes in saying they are dizzy, don't panic! Use the resources and thought processes herein.

Sujana S. Chandrasekhar, MD, FACS, FAAOHNS
Consulting Editor
Otolaryngologic Clinics of North America
Past President
American Academy of Otolaryngology–
Head and Neck Surgery
Secretary-Treasurer, American Otological Society
Partner, ENT & Allergy Associates LLP
18 East 48th Street, 2nd Floor
New York, NY 10017, USA

Clinical Professor, Department of Otolaryngology–
Head and Neck Surgery
Zucker School of Medicine at Hofstra-Northwell
Hempstead, NY, USA

Clinical Associate Professor
Department of Otolaryngology–
Head and Neck Surgery
Icahn School of Medicine at Mount Sinai
New York, NY, USA

E-mail address:
ssc@nyotology.com

Website:
http://www.ears.nyc

REFERENCES

1. Neuhauser HK. The epidemiology of dizziness and vertigo. Handb Clin Neurol 2016;137:67–82.
2. Murdin L, Schilder AG. Epidemiology of balance symptoms and disorders in the community: a systematic review. Otol Neurotol 2015;36(3):387–92.
3. Newman-Toker DE, Hsieh YH, Camargo CA Jr, et al. Spectrum of dizziness visits to US emergency departments: cross-sectional analysis from a nationally representative sample. Mayo Clin Proc 2008;83(7):765–75.
4. Post RE, Dickerson LM. Dizziness: a diagnostic approach. Am Fam Physician 2010;82(4):361–8, 369.

Preface
Rollercoaster of a Ride: More Effective, Efficient, and Rewarding Care for the Dizzy Patient

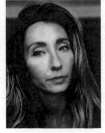
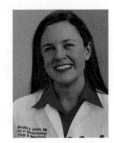

Maja Svrakic, MD, MSEd   Meredith E. Adams, MD, MS

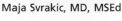

Editors

With its broad differential diagnosis and significant impact on quality of life, dizziness is a common symptom that presents substantial diagnostic and therapeutic challenges. This issue focuses on the clinical evaluation and management of the broad range of dizziness symptoms and syndromes. A multidisciplinary and interprofessional approach is promoted, supported by diverse authorship by specialists from the fields of otolaryngology, neurology, audiology, physical therapy, neuroradiology, and internal and emergency medicine. As accurate and efficient diagnosis is often the most challenging aspect of care for the dizzy patient, the issue delves deeply into evidence-based recommendations for the systematic evaluation of dizziness, best practices for clinic triage and multidisciplinary care, counseling, and assessment of quality of life. This edition then features not only the "classic" vestibular disorders in adults and children (eg, acute vestibular syndrome, positional vertigo, progressive and degenerative peripheral disorders) but also important neurologic and nonvestibular dizziness syndromes, which may be less familiar (although no less important) to the otolaryngologist (eg, vestibular migraine, chronic central vestibulopathies, and cardiac, ophthalmologic, orthopedic, and metabolic disorders). As common comorbidities and the interplay of psychiatric and neurologic factors add additional diagnostic, treatment, and prognostic challenges, the neuropsychology of dizziness and related disorders is also highlighted. In addition to learning the most up-to-date approaches to medical management and vestibular therapy, readers are also given a look into the future of vestibular medicine and surgery, and a valuable perspective on the use of complementary and alternative medicine. Ultimately, the issue aims to

Otolaryngol Clin N Am 54 (2021) xv–xvi
https://doi.org/10.1016/j.otc.2021.06.005
0030-6665/21/© 2021 Published by Elsevier Inc.

provide clinicians with useful information that will turn office visits with dizzy patients—
which previously may have seemed cumbersome—into efficient, effective, and
rewarding interactions for patients and providers alike.

Maja Svrakic, MD, MSEd
Department of Otolaryngology
Northwell Health
Hearing & Speech Center
430 Lakeville Road
New Hyde Park, NY 11042, USA

Meredith E. Adams, MD, MS
Department of Otolaryngology–
Head and Neck Surgery
University of Minnesota
420 Delaware Street Southeast, MMC 396
Minneapolis, MN 55455, USA

E-mail addresses:
msvrakic@northwell.edu (M. Svrakic)
meadams@umn.edu (M.E. Adams)

Overview of Dizziness in Practice

Heather M. Weinreich, MD, MPH[a],*, Emma Martin, MD[a], Yuri Agrawal, MD, MPH[b]

KEYWORDS

- Vertigo • Screening questionnaire • Multidisciplinary clinic • Falls

KEY POINTS

- About 50% of patients presenting to an otolaryngology clinic have a neuro-otologic condition.
- Evidence-based screening tools and questionnaires should be used to efficiently categorize patients based on symptoms.
- Vestibular testing is not diagnostic but can be used to evaluate the function of the semicircular canals and otolith organs as well as compensation for any loss of function.
- The creation of a multidisciplinary clinic to aid in diagnosis and management of dizzy patients is recommended.
- High-risk patients should be screened for falls.

INTRODUCTION

Dizziness can be a challenging chief complaint for many clinicians, including otolaryngologists. The key to seeing these patients is to have a plan. This article provides an overview of evidence-based practices on how to screen dizzy patients before being scheduled, how to efficiently move patients through the clinic, and strategies for managing a dizzy clinic.

PREVALENCE/INCIDENCE

Annually, 3% to 4% of all patients who present to an emergency department (ED) have a chief complaint of dizziness,[1] whereas for primary care, annual visits range from 1% to 15.5%.[2] For emergency medicine alone, this translates to between 3.9 million and 5.2 million visits per year.[3]

[a] Department of Otolaryngology Head and Neck Surgery, University of Illinois at Chicago, 1855 West Taylor Street, Chicago, IL 60612, USA; [b] Department of Otolaryngology Head and Neck Surgery, Johns Hopkins University, 601 North Caroline Street, 6th Floor JHOC, Baltimore, MD 21287, USA
* Corresponding author.
E-mail address: hweinre1@uic.edu
Twitter: @yuriagrawal (Y.A.)

Otolaryngol Clin N Am 54 (2021) 839–852
https://doi.org/10.1016/j.otc.2021.05.008
0030-6665/21/© 2021 Elsevier Inc. All rights reserved.

Between 9% and 13% of dizzy patients seen in general practice are referred to specialty clinics.[4] Of those dizzy patients, 48% to 50% have an ear-related diagnosis, whereas the rest are neurologic, medical, psychological, or unknown.[5,6]

NATURE OF THE PROBLEM

Approximately 50% of dizzy patients evaluated in an otolaryngology clinic are true neuro-otologic patients.[5,6] For many clinicians, the vestibular system is considered almost like a mysterious organ, perceived as too complicated to understand and poorly taught in medical school and residencies.

In many cases, vertigo is incorrectly considered a diagnosis, not a symptom. There are also many common misconceptions regarding dizziness, as noted in **Table 1**.[7] Inappropriate imaging is often obtained and patients are started on antiemetics such as meclizine. Even though noncontrast head computed tomography (CT) scans have low sensitivity in detecting ischemic strokes and are not recommended for ruling out stroke in patients presenting with vertigo,[8] the use of CT imaging in evaluating dizzy patients presenting to an ED has increased from 9.4% to 37.4%.[9]

Meclizine, an antiemetic thought to work through antagonism of H1 receptors, is a commonly prescribed drug for dizziness. However, this drug has the potential for consequences, with more than 50 drug interactions, and, for patients older than 65 years old, Beers criteria should be applied.[10] These criteria include lists of medications for which the potential risks may be greater than the potential benefits for people aged 65 years and older. In addition, meclizine is prescribed in cases where a diagnosis is unknown or inappropriately in cases where the diagnosis is known, such as benign paroxysmal positional vertigo (BPPV). One author (H.W.) reviewed more than 1000 patients diagnosed with BPPV at her institution, and 55% of patients received at least 1 prescription for meclizine.

Therefore, given these misconceptions, the medical community sends dizzy patients to otolaryngology. Therefore, the otolaryngologist's job is to:

1. Ensure the patient is not having a critical issue such as a stroke or cardiac arrhythmia
2. Rule in all the neuro-otologic diseases such as BPPV, Meniere disease, vestibular neuritis, and labyrinthitis
3. Refer to the appropriate specialty if not neuro-otology (eg, neurology)
4. Further work up, manage, and treat neuro-otologic conditions

DISCUSSION

Clinic workflows and options vary based on available personnel, testing, and associated specialists (**Fig. 1**).

Creating a High-Yield Patient Population

Screening is a critical step in ensuring neuro-otologic patients are being appropriately scheduled. If possible, screen referrals for vertigo and dizziness before scheduling. Although system dependent, the neuro-otologist or a team can perform this. Reviewing documentation to ensure neurologic or cardiac causes have been ruled out, discussing the patient with the referring clinician, or requiring completion of screening questionnaires can help facilitate getting the patient to the right specialist. These questionnaires may include demographic data; description of the dizzy episodes, including when and how long episodes last; otologic and migraine symptoms; and prior testing. Zhao and colleagues[11] provide an example.

Table 1
Ten pitfalls and pearls in the diagnosis of stroke in acute dizziness and vertigo

Pitfall	Pearl	Notes
True vertigo implies an inner ear disorder	Focus on timing and triggers, rather than type	Cerebrovascular disorders frequently present with true vertigo symptoms[33,34]
Worse with head movement implies peripheral	Differentiate triggers from exacerbating factors	Acute dizziness/vertigo is usually exacerbated by head movement, whether peripheral or central[35]
Auditory symptoms imply a peripheral cause	Beware auditory symptoms of vascular cause	Lateral pontine and inner ear strokes often cause tinnitus or hearing loss[36–38]
Diagnose vestibular migraine when headaches accompany dizziness	Inquire about headache characteristics and associated symptoms	Sudden, severe, or sustained pain in the head or neck may indicate aneurysm, dissection, or other vascular disorder[35]; photophobia may point to migraine[39]
Isolated vertigo is not a TIA symptom	Some TIA definitions do not recognize certain transient vertebrobasilar neurologic symptoms (including isolated vertigo) as TIAs	Isolated vertigo is the most common vertebrobasilar warning symptom before stroke[11,40]; it is rarely diagnosed correctly as a vascular symptom at first contact[7,11]
Strokes causing dizziness or vertigo have limb ataxia or other focal signs	Focus on eye examinations: VOR by head impulse test, nystagmus, eye alignment	Fewer than 20% of patients with stroke presenting with AVS have focal neurologic signs.[41,42] NIH stroke scales of 0 occur with posterior circulation strokes
Young patients have migraine rather than stroke	Do not overfocus on age and vascular risk factors. Consider vertebral artery dissection in young patients	Vertebral artery dissection mimics migraine closely[43]; young patients aged 18–44 y with stroke are 7-fold more likely to be misdiagnosed than patients aged >75 y[9]
CT is needed to rule out cerebellar hemorrhage in patients with isolated acute dizziness or vertigo	Intracerebral hemorrhage rarely mimics benign dizziness or vertigo presentations	Only 2.2% (n = 13/595) of intracerebral hemorrhages presented with dizziness or vertigo and only 0.2% (n = 1 out of 595) presented with isolated dizziness[44]
CT is useful to search for acute posterior fossa stroke	Recognize the limitations of imaging, especially CT	Although some retrospective studies[45,46] suggest CT may be up to 42% sensitive, prospective studies suggest the sensitivity is no higher than 16%[13,47]

(continued on next page)

Table 1 (continued)		
Pitfall	**Pearl**	**Notes**
A negative MRI-DWI scan rules out posterior fossa stroke	Recognize the limitations of imaging, even MRI-DWI	MRI-DWI in the first 24 h misses 15% to 20% of posterior fossa infarctions.[12] MRI-DWI sensitivity for brain stem stroke is maximal 72–100 h after infarction.[48] Labyrinthine strokes are not visible

Abbreviations: AVS, acute vestibular syndrome; CT, computed tomography; DWI, diffusion-weighted imaging; NIH, National Institutes of Health; TIA, transient ischemic attack; VOR, vestibulo-ocular reflex.

From Saber Tehrani AS, Kattah JC, Kerber KA, et al. Diagnosing stroke in acute dizziness and vertigo: Pitfalls and pearls. *Stroke.* 2018;49(3):788-795. https://doi.org/10.1161/STROKEAHA.117.016979 [doi], with permission.

Several studies have shown the predictive power in using such tools. Zhao and colleagues[11] found that certain questions provide highly predictive accuracies in diagnosing migraine, BPPV, and Meniere disease.[11] In a similar study, Friedland and colleagues[6] found a predictive accuracy of 71% in using a subset of questions to create a model for BPPV, Meniere disease, and vestibular migraine. Using this published formula, Britt and colleagues[12] validated this in a separate population showing predication of BPPV. Even using a simple 2 × 2 algorithm, Kentala and Rauch[13] showed that almost 60% of neuro-otologic diagnoses can be identified by assessing the association of hearing loss and duration of vertigo episode. Given the high predictability for identifying BPPV, clinic workflow could include sending these patients to physical therapy for repositioning maneuvers before requiring a visit with the otolaryngologist (see **Fig. 1**). Given the labor-intensive nature of screening, groups are trying to put this into artificial intelligence and integrate it into electronic medical records.[14]

Schedule Appropriately

Once an appropriate referral has been identified, the next step is to schedule. It would be difficult to get through a new dizzy patient visit in 5 minutes. Therefore, it is best to create a clinic schedule that allows adequate time with patients but not at the expense of running an efficient clinic. Suggestions include:

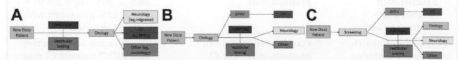

Fig. 1. Examples of clinic workflows. (*A*) Patient is scheduled for audiometric and vestibular testing before seeing otologist. Pending examination and testing, the otologist may refer to additional services. (*B*) The patient is evaluated first by the otologist. If examination and history are consistent with BPPV, patient is referred to physical therapy (PT). Audiometric and/or vestibular testing may be obtained or the patient may be referred to other services if diagnosis is not consistent with neuro-otologic condition. (*C*) Patient is screened. If history is consistent with BPPV, patient is referred to PT. Pending examination and history, audiometric and/or vestibular testing may be obtained, or the patient may be referred to other services if diagnosis is not consistent with neuro-otologic condition.

- Performing formal time studies on current workflows to capture the time it takes to evaluate and follow up new patients.
- Using tools such as process maps and value-stream maps to visualize where bottlenecks may occur or tasks that can be streamlined.
- Establishing blocks of time in schedules for patients specifically with dizzy complaints. This process can also include limiting the number of patients presenting with a complaint of dizziness.
- Creating a dizzy clinic that only evaluates or follows up with patients that have a complaint of dizziness.

Selectively Refer to Vestibular Testing

Once scheduled with an appointment, there are 2 schools of thought on whether to obtain vestibular testing before the visit or after being evaluated. One of the authors (Y.A.) obtains testing beforehand and the other (H.W.) determines the need for testing after evaluation. There are pros and cons to either approach (**Table 2**).

Regardless of when testing is obtained, clinicians should be thoughtful about why they are ordering testing. Vestibular testing is not diagnostic. Testing evaluates the status of the inner ear, which can be used to understand the disorder causing the patient's symptoms, examination findings, and can support or negate a diagnosis (**Table 3**).

Given the lack of evidence and guidelines for testing, there is significant variation in the use of vestibular testing. In a cross-sectional review of Medicare beneficiary claims, Adams and colleagues[15] found that most caloric tests were billed by audiologists and otolaryngologists, whereas primary care physicians and neurologists billed the largest proportion of rotary chair tests compared with other specialists. Within otolaryngology, academic practices are 15 times more likely to obtain vestibular testing at the initial visit compared with nonacademic practices.[16]

Table 2
The pros and cons to obtaining vestibular testing before or after clinical evaluation

Testing Before Evaluation	Testing After Evaluation
Pros	Pros
• Status of inner ear known before the visit	• Improves access to clinic by avoiding bottleneck of testing
• Clinic visit: able to perform a directed history, physical examination	• Avoids unnecessary testing and costs
• More efficient for patient (does not have to return for testing)	• Patient may be more likely to complete testing after seeing clinician
• Determine need for imaging	
• Narrow differential before visit	
Cons	Cons
• Can create a bottleneck for scheduling and limit patient access	• Multiple visits for patient
• Insurance many not cover if no diagnosis	• May not want to come back for testing
• After testing, risk loss to follow up	
• Patients may also refuse testing	
• May obtain unnecessary testing and costs	

Table 3
Common types of vestibular test

Test	What Does It Test?	Physiology	Pathophysiology
cVEMPs	Saccule and inferior vestibular nerve	Measures EMG activity from the sternocleidomastoid muscles following vestibular stimulation with brief pulses of sound. Manifestation of the vestibulocollic reflex: from activation of the vestibular nerve, the vestibulospinal tract, the accessory nerve and, the sternocleidomastoid muscle. cVEMP is a measure of the inhibitory response on the ipsilateral side	SCDS
oVEMP	Utricle and superior vestibular nerve	Extraocular muscles are part of the VOR. Measures EMG activity of VOR following activation of the vestibular nerve, transmitted possibly via the medial longitudinal fasciculus, the oculomotor nuclei and nerves, and the extraocular muscles. oVEMP is a measure of the excitatory response and contralateral side	SCDS
Rotary chair	Horizontal semicircular SCCs (rotating in horizontal plane) and their contribution to the VOR	SCCs are arranged in push-pull pairs; eg, rotation to the right increases the firing rate of the right, whereas it decreases firing rate of left SCC. If the stimulus is fast enough, 1 SCC goes into an inhibitory cut off, whereas the other SCC further increases firing	Bilateral horizontal hypofunction

(continued on next page)

Table 3
(continued)

Test	What Does It Test?	Physiology	Pathophysiology
Head impulse test	VOR	SCCs send information on head movement (excitatory or inhibitory to vestibular nerve, which transmits to vestibular nucleus). Causes excitation of contralateral abducens nucleus and inhibition of ipsilateral abducens nucleus, which then communicate with lateral rectus muscles via abducens nerve and other EOM via medial longitudinal fasciculus and oculomotor nerve. Lateral and anterior canals send information via superior vestibular nerve. Posterior canals send information via inferior vestibular nerve	Vestibular hypofunction; SCDS
Calorics	Horizontal canal	Irrigation of warm or cold water or air into the external ear canal. When the endolymph is warmed (by air or water), an excitatory response occurs in the lateral SCC. When a cold temperature is applied, an inhibitory response occurs	Vestibular hypofunction; SCDS
Dix-Hallpike	Evaluate for BPPV; otoliths within posterior semicircular canal	Detached otoliths, free floating in endolymph of posterior semicircular canal, create movement within fluid as the head is tilted posterior, leading to deflection of the cupula	BPPV

Abbreviations: cVEMP, cervical evoked myogenic potentials; EMG, electromyography; EOM, extra-ocular muscles; oVEMP, ocular evoked myogenic potentials; SCC, semicircular canal; SCDS, superior semicircular canal dehiscence syndrome.

Obtain a History

Having a process to efficiently obtain a history is critical for time. The diagnosis lies in the history and where the clinician should spend time. It is also where a clinician can lose time. Strategies include:

- As discussed earlier, usage of questionnaire sent out before the appointment and review can help facilitate efficient information gathering. This approach allows review of the history as well as an interview that focuses on clarifying with a targeted examination.

- Asking high-yield evidence-based questions. Goebel[17] examined the grouping of symptoms with the highest predictive value (**Table 4**), including:
  - Establishing whether they truly have vertigo versus other sensations (eg, syncope). Vertigo is defined by the American Academy of Otolaryngology's Equilibrium Committee as the "sensation of motion when no motion is occurring relative to earth's gravity."[18]
  - How long the vertigo lasts: seconds, minutes, hours, or constant for days?
  - Is it triggered by head position?
  - Presence or absence of hearing loss or changes in hearing.
  - Associated symptoms: headaches, visual changes.
  - What makes it better worse: vestibular suppressants, sleep, busy visual fields?
- Focusing on getting the information needed to essentially place patients into 1 of 4 peripheral vestibular groups: BPPV, Meniere disease, vestibular migraine, and/or unilateral/bilateral vestibular loss. These elements of the history are important for:
  - BPPV: duration and positional nature
  - Meniere disease: associated or prior known sensorineural hearing loss and otologic symptoms
  - Vestibular migraine: personal and family history of migraine/headache, associated migraine symptoms (eg, photophobia/phonophobia), motion sickness
  - Superior canal dehiscence: dizziness associated with sound or pressure, ear fullness, and pulsatile tinnitus.

Clinicians also need to evaluate for red-flag symptoms and signs that can indicate a central process. These signs include, but are not limited to:

- Ataxic gait
- Diplopia, vision loss, or other visual changes
- Cranial nerve deficits
- Slurred speech
- Paresthesia of face, head, or body
- Muscle weakness, incoordination

Develop a Network of Collaborators and Specialists

Even with the best screening tools, patients with non–neuro-otologic disease processes may find their way into the otolaryngologist's clinic. Therefore, it is critical to develop a network of specialists to whom patients can be referred for definitive treatment. **Table 5** provides a brief list of specialists.

Multidisciplinary Teams and Falls Clinic

The authors strongly recommend a team approach and developing a multidisciplinary group to assist in evaluating and managing dizzy patients. The cause of the dizziness may not be clear, it may involve peripheral and central pathophysiology, and treatment may require rehabilitation or the need to address associated anxiety or depression. Between 42.5% and 68% of patients with vertigo may have an associated psychiatric comorbidity, including anxiety and depression.[19] Associated disorders can have an impact on therapy and recovery. Patients with anxiety and depression take longer to compensate with vestibular therapy and may not achieve outcomes as satisfactory as those without.[20]

Table 4
Predictive power of symptoms for the diagnosis of dizziness

Diagnosis	Percentage of Study Population with Diagnosis	Grouping of Symptoms with the Highest Positive Predictive Value	Odds Ratio	Positive Likelihood Ratio
Benign positional vertigo	24.3	No dizziness between attacks, positional	11.25	5.659
Migraine	17.4	Photophobia, worse in moments of stress, associated headache	87.75	70.4
Meniere	14.2	Hearing change during attack, aural fullness	8.645	4.75
Vestibular neuritis	8.1	Dizziness in attacks, nausea, attacks <20 min	2.565	1.804
Central	7.1	Constant dizziness, history of depression, neurologic comorbidity	26.607	22.72
Anxiety	5.3	Worse in moments stress, breathing quickly while dizzy, numbness in face/extremities	4.111	3.667
Cardiac	5.3	Confusion, history of fall, history of loss of consciousness	7.364	6.303
Postural	3.5	Weakness/clumsiness, age >60 y, difficulty hearing	5.084	3.808
Bilateral vestibular loss	3.3	Irregular heartbeat, difficulty walking in the dark, frequency (once a month)	18.36	15.467
Unilateral vestibular loss	3.1	Difficulty hearing. cardiac comorbidity, family history of deafness	5.729	4.637
Cervical	1.9	Weakness/clumsiness, slurred speech, facial weakness	19.020	15.016
Other	5.9	NA	NA	NA

Abbreviation: NA, not available.
Reprinted with permission from authors *From* Goebel JA. Evaluation of the dizzy patient: History and physical examination. *Research in Vestibular Science.* 2011;10:S107-S122, with permission.

Table 5	
List of specialists and conditions	
Specialty	**Diseases, Conditions, or Testing**
Cardiology	Arrhythmias, postural orthostatic tachycardia syndrome
Memory clinic	Neurocognitive assessment
Neurology	Central examination findings, abnormal oculomotor findings, vestibular migraine
Physical therapy	Posturography, vestibular rehabilitation
Psychiatry	Persistent postural-perceptual dizziness, anxiety disorders
Traumatic brain injury clinic	Comprehensive evaluation

Thus, having a team member who can help manage patients' anxiety may further help in the patients' recovery and compensation. A team may include otolaryngology/neuro-otology, neurology, neuro-ophthalmology, audiology, physical therapy, psychiatry/psychology, and social work. Formats can vary from true multidisciplinary clinics, to inclusion of group treatment, to a regularly scheduled vestibular conference.[21,22] In the experience of the Ottawa Hospital multidisciplinary clinic, the clinic screened patients, improved diagnostic accuracy, ensured appropriate diagnostic testing, and facilitated effective care plans for patients with dizziness in both acute and chronic settings.[22] Inclusion of interdisciplinary clinics with group treatment furthermore improved patient mood, physical and mental health, functionality, and satisfaction.[23]

A specific note regarding falls: one of the many realities of dizzy patients is that they may have a true vestibular loss. The cause of the loss may never be known; however, improving balance and preventing a fall may be the only option. In the United States, falls made up the greatest percentage of injuries in 2019, with an estimated 2.6 million nonfatal falls and 21,700 fatal falls.[24]

Vestibular patients should be screened for falls. The American Geriatrics Society recommends that all patients older than 65 years with a history of falls, balance, or gait disorder should undergo multifactorial falls risk evaluation.[25] Screening tools listed here measure the effect of imbalance and falls risk on functional status and patient quality of life:

- Falls Efficacy Scale[26]
- The Activities Balance Confidence Scale[27]
- Lawton Instrumental Activities of Daily Living Scale[28]

The development of a falls clinic can specifically target these at-risk patients. A team can include otolaryngologists, ophthalmologists, physical medicine and rehabilitation, geriatricians, neurologists, orthopedists, cardiologists, physiatrists, psychiatrists, and physical and occupational therapists.

In addition to a standardized physical examination, a falls examination should include evaluation of orthostatic vital signs, strength, sensory and reflex testing, and inclusion of the following tests:

- Mini-BEST (Balance Evaluations Systems Test)[29]
- SARA (Scale for the Assessment and Rating of Ataxia)[30]
- MOCA (Montreal Cognitive Assessment)[31]

QUALITY INDICTORS

Given the need for patient-reported outcomes, every clinician should strive to adhere to and track quality indicators. Published in 2017, a multidisciplinary work group provided recommendations regarding the following[32]:

- Quality of life for patients with neuro-otology disorders
- Vestibular rehabilitation for unilateral or bilateral vestibular hypofunction
- Dix-Hallpike maneuver performed for patients with BPPV
- Canalith repositioning procedure performed for patients with posterior canal BPPV
- Standard BPPV management

A validated quality improvement tool can provide objective data for patients and provide data for both clinician and patient about how the patient is responding to treatment. Several published tools exist.[32]

SUMMARY

In summary, dizzy patients can be challenging, but having a plan for how to screen and schedule, how to gather data, and how to develop a workflow for testing can improve efficiency. Development of a team approach can alleviate some of the burden and helps to provide better care. The bottom line is to be thoughtful about these patients. The reality is that if clinicians provide efficient and high-quality care, the successful management of dizzy patients can be rewarding.

CLINICS CARE POINTS

- Only 50% of patients presenting to an otolaryngology clinic have a neuro-otologic condition.
- Screening tools and questionnaires should be used to efficiently categorize patients based on evidence-based symptoms.
- Vestibular testing is not diagnostic.
- Create a multidisciplinary clinic.
- Screen high-risk patients for falls.

DISCLOSURE

The authors have nothing to disclose. H.W. Weinreich is funded by the University of Illinois at Chicago (UIC)'s Building Interdisciplinary Research Careers in Women's Health (BIRCWH) grant K12HD101373 from the National Institutes of Health (NIH) Office of Research on Women's Health. Y. Agrawal is funded by the National Institute on Aging R01 AG057667.

REFERENCES

1. Edlow JA. Diagnostic algorithm for patients presenting with acute dizziness: The ATTEST method. In: Micieli G, Cavallini A, Ricci S, et al, editors. Decision algorithms for emergency neurology. Springer-Cham; 2021. https://doi.org/10.1007/978-3-030-51276-7_9.
2. Bosner S, Schwarm S, Grevenrath P, et al. Prevalence, aetiologies and prognosis of the symptom dizziness in primary care - a systematic review. BMC Fam Pract 2018;19(1):33.
3. Centers for Disease Control and Prevention. Emergency department visits. 2021. Available at: https://www.cdc.gov/nchs/fastats/emergency-department.htm. Accessed February 26, 2021.

4. Jayarajan V, Rajenderkumar D. A survey of dizziness management in general practice. J Laryngol Otol 2003;117(8):599–604.

5. Arya AK, Nunez DA. What proportion of patients referred to an otolaryngology vertigo clinic have an otological cause for their symptoms? J Laryngol Otol 2008;122(2):145–9.

6. Friedland DR, Tarima S, Erbe C, et al. Development of a statistical model for the prediction of common vestibular diagnoses. JAMA Otolaryngol Head Neck Surg 2016;142(4):351–6.

7. Saber Tehrani AS, Kattah JC, Kerber KA, et al. Diagnosing stroke in acute dizziness and vertigo: Pitfalls and pearls. Stroke 2018;49(3):788–95.

8. Kattah JC, Talkad AV, Wang DZ, et al. HINTS to diagnose stroke in the acute vestibular syndrome: Three-step bedside oculomotor examination more sensitive than early MRI diffusion-weighted imaging. Stroke 2009;40(11):3504–10.

9. Saber Tehrani AS, Coughlan D, Hsieh YH, et al. Rising annual costs of dizziness presentations to U.S. emergency departments. Acad Emerg Med 2013;20(7): 689–96.

10. IBM Micromedex. Meclizine hydrochloride. Available at: www-micromedexsolutions-com. Accessed February 23, 2021.

11. Zhao JG, Piccirillo JF, Spitznagel EL, et al. Predictive capability of historical data for diagnosis of dizziness. Otol Neurotol 2011;32(2):284–90.

12. Britt CJ, Ward BK, Owusu Y, et al. Assessment of a statistical algorithm for the prediction of benign paroxysmal positional vertigo. JAMA Otolaryngol Head Neck Surg 2018;144(10):883–6.

13. Kentala E, Rauch SD. A practical assessment algorithm for diagnosis of dizziness. Otolaryngol Head Neck Surg 2003;128(1):54–9.

14. McCaslin DL. 20Q: Using artificial intelligence to triage and manage patients with dizziness - the mayo clinic experience. 2020. Available at: https://www.audiologyonline.com/articles/20q-using-artificial-intelligence-to-26880. Accessed February 26, 2021.

15. Adams ME, Yueh B, Marmor S. Clinician use and payments by medical specialty for audiometric and vestibular testing among US medicare beneficiaries. JAMA Otolaryngol Head Neck Surg 2020;146(2):143–9.

16. Piker EG, Schulz K, Parham K, et al. Variation in the use of vestibular diagnostic testing for patients presenting to otolaryngology clinics with dizziness. Otolaryngol Head Neck Surg 2016;155(1):42–7.

17. Goebel JA. Evaluation of the dizzy patient: History and physical examination. Res Vestib Sci 2011;10:S107–22.

18. Committee on hearing and equilibrium guidelines for the diagnosis and evaluation of therapy in meniere's disease. american academy of otolaryngology-head and neck foundation, inc. Otolaryngol Head Neck Surg 1995;113(3):181–5.

19. Lahmann C, Henningsen P, Brandt T, et al. Psychiatric comorbidity and psychosocial impairment among patients with vertigo and dizziness. J Neurol Neurosurg Psychiatry 2015;86(3):302–8.

20. MacDowell SG, Wellons R, Bissell A, et al. The impact of symptoms of anxiety and depression on subjective and objective outcome measures in individuals with vestibular disorders. J Vestib Res 2018;27(5–6):295–303.

21. Staibano P, Lelli D, Tse D. A retrospective analysis of two tertiary care dizziness clinics: A multidisciplinary chronic dizziness clinic and an acute dizziness clinic. J Otolaryngol Head Neck Surg 2019;48(1):11.

22. Bachmann K, Lavender V, Castiglione M. Development of a pediatric balance center: A multidisciplinary approach. Semin Hear 2018;39(3):243–56.

23. Naber CM, Water-Schmeder O, Bohrer PS, et al. Interdisciplinary treatment for vestibular dysfunction: The effectiveness of mindfulness, cognitive-behavioral techniques, and vestibular rehabilitation. Otolaryngol Head Neck Surg 2011; 145(1):117–24.

24. Centers for Disease Control and Prevention. Injury data 2019. Available at: https://www.cdc.gov/injury/wisqars/index.html. Accessed April 6, 2021.

25. Guideline for the prevention of falls in older persons. american geriatrics society, british geriatrics society, and american academy of orthopaedic surgeons panel on falls prevention. J Am Geriatr Soc 2001;49(5):664–72.

26. Tinetti ME, Richman D, Powell L. Falls efficacy as a measure of fear of falling. J Gerontol 1990;45(6):239.

27. Powell LE, Myers AM. The activities-specific balance confidence (ABC) scale. J Gerontol A Biol Sci Med Sci 1995;50A(1):28.

28. Lawton MP, Brody EM. Assessment of older people: Self-maintaining and instrumental activities of daily living. Gerontologist 1969;9(3):179–86.

29. Franchignoni F, Horak F, Godi M, et al. Using psychometric techniques to improve the balance evaluation systems test: The mini-BESTest. J Rehabil Med 2010; 42(4):323–31.

30. Schmitz-Hubsch T, du Montcel ST, Baliko L, et al. Scale for the assessment and rating of ataxia: Development of a new clinical scale. Neurology 2006;66(11): 1717–20.

31. Nasreddine ZS, Phillips NA, Bedirian V, et al. The montreal cognitive assessment, MoCA: A brief screening tool for mild cognitive impairment. J Am Geriatr Soc 2005;53(4):695–9.

32. Neurology Quality Measurement Work Group (authors). Universal Neurology Quality Measurement Set. American Academy of Neurology Institute: American Medical Association; 2019. p. 1–69.

33. Newman-Toker DE, Cannon LM, Stofferahn ME, et al. Imprecision in patient reports of dizziness symptom quality: a cross-sectional study conducted in an acute care setting. Mayo Clin Proc 2007;82:1329–40.

34. Lee H, Sohn SI, Cho YW, et al. Cerebellar infarction presenting isolated vertigo: frequency and vascular topographical patterns. Neurology 2006;67:1178–83.

35. Neuro-otologic disorders. Continuum (Minneap Minn) 2012;18(5 Neuro-otology): 1016–40.

36. Häusler R, Levine RA. Auditory dysfunction in stroke. Acta Otolaryngol 2000;120: 689–703.

37. Chang TP, Wang Z, Winnick AA, et al. Sudden hearing loss with vertigo portends greater stroke risk than sudden hearing loss or vertigo alone. J Stroke Cerebrovasc Dis 2018;27:472–8.

38. Newman-Toker DE, Kerber KA, Hsieh YH, Pula JH, Omron R, Saber Tehrani AS, et al. HINTS outperforms ABCD2 to screen for stroke in acute continuous vertigo and dizziness. Acad Emerg Med 2013;20:986–96.

39. Lempert T, Neuhauser H, Daroff RB. Vertigo as a symptom of migraine. Ann N Y Acad Sci 2009;1164:242–51.

40. Hoshino T, Nagao T, Mizuno S, et al. Transient neurological attack before vertebrobasilar stroke. J Neurol Sci 2013;325:39.

41. Tarnutzer AA, Berkowitz AL, Robinson KA, et al. Does my dizzy patient have a stroke? A systematic review of bedside diagnosis in acute vestibular syndrome. CMAJ 2011;183:E571–92.

42. Kattah JC, Talkad AV, Wang DZ, et al. HINTS to diagnose stroke in the acute vestibular syndrome: threestep bedside oculomotor examination more sensitive than early MRI diffusion-weighted imaging. Stroke 2009;40:3504–10.

43. Gottesman RF, Sharma P, Robinson KA, et al. Clinical characteristics of symptomatic vertebral artery dissection: a systematic review. Neurologist 2012;18:245–54.

44. erber KA, Burke JF, Brown DL, et al. Does intracerebral haemorrhage mimic benign dizziness presentations? A population based study. Emerg Med J 2012;29:43–6.

45. Hwang DY, Silva GS, Furie KL, Greer DM. Comparative sensitivity of computed tomography vs. magnetic resonance imaging for detecting acute posterior fossa infarct. J Emerg Med 2012;42:559–65.

46. Lawhn-Heath C, Buckle C, Christoforidis G, et al. Utility of head CT in the evaluation of vertigo/dizziness in the emergency department. Emerg Radiol 2013; 20:45–9.

47. Ozono Y, Kitahara T, Fukushima M, et al. Differential diagnosis of vertigo and dizziness in the emergency department. Acta Otolaryngol 2014;134:140–5.

48. Axer H, Grässel D, Brämer D, et al. Time course of diffusion imaging in acute brainstem infarcts. J Magn Reson Imaging 2007;26:905–12.

Interviewing and Counseling the Dizzy Patient with Focus on Quality of Life

Habib G. Rizk, MD[a],*, Yuan F. Liu, MD[b]

KEYWORDS

- Sleep Disturbances • Counseling • Quality of life (QOL) • Dizziness
- Vestibular disorders • Cognitive function • Multidisciplinary treatment
- Psychiatric comorbidities

KEY POINTS

- Patients with dizziness experience a negative effect in their cognitive function, sleep function and mental health.
- Patients with dizziness report a decrease in their general quality of life and productivity.
- Initial and subsequent patient interviews should include an assessment of the impact of dizziness on the patient's quality of life, specifically on work performance, productivity, cognitive functioning, sleep disturbances, and mental health.
- Counseling and tracking treatment progress for a patient with dizziness should focus on preferably measurable and realistic functional outcomes.
- Multidisciplinary treatment approaches improve quality of life and patients' outcomes as well as health care utilization while minimizing the burden on one practitioner managing this multifactorial disease.

INTRODUCTION

Dizziness and vertigo affect a staggering 15% to 20% of adults every year,[1] accounting for 2% to 3% of all emergency department consultations in the United States.[2] Unfortunately, this common presenting symptom can be complex to diagnose and manage appropriately, and consequently, many practitioners lack the willingness or expertise to treat patients with dizziness. Approximately 45% to 55% of patients with dizziness in the United States are initially seen by primary care physicians,[2,3] yet a systematic review in 2016 revealed that many studies failed to show significant

The authors have nothing to disclose.
[a] Department of Otolaryngology, Medical University of South Carolina, Otolaryngology H&N Surgery, 135 Rutledge Avenue, MSC 550, Charleston, SC 29425, USA; [b] Department of Otolaryngology, Loma Linda University Health, 11234 Anderson Street, Room: 2586A, Loma Linda, CA 92354, USA
* Corresponding author.
E-mail address: rizkh@musc.edu

Otolaryngol Clin N Am 54 (2021) 853–861
https://doi.org/10.1016/j.otc.2021.05.009
0030-6665/21/© 2021 Elsevier Inc. All rights reserved.

or clinically relevant improvement in functioning when these patients are treated in the primary care setting.[4] Due to the anatomic location of the balance sensory organ in the inner ear, otolaryngologists (especially otologists) and neurologists, have inherited this group of patients, who frequently present to clinics discouraged and frustrated after less-than-productive past visits to doctors' offices and/or having lived with dizziness for an extended time without proper treatment. However, one must bear in mind that dizziness can encompass many organ systems, and although the ultimate goal is to provide appropriate treatment following an accurate diagnosis, physicians of various specialties can make dramatic differences in the quality of life of patients with dizziness through interviews focused on an evaluation of functional impact of their symptoms. This type of approach leads to more judicious decision-making guided by diagnostic and therapeutic algorithms. A recent joint American Academy of Otolaryngology-Head and Neck Surgery/American Academy of Neurology task force established that the quality of life of patients with neurotology disorders should be a key quality measure to improve outcomes of this patient population.[5]

DISCUSSION
Absenteeism and General Well-Being

Over the years, we have received a disproportionate number of disability form requests from patients with dizziness rather than from those with other otologic disorders. This attests to the disturbance dizziness inflicts on day-to-day life. To put things in perspective, a study examining patients with dizziness presenting to clinics in London and Siena found that 27% reported changing their jobs and 21% gave up work as a direct result of dizziness.[6] Furthermore, a mean of 7 days of work were missed in the 6 months before their visit and 50% reported a significant drop in work efficiency because of dizziness.[6] Although more difficult to quantify, 57% of patients with dizziness reported disruptions in social life.[6] Similarly in Belgium, a study of patients referred to a tertiary care facility for dizziness showed 51% had to miss work because of dizziness and 12% were disabled and could no longer return to work.[7] Even in elderly individuals, in whom work is less of a concern, dizziness decreases social, functional, and psychological well-being, and has been linked to isolation, depression, and diminished autonomy.[8] A decrease in health-related quality of life has also been demonstrated in children ages 8 through 18, in whom physical well-being, psychological well-being, and autonomy were significantly reduced compared with the healthy population.[9]

In terms of general health status as measured by the Health Utility Index Mark 3 questionnaire (HUI3), which examines health-related quality of life in 8 functional domains (vision, hearing, speech, ambulation, dexterity, emotion, cognition, and pain), patients with vestibular loss score significantly lower than healthy individuals.[10] HUI3 domain scores range from 0 ("death") to 1 ("perfect health"), and patients with vertigo have a mean overall score of 0.53 for male individuals (vs 0.81 for the general population) and 0.44 for female individuals (vs 0.77 for the general population).[10] Agrawal and colleagues[11] estimated that this amounts to 1.3 lifetime quality-adjusted life years lost per person, or a mean of $64,929 of individual economic burden for those older than 60. Interestingly, and perhaps not unexpectedly given the broad impact of dizziness on function, patients reported deficits in the speech, dexterity, and emotion domains outside the expected vision and ambulation domains of the HUI3.[10]

- Ask the patient what is their professional occupation. In addition to looking for potential triggers, it will help identify specific risks related to their occupation in the setting of their symptoms.

- Ask the patient if they are currently working, on FMLA (family medical leave act) or on disability. The financial burden of the vestibular pathology may be an additional issue to address to help patients get maximum improvement by attending physical therapy sessions or have access to medication or in some cases surgical procedures.
- In patients with chronic symptoms and inability to go back to their current occupation, suggest vocational rehabilitation referrals. These are usually state-sponsored programs.

Cognitive Dysfunction

The impact of dizziness on cognition has become increasingly recognized over time, but studies are still lacking. Vestibular migraine (VM), the most common cause of dizziness,[12] affects 2.7% of the US population and approximately 10% to 15% of patients presenting with dizziness,[13] Yet, a query of PubMed and Scopus for the topic "vestibular migraine" resulted in more than 1000 articles, and only 2 of those studies looked into cognitive changes in patients with VM.[14] One study found that, using a test based on the Stroop effect (interference with reaction time, eg, naming a font color of a word that spells out a different color), patients with VM and migraine demonstrated worse performance compared with healthy subjects.[14] Another study found that cognitive test scores (Mini-Mental State Examination, tracing, memory, and verbal fluency tests) in VM were significantly worse than those with simple migraine and healthy controls.[15] The incidence of deep brain, peripheral lateral ventricle, and total white matter lesions were also higher in patients with VM than patients with migraine.[15] A cross-sectional survey of the US population in 2008 found that adults with vestibular vertigo had an eightfold higher odds of "serious difficulty concentrating or remembering" and a four-fold higher odds of activity limitation from difficulty remembering or confusion.[16] A major reason that subjective cognitive dysfunction is often not assessed in patients with dizziness is that there is a lack of available tools to quantify the impairment. The Dizziness Handicap Inventory (DHI), a popular and widely used instrument to measure how much functional impact dizziness has on patients' lives,[17] is not very sensitive to differences in cognitive dysfunction among patients with different vestibular diagnoses. However, it does correlate moderately with general cognitive instruments, such as the Cognitive Failure Questionnaire.[18,19]

A recent cross-sectional analysis of cognitive dysfunction in patients with vestibular disorders using the Cognitive Failure Questionnaire showed that this patient group had higher levels of cognitive impairment than similarly aged published controls.[20] Furthermore, the degree of impairment is associated with the duration of symptoms before diagnosis and treatment as well as by specific etiology. Patients with persistent postural perceptual dizziness concurrently with VM and Meniere disease had the most cognitive complaints. In addition, patients with Meniere disease (a peripheral vestibular disorder) performed similarly to patients with VM (a central disorder), suggesting that some peripheral vestibulopathies may affect the central vestibular system and cause symptoms beyond dizziness and hearing loss.[20]

Some researchers have attempted to fill in this knowledge gap by developing instruments more suited for detecting cognitive dysfunction specifically in patients with dizziness, such as the Neuropsychiatric Vertigo Inventory (NVI).[21] Using the NVI, we found that patients with VM and Meniere disease had similar levels of cognitive dysfunction, but significantly more than that of patients with benign paroxysmal positional vertigo.[18] However, there is much work to be done. The effect of different treatments on cognitive function in patients with dizziness is largely unknown. One could speculate that improvement in dizziness would lead to improvement in cognition, but that may not always be the case. For example, in patients with Meniere disease and concurrent migraine, intratympanic gentamicin injections helped with preventing further drop attacks and decreased episodes of dizziness, but there was limited functional improvement compared with patients with only Meniere disease who received gentamicin.[22] Lacroix and colleagues[21] have shown that the space perception, attention, time perception, memory, emotional, visual/oculomotor, and motor domains of cognition are all implicated in complaints from patients with dizziness. With more data we would be able to parse out which domains are affected in various vestibulopathies and perhaps even alter treatment to address impairment in specific cognitive domains.

- In the absence of a disease-specific cognitive questionnaire, the physician/ vestibular clinician should rely on subjective report regarding executive functions such as memory, attention, and concentration.
- The cognitive failure questionnaire, although not validated for vestibular pathologies, can help identify problems in some of those areas and is used by the senior author to have a quantitative idea of how much the patient is prone to error in simple, daily life tasks.

Psychiatric Comorbidities

Unlike cognitive dysfunction, psychiatric comorbidities such as anxiety and depression are well-established in patients with dizziness. The 2008 National Health Interview Survey revealed that the odds of depression, anxiety, and panic disorder are approximately 3 times higher in those with vestibular vertigo compared with the general US population.[16] Comorbid psychiatric disorders are especially pronounced in VM as well as in Meniere disease. Anxiety is found in 25.9% to 70.2%[23–26] and depression in 14.6% to 40.5% of patients with VM.[23–25,27] Conversely, Teggi and colleagues[28] found that between 13.3% and 34.6% of patients with panic disorders, and 10% of patients with depression have VM. Several groups have found that patients with VM have significantly greater anxiety and depression than healthy controls and those with Meniere disease, benign paroxysmal positional vertigo (BPPV), and vestibular neuritis.[24,25,29–31] That being said, a recent systematic review found that the prevalence of depression and mood disorders was nearly 50% in patients with Meniere disease.[32] Best and colleagues[30] found that patients with VM had persistently elevated anxiety over a 1-year period, whereas those with BPPV, Meniere disease, and vestibular neuritis did not. Furthermore, Staab and colleagues[33] found that VM could trigger major anxiety disorders or worsen preexisting psychiatric disorders. Best and colleagues[30] similarly reported that a history of psychiatric disorders was a predictor for the development of psychiatric disorders after VM. Interestingly, severity of dizziness did not correlate with psychometric scores or the development of psychiatric disorders, suggesting that VM in itself, as opposed to the dizziness caused by VM, is the culprit in triggering or worsening anxiety and depression.[30,34]

This is another reason for eliciting information about psychiatric comorbidities aside from presence and severity of simply dizziness itself. Greater anxiety and depression are associated with greater handicap from dizziness.[24,26,30] Patients with VM were found to have the highest rates of vertigo-related handicap compared with those with BPPV, Meniere disease, and vestibular neuritis.[31,34] In terms of DHI scores, disability levels were low in 38.7%, moderate in 51.6%, and severe in 9.7% of patients with VM. Weidt and colleagues[35] found that patients with dizziness had worse Hospital Anxiety and Depression Scale scores, which correlated with worse scores on the Mental Component Summary and Physical Component Summary portions of the

Short-Form 36 questionnaire (a health-related quality-of-life survey). The investigators advocated for basic psychological examinations to be performed alongside routine dizziness examinations because psychosocial factors play such a large role in the mental health of patients with dizziness.[35] We have found that at times, patients are equally or more debilitated by their psychiatric disorders than the physical manifestations of dizziness, and concurrent treatment may be necessary to achieve true improvement in quality of life. For instance, fear of social stigmatization elicited on one of the emotional domain questions of the DHI was correlated with failure of pharmacologic treatment in VM.[36]

Fortunately, some medications used to treat VM, such as venlafaxine and nortriptyline, can help with anxiety and depression. Some researchers have already attempted an integrated approach and early evidence has shown that nursing and psychiatry included in a multidisciplinary neurotology clinic led to greater improvement in DHI scores than when they were not used.[37] We have incorporated a vestibular physical therapist and dietician in our multidisciplinary neurotology clinic, and early anecdotal evidence suggests greater improvement in quality of life from what we suspect is a more comprehensive management of underlying factors associated with dizziness.

- There is a variety of validated instruments that could help identify a mood disorder such as depression or an anxiety disorder. The Patient Health Questionnaire-9 to screen for depression and the Generalized Anxiety Disorder-7 to screen for a generalized anxiety disorder are readily available instruments. However, the Beck depression inventory and the Penn State Worry Questionnaire are also useful tools that could guide the clinician to suggest a referral.
- Even if the preceding instruments do not give a clear-cut indication for depression and anxiety, suggesting to the patient participation in support groups and patient advocacy organizations and even discussing with a counselor in the context of chronic dizziness diagnoses may prove helpful.

Sleep Disturbance

Drowsiness, a common side effect of VM medications, may actually be beneficial for many patients. Associations have been found between subtypes of dizziness, especially VM, and sleep disturbance.[38] Approximately 30% of individuals suffering from vestibular vertigo were found to have abnormal sleep duration in a large population survey of the United States.[39] As high as 65% of patients with chronic dizziness have been found to have sleep disturbance, which was significantly associated with poorer DHI scores.[40] In fact, obstructive sleep apnea (OSA) has been associated with dizziness and may be a causative or exacerbating factor.[41–43] In a Dutch cross-sectional study, 20% of patients with dizziness were at high risk for OSA, and male patients at high risk for OSA scored 9 points worse on the DHI than those at low risk for OSA.[42] When videonystagmography and caloric response tests were performed on patients with OSA, there was evidence of vestibular asymmetry, which the investigators interpreted as possible hypoxic injury from OSA leading to vestibular dysfunction.[41] However, this was a retrospective study so a causative link could not be drawn.

Some researchers have demonstrated change in dizziness symptoms with OSA treatment. One group found that of patients with both OSA and dizziness, 36% of those treated for OSA had complete resolution of dizziness symptoms (this group consisted of the following: 37% brief spells of dizziness, 32% VM, 16% Meniere disease, 11% sudden hearing loss with vertigo, and 11% persistent postural perceptual dizziness).[43] Another group explored change in sleep disturbance with vestibular rehabilitation and found that approximately 20% of patients with sleep disturbance normalized their sleep after treatment.[40] Sleep quality should be routinely assessed as part of the dizziness interview, as in some cases it may play a large part in exacerbating dizziness during waking hours. Integrating a sleep specialist into a vestibular clinic would benefit the patients and the treatment team.

- Asking about sleep disturbances should be implemented in every encounter with a patient with dizziness. To screen for OSA, one may ask about snoring, frequent nighttime awakening, polyuria, and fatigue despite adequate number of sleeping hours this is especially pertinent in the setting of a high body mass index or suggestive body habitus.
- For patients who admit they have a diagnosis of OSA, inquire about their compliance with the continuous positive airway pressure machine and suggest follow-up with their sleep medicine specialist.
- One can also screen for OSA using validated questionnaires, such as the Epworth Sleepiness Scale, and refer patients accordingly.
- In the absence of OSA, inquiring about sleep hygiene would detect other sleep issues that could interfere with compensation processes in vestibular hypofunction as well as to educate patients about the effects of certain medications that could cause insomnia or fatigue and sedation.

Integrated Treatment of Patients with Vestibular Disorders

The concept of a multidisciplinary assessment of dizziness is not novel.[44] Studies have consistently shown that this approach leads to better diagnoses, improved management, and reduction in health care utilization and unnecessary testing.[44–46] By endeavoring to highlight the impact of the vestibular problem on a patient's quality of life beyond the specific symptom addressed within one consultant's specialty/expertise, the stage is set for implanting an integrated, holistic approach to management. For instance, integrating nursing and psychiatry in a multidisciplinary clinic allows better reduction in DHI scores by taking away the stigma of referring to psychiatry from the equation. Instead of relying on patients to accept the possibility of a psychosomatic diagnosis or to wait for their buy-in into counseling, the psychiatrist would be available to deliver an assessment at the point of care that will help with ultimate management.[32] The addition of behavioral therapy (cognitive behavioral therapy or acceptance and commitment therapy) or group therapy to a regimen of vestibular rehabilitation also seems to help with chronic disorders such as persistent postural perceptual dizziness.[47,48] Another example of an integrated approach is the addition of a nutritionist for dietary counseling and compliance with dietary modifications needed for VM and Meniere disease.[49] Especially in patients with multiple comorbidities and dietary requirements, managing yet another aspect of their lifestyle may improve their quality of life substantially and reduce noncompliance with the treatment plan.

SUMMARY

As our understanding of dizziness in general and vestibular disorders in particular improves, we realize that the repercussions of these pathologies goes beyond their physical and anatomic impact. An understanding of the extent of injury to the functional status and quality of life of patients suffering from dizziness allows for a more empathetic approach. In addition, this understanding may alter the treatment plan to be more or less conservative depending on the degree of dysfunction or disability. Ultimately, a comprehensive management initiative is more likely to enhance patients' commitment to their treatment plan, which in most vestibular disorders is a primary component for successful recovery.

CLINICS CARE POINTS

- Vestibular disorders are an invisible injury that can lead to significant disability and reduced productivity.

- Vestibular disorders can be associated with cognitive dysfunction. We currently lack appropriate tools to adequately measure this aspect of the patients' symptoms.

- Vestibular disorders are associated with psychiatric comorbidities and sleep disturbances that influence overall prognosis and need to be detected and addressed.

- Addressing the quality of life and functional impact of a patient's condition allows for a more integrated approach, which has been shown to improve long-term outcomes and reduce health care utilization.

DISCLOSURE

This publication was supported, in part, by the National Center for Advancing Translational Sciences of the National Institutes of Health under Grant Number UL1 TR001450. The content is solely the responsibility of the authors and does not necessarily represent the official views of the National Institutes of Health.

REFERENCES

1. Neuhauser HK. The epidemiology of dizziness and vertigo. Handb Clin Neurol 2016;137:67–82.
2. Sloane PD. Dizziness in primary care. J Fam Pract 1989;29(1):33–8.
3. Yardley L, Barker F, Muller I, et al. Clinical and cost effectiveness of booklet based vestibular rehabilitation for chronic dizziness in primary care: single blind, parallel group, pragmatic, randomised controlled trial. BMJ 2012;344:e2237.
4. Grill E, Penger M, Kentala E. Health care utilization, prognosis and outcomes of vestibular disease in primary care settings: systematic review. J Neurol 2016; 263(1):36–44.
5. Rizk H, Agrawal Y, Barthel S, et al. Quality improvement in neurology: neurotology quality measurement set. Otolaryngol Head Neck Surg 2018;159(4):603–7.
6. Bronstein AM, Golding JF, Gresty MA, et al. The social impact of dizziness in London and Siena. J Neurol 2010;257(2):183–90.
7. Van der Zaag-Loonen H, van Leeuwen R. Dizziness causes absence from work. Acta Neurol Belgica 2015;115(3):345–9.
8. Ciorba A, Bianchini C, Scanelli G, et al. The impact of dizziness on quality-of-life in the elderly. Eur Arch Otorhinolaryngol 2017;274(3):1245–50.
9. Deissler A, Albers L, von Kries R, et al. Health-related quality of life of children/adolescents with vertigo: retrospective study from the German Center of Vertigo and Balance Disorders. Neuropediatrics 2017;48(02):091–7.
10. Agrawal Y, Carey JP, Della Santina CC, et al. Disorders of balance and vestibular function in US adults: data from the National Health and Nutrition Examination Survey, 2001-2004. Arch Intern Med 2009;169(10):938–44.
11. Agrawal Y, Pineault KG, Semenov YR. Health-related quality of life and economic burden of vestibular loss in older adults. Laryngoscope Invest Otolaryngol 2018; 3(1):8–15.

12. Lempert T, Neuhauser H. Epidemiology of vertigo, migraine and vestibular migraine. J Neurol 2009;256(3):333–8.
13. Formeister EJ, Rizk HG, Kohn MA, et al. The epidemiology of vestibular migraine: a population-based survey study. Otol Neurotol 2018;39(8):1037–44.
14. Balci B, Şenyuva N, Akdal G. Definition of balance and cognition related to disability levels in vestibular migraine patients. Arch Neuropsychiatry 2018; 55(1):9.
15. Wang N, Huang H, Zhou H, et al. Cognitive impairment and quality of life in patients with migraine-associated vertigo. Eur Rev Med Pharmacol Sci 2016;20(23): 4913–7.
16. Bigelow RT, Semenov YR, du Lac S, et al. Vestibular vertigo and comorbid cognitive and psychiatric impairment: the 2008 National Health Interview Survey. J Neurol Neurosurg Psychiatry 2016;87(4):367–72.
17. Jacobson GP, Newman CW. The development of the dizziness handicap inventory. Arch Otolaryngol Head Neck Surg 1990;116(4):424–7.
18. Liu YF, Locklear TD, Sharon JD, et al. Quantification of cognitive dysfunction in dizzy patients using the neuropsychological vertigo inventory. Otol Neurotol 2019;40(7):e723–31.
19. Broadbent DE, Cooper PF, FitzGerald P, et al. The cognitive failures questionnaire (CFQ) and its correlates. Br J Clin Psychol 1982;21(1):1–16.
20. Rizk HG, Sharon JD, Lee JA, et al. Cross-sectional analysis of cognitive dysfunction in patients with vestibular disorders. Ear Hear 2019;41(4):1020–7.
21. Lacroix E, Deggouj N, Salvaggio S, et al. The development of a new questionnaire for cognitive complaints in vertigo: the Neuropsychological Vertigo Inventory (NVI). Eur Arch Otorhinolaryngol 2016;273(12):4241–9.
22. Liu YF, Renk E, Rauch SD, et al. Efficacy of intratympanic gentamicin in Ménière's disease with and without migraine. Otol Neurotol 2017;38(7):1005–9.
23. Beh SC, Masrour S, Smith SV, et al. The spectrum of vestibular migraine: clinical features, triggers, and examination findings. Headache 2019;59(5):727–40.
24. Kim SK, Kim YB, Park I-S, et al. Clinical analysis of dizzy patients with high levels of depression and anxiety. J Audiol otology 2016;20(3):174.
25. Eckhardt-Henn A, Best C, Bense S, et al. Psychiatric comorbidity in different organic vertigo syndromes. J Neurol 2008;255(3):420–8.
26. Lahmann C, Henningsen P, Brandt T, et al. Psychiatric comorbidity and psychosocial impairment among patients with vertigo and dizziness. J Neurol Neurosurg Psychiatry 2015;86(3):302–8.
27. Warninghoff JC, Bayer O, Ferrari U, et al. Co-morbidities of vertiginous diseases. BMC Neurol 2009;9(1):29.
28. Teggi R, Caldirola D, Colombo B, et al. Dizziness, migrainous vertigo and psychiatric disorders. J Laryngol Otol 2010;124(3):285–90.
29. Kutay Ö, Akdal G, Keskinoğlu P, et al. Vestibular migraine patients are more anxious than migraine patients without vestibular symptoms. J Neurol 2017; 264(1):37–41.
30. Best C, Tschan R, Eckhardt-Henn A, et al. Who is at risk for ongoing dizziness and psychological strain after a vestibular disorder? Neuroscience 2009; 164(4):1579–87.
31. Best C, Eckhardt-Henn A, Diener G, et al. Interaction of somatoform and vestibular disorders. J Neurol Neurosurg Psychiatry 2006;77(5):658–64.
32. Patel J, Levy D, Nguyen S, et al. Depression in Ménière's disease: a systematic review and meta-analysis. J Laryngol Otol 2020;134(4):293–301.

33. Staab JP, Ruckenstein MJ. Which comes first? Psychogenic dizziness versus oto-genic anxiety. Laryngoscope 2003;113(10):1714–8.
34. Best C, Eckhardt-Henn A, Tschan R, et al. Psychiatric morbidity and comorbidity in different vestibular vertigo syndromes. J Neurol 2009;256(1):58–65.
35. Weidt S, Bruehl AB, Straumann D, et al. Health-related quality of life and emotional distress in patients with dizziness: a cross-sectional approach to disentangle their relationship. BMC Health Serv Res 2014;14(1):317.
36. Liu Y, Macias D, Donaldson L, et al. Pharmacotherapy failure and progression to botulinum toxin injection in vestibular migraine. J Laryngol Otol 2020;134(7): 586–91.
37. Gerretsen P, Shah P, Logotheti A, et al. Interdisciplinary integration of nursing and psychiatry (INaP) for the treatment of dizziness. Laryngoscope 2020;130(7): 1792–9.
38. Kim SK, Kim JH, Jeon SS, et al. Relationship between sleep quality and dizziness. PLoS One 2018;13(3):e0192705.
39. Albathi M, Agrawal Y. Vestibular vertigo is associated with abnormal sleep duration. J Vestib Res 2017;27(2–3):127–35.
40. Sugaya N, Arai M, Goto F. The effect of sleep disturbance in patients with chronic dizziness. Acta Otolaryngol 2017;137(1):47–52.
41. Gallina S, Dispenza F, Kulamarva G, et al. Obstructive sleep apnoea syndrome (OSAS): effects on the vestibular system. Acta Otorhinolaryngol Itál 2010;30(6): 281–4.
42. Maas BD, Bruintjes TD, van der Zaag-Loonen HJ, et al. The relation between dizziness and suspected obstructive sleep apnoea. Eur Arch Otorhinolaryngol 2020;277(5):1537–43.
43. Foster CA, Machala M. The clinical spectrum of dizziness in sleep apnea. Otol Neurotol 2020;41(10):1419–22.
44. Bath AP, Walsh RM, Ranalli P, et al. Experience from a multidisciplinary "dizzy" clinic. Otol Neurotol 2000;21(1):92–7.
45. Staibano P, Lelli D, Tse D. A retrospective analysis of two tertiary care dizziness clinics: a multidisciplinary chronic dizziness clinic and an acute dizziness clinic. J Otolaryngol Head Neck Surg 2019;48(1):1–8.
46. Rodriguez AI, Zupancic S, Song MM, et al. Importance of an interprofessional team approach in achieving improved management of the dizzy patient. J Am Acad Audiol 2017;28(3):177–86.
47. Kuwabara J, Kondo M, Kabaya K, et al. Acceptance and commitment therapy combined with vestibular rehabilitation for persistent postural-perceptual dizziness: a pilot study. Am J Otolaryngol 2020;41(6):102609.
48. Naber CM, Water-Schmeder O, Bohrer PS, et al. Interdisciplinary treatment for vestibular dysfunction: the effectiveness of mindfulness, cognitive-behavioral techniques, and vestibular rehabilitation. Otolaryngol Head Neck Surg 2011; 145(1):117–24.
49. Luxford E, Berliner KI, Lee J, et al. Dietary modification as adjunct treatment in Ménière's disease: patient willingness and ability to comply. Otol Neurotol 2013;34(8):1438–43.

The Efficient Dizziness History and Exam

Divya A. Chari, MD[a,b], Steven D. Rauch, MD[a,b,*]

KEYWORDS

- Dizziness • Dizziness evaluation • Gait tests • Head impulse test • Nystagmus
- Physical examination • Vertigo

KEY POINTS

- Dizziness is diagnostically challenging, but a careful history and physical examination are often sufficient to reach a reasonable diagnosis to explain the patient's symptoms.
- Differentiation of otologic and nonotologic causes of dizziness is one of the first branch points in the diagnostic algorithm.
- Otologic forms of dizziness often result in acute onset vertigo and may exhibit laterality of auditory or vestibular symptoms (eg, tendency to drift or fall to one side or unilateral hearing loss, tinnitus, or aural fullness). Nonotologic causes of dizziness tend to be more insidious in onset, and triggers include dietary, environmental, or hormonal changes.
- In some cases, vestibular testing or imaging is necessary. Imaging is required for the evaluation of tumors, cerebrovascular conditions, and neurologic disorders.

INTRODUCTION

Dizziness accounts for an estimated 3% to 5% of visits to emergency departments and primary care clinics and is a common complaint in the otolaryngology clinic.[1,2] Despite the widespread prevalence of this symptom, however, the dizzy patient often presents a diagnostic challenge. Accurate identification of the underlying etiology of dizziness is difficult largely because dizziness is a general term used to describe 1 or more of the following sensations: (1) presyncope, (2) spinning or nonspinning vertigo, (3) disequilibrium, and (4) lightheadedness. Dizziness may be attributed to otologic or nonotologic causes. Otologic, or peripheral, vestibular disorders include benign paroxysmal positional vertigo (BPPV), labyrinthitis, vestibular neuritis, Meniere's disease, and superior semicircular canal dehiscence (SSCD). Nonotologic, or central, causes of dizziness comprise neurologic (eg, migraine-associated dizziness, postconcussion syndromes, multiple sclerosis, Parkinson disease,

[a] Department of Otolaryngology–Head and Neck Surgery, Massachusetts Eye and Ear, 243 Charles Street, Boston, MA 02114, USA; [b] Department of Otolaryngology–Head and Neck Surgery, Harvard Medical School, 243 Charles Street, Boston, MA 02114, USA
* Corresponding author.
E-mail address: Steven_Rauch@meei.harvard.edu

Otolaryngol Clin N Am 54 (2021) 863–874
https://doi.org/10.1016/j.otc.2021.05.010
0030-6665/21/© 2021 Elsevier Inc. All rights reserved.

oto.theclinics.com

Abbreviations	
BPPV	Benign paroxysmal positional vertigo
SSCD	Superior semicircular canal dehiscence

dysautonomia), cerebrovascular (eg, vertebrobasilar ischemia), cardiovascular (eg, orthostatic hypotension, myocardial infarction), and psychiatric etiologies.

Evaluation of the dizzy patient involves a detailed history followed by a comprehensive otologic and neurologic physical examination. However, given the fairly short list of common diagnostic possibilities and the long history of an algorithmic approach to diagnosis, the clinician may tailor the interview and examination to efficiently evaluate the patient. While imaging is required to detect concerning pathologies such as tumors, cerebrovascular disorders, and multiple sclerosis, many dizzy patients will have no identifiable pathology on imaging studies. For example, 1 prospective study noted that only 24% of patients with vestibular migraine had an identifiable abnormality on imaging.[3] Indeed, in some patients with dizziness, the symptoms have subsided by the time they are seen by a physician, and physical examination and laboratory testing may show no abnormalities. Vestibular function tests are used to confirm a suspected diagnosis, aid in preoperative evaluation, and determine recovery after unilateral injury. However, at present, many vestibular disorders cannot be diagnosed with a simple laboratory test, serum blood test, or imaging study. A notable exception is SSCD syndrome, which is diagnosed with radiologic evidence of dehiscence of the superior semicircular canal and confirmed with cervical and ocular vestibular-evoked myogenic potential testing and suprathreshold bone conduction hearing levels on audiogram. Vestibular function tests can confirm a suspected diagnosis (eg, vestibular neuritis), provide preoperative evaluation, and offer an objective measurement of the patient's vestibular function.

The history and physical examination are critical in the diagnostic evaluation of the dizzy patient. Herein, we discuss efficient evaluation of the dizzy patient by identifying clinically relevant questions and physical examination tests to guide the diagnostic approach and determine the next steps in management. The primary goals of this review are as follows:

1. Outline a systematic approach to interview the patient with dizziness or imbalance
2. Discuss physical examination findings that are useful in clinical practice for making a diagnosis

CLINICAL EVALUATION
Patient History

A meticulous and thoughtful patient history is required. The first step in the diagnostic evaluation of the dizzy patient is to assess the patient for life-threatening causes of dizziness. Patients suffering from strokes or transient ischemic attacks or those with cardiovascular causes of dizziness such as arrhythmias or myocardial infarctions may present with acute dizziness, although most of these patients have other symptoms or neurologic findings.[4] Symptoms, including altered mental status, loss of consciousness, sensory/motor disturbances of the face or extremities, visual disturbances, respiratory difficulties, or chest pain, require emergent evaluation, as patients may be at risk for permanent disability or even death. In general, most patients presenting to otolaryngology clinics report a chronic form of dizziness or imbalance, which is less likely to represent critical neurologic or cardiovascular disorders.

The clinician should inquire about the quality of the dizziness sensation. The patient may describe a sensation of spinning, tilting, swaying, or falling and may perceive the motion of oneself or surroundings. It is not uncommon for patients with dizziness to have difficulty describing their symptoms; moreover, recent studies suggest that the quality of the dizzy symptom does not reliably predict etiology.[5] By contrast, assessing characteristics such as onset, duration, the evolution of symptoms, exacerbating and alleviating factors, and persistence (constant vs intermittent) tends to guide the diagnostic evaluation more reliably. Selected causes of dizziness are listed with associated symptoms in **Table 1**.

A complete otologic history should be obtained, including the presence or absence of hearing loss, otalgia, otorrhea, aural fullness, tinnitus (pulsatile vs continuous), autophony, sound-induced or pressure-induced vertigo, childhood ear infections, noise exposure, prior otologic or neurotologic surgeries, and family history of hearing and balance disorders. Current or previous medications should be reviewed, as dizziness is a well-known adverse effect of many drugs.[6,7] Aminoglycosides, furosemide, quinine, cisplatin, and aspirin, among others, can lead to ototoxicity.[1,8] Antihypertensives can cause orthostatic hypotension, and sedating medications can exacerbate dizzy symptoms, particularly in elderly populations. A history of head or cervical spine trauma or repetitive stress may cause various dizzy symptoms even years after the initial injury.[9] As balance function is affected not only by abnormalities in the vestibular system but also by aberrant sensory inputs from the visual and proprioceptive systems, the patient should be asked about visual disturbances, musculoskeletal problems (eg, history of joint replacement), and peripheral neuropathy. Screening for anxiety and depression during the interview is critical, as these psychiatric disorders may exacerbate underlying vestibular disorders.[10]

A headache history should be obtained in all patients presenting with dizziness. Patients with muscle tension-type headaches may suffer from neck dysfunction that can aggravate cervicogenic dizziness.[9,11] If the history suggests migraine or migraine-like features (eg, photophobia, phonophobia, visual aura), a detailed migraine history is warranted (**Table 2**). In patients with suspected vestibular migraine, the role of possible food triggers, such as caffeine, red wine, chocolate, and cheese, should be evaluated.

Here we present an algorithm to help guide the diagnostic workup for dizziness (**Fig. 1**).

Otologic Versus Nonotologic Causes of Dizziness

One of the first and perhaps most important branch points in the diagnostic algorithm of dizziness is the discernment of whether the symptoms arise from an otologic or nonotologic etiology. Making this determination early in the interview can help efficiently guide the diagnostic workup. Often, patients are able to identify a "sidedness" to their vestibular symptoms, such as a tendency to drift or fall to one side or increased or decreased discomfort with movement to one side. Patients may notice asymmetry of associated symptoms, such as hearing loss or tinnitus. While lateralization of symptoms does not absolutely distinguish otologic from nonotologic disease, it can help narrow the differential diagnosis. Of note, while some patients with nonotologic disease occasionally experience unilateral symptoms, they also tend to describe other accompanying symptoms. For example, a vestibular migraine patient may suffer from unilateral tinnitus and aural fullness or pressure but report associated headaches and visual or sensory disturbances.[12]

Occasionally, the patient is able to identify certain triggers that exacerbate their symptoms. When movement or loud sound or pressure changes elicit immediate

Table 1
Selected causes of dizziness

Causes of Dizziness	Length of Time of Dizzy Symptoms	Sidedness	Associated Symptoms	Physical Examination Findings
Benign paroxysmal positional vertigo	Seconds to minutes	Yes	None	Torsional, upbeat nystagmus on Dix-Hallpike maneuver
Vestibular neuritis	Hours to days with gradual recovery over weeks to months	Yes	None	Catch up saccades present on head impulse test with head rotated to the side of the lesion; may fall to the affected side
Labyrinthitis	Hours to days with gradual recovery over weeks to months	Yes	Hearing loss, tinnitus, and aural fullness	Catch up saccades present on head impulse test with head rotated to the side of the lesion; may fall to the affected side; hearing loss
Meniere's disease	Minutes to hours	Yes	Hearing loss, tinnitus, and aural fullness	May not have interictal symptoms
Vestibular migraines	Hours to days	No	Personal history of family history of migraine, aura, photophobia, phonophobia, sensory disturbances	May not have interictal symptoms
Cerebrovascular disease or tumor	Variable	Possibly	Coordination deficits, motor weakness, neuropathy	Abnormal neurologic exam findings
Neurologic (eg, multiple sclerosis or Parkinson's)	Variable	Possibly	Resting tremor, vision changes, impaired coordination	Abnormal neurologic exam findings
Cardiovascular (eg, orthostatic hypotension, carotid artery stenosis, arrhythmias)	Seconds to minutes	No	Palpitations or arrhythmias	Provoked hypotension with standing

Table 2
Diagnostic criteria for migraine headache[32]

Migraine without aura	• At least 5 attacks fulfilling B-D
	• Headache attacks lasting 4–72 h
	• Headache has at least 2 of the following characteristics
	  ○ Unilateral location
	  ○ Pulsating quality
	  ○ Moderate or severe intensity (inhibits or prohibits daily activities)
	  ○ Aggravation by routine physical activity
	• During headache at least 1 of the following:
	  ○ Nausea and/or vomiting
	  ○ Photophobia and phonophobia
	• Not attributed to another disorder

Migraine with aura	• At least 2 attacks fulfilling B-D
	• One or more of the following fully reversible aura symptoms:
	  ○ Visual
	  ○ Sensory
	  ○ Speech and/or language
	  ○ Motor
	  ○ Brainstem
	  ○ Retinal
	• At least 3 of the following 6 characteristics
	  ○ At least 1 aura symptom spreads gradually over 5 or more minutes
	  ○ Two or more aura symptoms occur in succession
	  ○ Each individual aura symptom lasts 5–60 min
	  ○ At least 1 aura symptom is unilateral
	  ○ At least 1 aura symptom is positive
	  ○ The aura is accompanied, or followed within 60 min, by headache
	• Not attributed to another disorder

Data from IHS. The International Classification of Headache Disorders, 3rd edition (beta version), Headache Classification Committee of the International Headache Society. Cephalalgia. 2013. https://doi.org/10.1177/0333102413485658.

auditory or vestibular symptoms, the etiology is almost certainly otologic. Alternatively, if dietary, environmental, or hormonal changes lead to the onset of symptoms in minutes to hours following exposure, vestibular migraine is far more likely to be the cause.

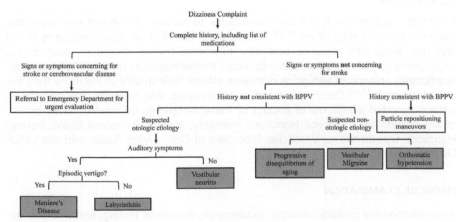

Fig. 1. Algorithm for the management of patients with dizzy complaints.

Episodic Versus Nonepisodic

The nature of the dizziness and whether it is episodic or persistent should be determined. Chronic episodic vertigo could indicate BPPV, Meniere's disease, or vestibular migraine. Nonepisodic forms of vertigo include vestibular neuritis, labyrinthitis, and progressive disequilibrium of aging. Patients with vestibular neuritis and labyrinthitis present with an acute attack of vertigo followed by gradual recovery; in addition to symptoms of vertigo, the latter group suffers from associated sudden unilateral hearing loss.[7]

Duration, Position, and Association

Vertigo of short duration (eg, less than a minute) and provoked by positional changes may indicate BPPV. Typically, patients with BPPV experience vertigo with associated nystagmus upon lying down, rolling over in bed, or bending over/reaching up. Vertigo at rest is uncommon in these patients. While positional nystagmus is not unique to BPPV, the absence of vertigo at rest and short duration of symptoms along with characteristic and stereotyped, reproducible, position-induced vertigo should increase suspicion for BPPV. Of note, patients with BPPV can suffer from residual disequilibrium for weeks after an acute episode, with patients older than 65 at higher risk for residual symptoms.[13]

Associated otologic symptoms, such as hearing loss, tinnitus, and aural fullness, occur in conjunction with vertigo in Meniere's disease and labyrinthitis. The duration of the vertigo attack differentiates these 2 conditions. Recurrent vertigo attacks lasting for 20 minutes to 12 hours are consistent with Meniere's disease. A severe episode of vertigo lasting 24 to 72 hours followed by several weeks of lingering, gradually improving disequilibrium suggests a diagnosis of labyrinthitis.[7] Patients with vestibular migraine often have accompanying photophobia, phonophobia, aura, and motion sensitivity as well as a personal or family history of migraine.[14] Adjunctive complaints of extreme intolerance of visual stimuli, such as visual flow or flicker or complex and chaotic visual fields from carpet and tile patterns or grocery store aisles, and cognitive dysfunction or "brain fog" are much more common in migraineurs than patients with other causes of peripheral or central vestibulopathy. Cranial nerve deficits, ataxia, seizures, or other neurologic symptoms typically arise from central pathologic conditions and warrant further workup with neuroimaging and neurologic consultation.

Quality of Life

Vestibular dysfunction is a major contributor to patient discomfort and disability, resulting in low quality of life.[15,16] Subjective perception of dizzy symptoms is not well correlated with objective vestibular functional testing. Moreover, even during asymptomatic periods, some patients report that anticipatory anxiety of the next unpredictable episode of vertigo or dizziness affects their quality of life more than the symptom itself.[17,18] Commonly used questionnaires that measure the severity of patient-reported symptoms or impact of these symptoms on health-related quality of life include the Dizziness Handicap Inventory, Vertigo Symptom Scale, Vertigo Handicap Questionnaire, Vestibular Disorders of Daily Living Scale, and the UCLA Dizziness Questionnaire.[19]

PHYSICAL EXAMINATION

A comprehensive bedside otologic, oculomotor, positional testing, and postural examination is required for the workup of patients with dizziness or imbalance.

Mental Status

Dizziness may arise from a lesion of the cerebral cortex or from an inability to integrate multisensory information. Abnormal cognitive behaviors such as repetitive questioning, memory lapses, inattention, and declining executive function should be noted and may necessitate referral to a neurologist for additional cognitive and neuropsychiatric testing.

Orthostatic Vital Signs

Orthostatic hypotension may manifest as dizziness. When assessing postural hypotension, vital signs should be checked while the patient is lying down, sitting up, and standing. Sufficient time must be allowed to cause enough pooling of blood below the heart to elicit orthostatic intolerance. The examiner should inquire about associated symptoms such as visual change or palpitations. A sustained drop in systolic pressure of at least 20 mm Hg and at least 10 mm Hg in diastolic pressure within 3 minutes of postural change is diagnostic for orthostatic hypotension.[20]

Otoscopic and Focused Head and Neck Examination

An otoscopic examination with pneumatic insufflation is necessary for evaluating the vertiginous patient. Fluid within the tympanic cavity or perforation of the tympanic membrane can contribute to vertigo symptoms. In cases of SSCD syndrome, the application of pneumatic pressure during otoscopy can elicit dizziness. An audiogram should be performed if the patient complains of hearing impairment, and a bedside tuning fork exam may be used to distinguish between conductive or sensorineural hearing loss.

Cranial nerve function should be assessed, with particular attention paid to the oculomotor function (CNs III, IV, and VI), trigeminal (CN V), and facial (CN VII) nerves. Central pathology may result in deficits of 1 or more cranial nerves along with symptoms of dizziness. Ramsay Hunt syndrome and neurosyphilis can result in vertigo and associated cranial nerve deficits.[21,22] Lyme disease, caused by the spirochete *Borrelia burgdorferi*, is often associated with a characteristic rash, erythema migrans, but patients may also present with a variety of otolaryngologic complaints.[23] While the pathophysiology of vestibular dysfunction due to Lyme disease is not well-characterized, there have been case reports of neuroborreliosis with accompanying vertigo, imbalance, or dizziness have been described.[24]

Ocular Examination and Nystagmus

A thorough physical examination involves a complete ocular examination, including pupillary reactivity and oculomotor movements. The examiner should be able to evaluate pupillary reactivity, smooth pursuit, saccadic eye movement, and the ability to keep the eyes stable in different positions of gaze. Smooth pursuit may be tested by asking the patient to follow a finger to the right and left and up and down, noting smoothness of eye movements. Saccadic eye movement may be tested by asking the patient to alternately fixate on 2 widely spaced objects.

Jerk nystagmus is a common type of rhythmic eye movement with well-defined slow and fast phases. Spontaneous nystagmus may be observed with the patient's gaze straight ahead. In cases of unilateral peripheral vestibulopathy, vestibular neuritis, or labyrinthitis, spontaneous nystagmus is predominantly horizontal and unidirectional, with the fast phase away from the side of the lesion. The amplitude of spontaneous, unidirectional nystagmus typically increases with the gaze in the direction of the fast phase. In peripheral vestibular injury, nystagmus may be suppressed after a few days. However, nystagmus can be "unmasked" by headshaking, hyperventilation, or the Jendrassik maneuver.[25] Visual fixation should decrease nystagmus over time; the inability to suppress nystagmus suggests a central cause. Gaze-evoked nystagmus, direction-switching nystagmus (ie, right beating with right gaze and left beating with left gaze), and pure vertical nystagmus are concerning for a possible brain lesion and should prompt appropriate in-person patient evaluation, including neuroimaging.

Positional Testing

The hallmark nystagmus of BPPV occurs within seconds after moving into a provocative position. Nystagmus may be reproduced with the Dix-Hallpike maneuver or the roll test.[26,27] In the most common form of BPPV, where debris is trapped in the posterior semicircular canal, the nystagmus is a combination of upbeat and torsional when the patient is placed into a supine position with the head turned 45° toward the affected side and extend approximately 20° backward.

Vestibulo-Ocular Reflex Tests

Assessment of semicircular canal function is performed with the head impulse test. The patient is asked to fix their gaze at a target point about 1 m away, and the head is quickly rotated in an unpredictable direction by 10° to 20°.[28] For the lateral semicircular canals, the head impulse is applied horizontally, and for the vertical semicircular canals, the head is rotated vertically after turning the head 30° to the right or left to stimulate the coplanar canals.[29] In a normally functioning VOR, the patient's eyes remain fixed on the target. However, in vestibular hypofunction, the patient will exhibit a corrective catch-up saccade that is more prominent when the head is turned toward the side of the lesion.[30]

Balance and Gait Tests

The Romberg sign is a well-known indicator of visual dependence that implies abnormal proprioception or loss of peripheral vestibular function. Inability to maintain a straight posture or occurrence of sway suggests a pathologic condition. The Romberg test may show abnormal findings in a variety of patients, including those with vestibular hypofunction, peripheral neuropathy, cerebellar lesions, tabes dorsalis (demyelination of the dorsal spinal columns due to neurosyphilis), vitamin B12 deficiency, or copper deficiency, among other causes.[31] Variations of the Romberg test have been proposed, such as performing the test with eyes closed and standing in tandem with and without eyes closed. While these modifications make the test more challenging, the Romberg test remains imperfect, as it cannot localize the lesion. An isolated abnormality of the Romberg test must be interpreted with caution, but when combined with other tests, this test increases the sensitivity of the neurologic examination. For example, a patient who presents after an acute vertiginous illness falls strongly to the left on the Romberg test and has right-beating nystagmus on rightward gaze may be suspected to have suffered from left-sided vestibular neuritis.

In the Fukuda stepping test, the patient is asked to march in place with arms outstretched and eyes closed for about 1 minute. The examiner observes the patient for abnormal turning toward the right or left greater than 20°. As in the Romberg test, patients with peripheral vestibular hypofunction tend to rotate, drift, or fall toward the affected side. Again, if used in isolation, the Fukuda test is nonspecific, but when combined with other neurologic tests, the Fukuda test increases the likelihood of recognition of a diagnostically useful pattern.

Balance and gait testing should be performed in patients complaining of vertigo, dizziness, or imbalance. A simple task includes the tandem gait test, in which the patient is asked to walk in a straight line with the toes of the back foot touching the heel of the front foot at each step. In patients with peripheral hypofunction, there is a tendency to consistently fall or drift to the affected side. In contrast, patients with lower extremity neuropathy or central gait ataxias stagger or fall to both sides.

SUMMARY

Evaluation of dizzy patients can be diagnostically challenging. Differentiation of otologic and nonotologic causes of dizziness is one of the first branch points in the diagnostic algorithm and will allow the physician to appropriately triage the patient and determine the next steps in the workup and management. Otologic forms of dizziness often result in vertigo and may be associated with unilateral symptoms of hearing loss, aural fullness, or tinnitus. Central dizziness is more often constant and insidious.

A thoughtful and careful history and physical examination are often sufficient to reach a plausible diagnosis to explain the patient's dizziness. However, in certain cases, vestibular testing and imaging may be required. MRI with contrast is necessary for the evaluation of tumors, cerebrovascular conditions, and neurologic disorders, such as multiple sclerosis. Vestibular testing can confirm unilateral hypofunction and provide an assessment of the patient's vestibular function.

CLINICS CARE POINTS

- Stereotyped repetitive bouts of short duration (<60 sec) episodic vertigo triggered by change of head position relative to gravity – especially anterior or posterior pitch (tipping the head to look down or up) or rolling over in bed toward the affected side – should be considered BPPV until proven otherwise.

- Apparent BPPV that (1) is resistant to particle repositioning treatment, (2) repeatedly relapses within days of successful particle repositioning, or (3) changes sides with frequent relapses should be considered vestibular migraine until proven otherwise. A more detailed assessment for migraine indicators should be undertaken.

- Recurrent vertigo attacks lasting 20 minutes to 12 hours associated with unilateral hearing loss, aural fullness, and tinnitus in the absence of migraine are diagnostic of Meniere's disease.

- Patients meeting diagnostic criteria for Meniere's disease who have *any* history of migraine headache, ocular migraine, or a first-degree family member with migraine should receive a more detailed assessment for migraine indicators that are temporally associated with the Meniere attacks. If found, the patient should be treated for vestibular migraine.

- In patients who suffer from concurrent vestibular migraine and Meniere's disease, migraine should be treated first. Once migraine is under control, the patient can be assessed to judge if any Meniere treatment is needed.

- Patients with vertigo of "the Meniere type" who have no auditory symptoms (the presentation formerly known as "vestibular Meniere's disease") or who are unable to localize which is the affected ear should be considered vestibular migraine until proven otherwise. Detailed assessment of family migraine history and patient assessment for migraine indicators should be undertaken.

- Patients with active migraine symptoms or any prior history of migraine headache or ocular migraine who have unexplained vestibular symptoms should be considered to have a possible vestibular migraine. Detailed assessment of family migraine history and patient assessment for migraine indicators should be undertaken.

- Acute onset of severe vertigo lasting 24 to 72 hours followed by several weeks-months of disequilibrium and gradual recovery strongly suggests a diagnosis of vestibular neuritis.

The exact same vestibular symptoms accompanied by concurrent acute onset of unilateral sensorineural hearing loss are strongly suggestive of labyrinthitis.

- Approximately 50% of vestibular neuritis patients develop secondary BPPV on the affected side 2 to 4 months after the onset of the neuritis. They can be warned about this and be prepared to seek prompt particle repositioning.

- Meniere's disease is an ear disease, and therefore the peri-ictal clinical presentation is confined to unilateral ear symptoms plus nausea and vomiting. In contrast, vestibular migraine is a neurologic disease. Therefore, it is typically associated with other peri-ictal neurologic symptoms, such as profound headache, photophobia, osmophobia, "brain fog," lethargy and fatigue, or other sensory or motor disturbances.

- Obstructive sleep apnea is an under-appreciated but extremely potent trigger for both Meniere attacks and vestibular migraine attacks. Uncontrolled OSA is likely to prevent adequate treatment response of the vestibulopathy. Patients with either of these diagnoses should be thoroughly evaluated and, if necessary, treated for OSA.

DISCLOSURE

The authors have no disclosures to report.

REFERENCES

1. Sorathia S, Agrawal Y, Schubert MC. Dizziness and the otolaryngology point of view. Med Clin North Am 2018. https://doi.org/10.1016/j.mcna.2018. 06.004.

2. Kutz JW. The dizzy patient. Med Clin North Am 2010. https://doi.org/10.1016/j. mcna.2010.05.011.

3. Lepcha A, Tyagi AK, Ashish G, et al. Audiovestibular and radiological findings in patients with migrainous vertigo. Neurol Asia 2015;20(4): 367–73.

4. Kerber KA, Brown DL, Lisabeth LD, et al. Stroke among patients with dizziness, vertigo, and imbalance in the emergency department: a population-based study. Stroke 2006. https://doi.org/10.1161/01.STR.0000240329. 48263.0d.

5. Newman-Toker DE, Cannon LM, Stofferahn ME, et al. Imprecision in patient reports of dizziness symptom quality: a cross-sectional study conducted in an acute care setting. Mayo Clin Proc 2007. https://doi.org/10.4065/82.11. 1329.

6. Gupta V, Lipsitz LA. Orthostatic hypotension in the elderly: diagnosis and treatment. Am J Med 2007. https://doi.org/10.1016/j.amjmed.2007.02.023.

7. Muncie HL, Sirmans SM, James E. Dizziness: approach to evaluation and management. Am Fam Physician 2017;95(3):154–62.

8. Chawla N, Olshaker JS. Diagnosis and management of dizziness and vertigo. Med Clin North Am 2006. https://doi.org/10.1016/j.mcna.2005.11.003.

9. Hain TC. Cervicogenic causes of vertigo. Curr Opin Neurol 2015. https://doi.org/ 10.1097/WCO.0000000000000161.

10. Yuan Q, Yu L, Shi D, et al. Anxiety and depression among patients with different types of vestibular peripheral vertigo. Medicine (Baltimore) 2015. https://doi.org/ 10.1097/MD.0000000000000453.

11. Takahashi S. Importance of cervicogenic general dizziness. J Rural Med 2018. https://doi.org/10.2185/jrm.2958.

12. Liu YF, Xu H. The intimate relationship between vestibular migraine and meniere disease: a review of pathogenesis and presentation. Behav Neurol 2016. https://doi.org/10.1155/2016/3182735.

13. Vaduva C, Estéban-Sánchez J, Sanz-Fernández R, et al. Prevalence and management of post-BPPV residual symptoms. Eur Arch Oto-rhino-laryngology 2018. https://doi.org/10.1007/s00405-018-4980-x.

14. Lempert T, Olesen J, Furman J, et al. Vestibular migraine: diagnostic criteria. J Vestib Res Equilib Orientat 2012. https://doi.org/10.3233/VES-2012-0453.

15. Neuhauser HK, Radtke A, Von Brevern M, et al. Burden of dizziness and vertigo in the community. Arch Intern Med 2008. https://doi.org/10.1001/archinte.168.19.2118.

16. Ten Voorde M, Van Der Zaag-Loonen HJ, Van Leeuwen RB. Dizziness impairs health-related quality of life. Qual Life Res 2012. https://doi.org/10.1007/s11136-011-0001-x.

17. Jacobson GP, Newman CW. The development of the dizziness handicap inventory. Arch Otolaryngol Neck Surg 1990. https://doi.org/10.1001/archotol.1990.01870040046011.

18. Yardley L, Masson E, Verschuur C, et al. Symptoms, anxiety and handicap in dizzy patients: development of the Vertigo symptom scale. J Psychosom Res 1992. https://doi.org/10.1016/0022-3999(92)90131-K.

19. Duracinsky M, Mosnier I, Bouccara D, et al. Literature review of questionnaires assessing vertigo and dizziness, and their impact on patients' quality of life. Value Heal 2007. https://doi.org/10.1111/j.1524-4733.2007.00182.x.

20. Joseph A, Wanono R, Flamant M, et al. Orthostatic hypotension: a review. Nephrol Ther 2017. https://doi.org/10.1016/j.nephro.2017.01.003.

21. Sweeney CJ, Gilden DH. Ramsay hunt syndrome. J Neurol Neurosurg Psychiatry 2001. https://doi.org/10.1136/jnnp.71.2.149.

22. Smith MM, Anderson JC. Neurosyphilis as a cause of facial and vestibulocochlear nerve dysfunction: MR imaging features. Am J Neuroradiol 2000.

23. Moscatello AL, Worden DL, Nadelman RB, et al. Otolaryngologic aspects of lyme disease. Laryngoscope 1991. https://doi.org/10.1288/00005537-199106000-00004.

24. Jozefowicz-Korczynska M, Zamyslowska-Szmytke E, Piekarska A, et al. Vertigo and severe balance instability as symptoms of lyme disease—literature review and case report. Front Neurol 2019. https://doi.org/10.3389/fneur.2019.01172.

25. Roberts L, Cacace AT. Jendrassik maneuver facilitates cVEMP amplitude: Some preliminary observations. J Am Acad Audiol 2014. https://doi.org/10.3766/jaaa.25.3.2.

26. Bhattacharyya N, Gubbels SP, Schwartz SR, et al. Clinical Practice Guideline: Benign Paroxysmal Positional Vertigo (Update). Otolaryngol Head Neck Surg 2017. https://doi.org/10.1177/0194599816689667.

27. Hornibrook J. Benign Paroxysmal Positional Vertigo (BPPV): history, pathophysiology, office treatment and future directions. Int J Otolaryngol 2011. https://doi.org/10.1155/2011/835671.

28. Ulmer E, Chays A. Curthoys and Halmagyi Head Impulse test: an analytical device. Ann Otolaryngol Chir Cervicofac 2005. https://doi.org/10.1016/s0003-438x(05)82329-1.

29. Migliaccio AA, Cremer PD. The 2D modified head impulse test: A 2D technique for measuring function in all six semi-circular canals. J Vestib Res Equilib Orientat 2011. https://doi.org/10.3233/VES-2011-0421.

30. Schubert MC, Tusa RJ, Grine LE, et al. Optimizing the Sensitivity of the Head Thrust Test for Identifying Vestibular Hypofunction. Phys Ther 2004. https://doi.org/10.1093/ptj/84.2.151.

31. Verma R, Praharaj HN, Khanna VK, et al. Study of micronutrients (copper, zinc and vitamin B12) in posterolateral myelopathies. J Neurol Sci 2013. https://doi.org/10.1016/j.jns.2013.03.004.

32. IHS. The International Classification of Headache Disorders, 3rd edition (beta version). Cephalalgia 2013. https://doi.org/10.1177/0333102413485658.

Efficient Use of Vestibular Testing

Steven A. Zuniga, MD*, Meredith E. Adams, MD, MS

KEYWORDS

- Balance • Dizziness • Vertigo • Vestibular disorders • Vestibular testing

KEY POINTS

- The majority of vestibular disorders may be readily diagnosed from a thorough clinical history and physical exam.
- Objective assessment of vestibular function may provide insights that facilitate diagnostic refinement and inform management decisions in specific clinical scenarios.
- An understanding of the data provided by vestibular tests, as well as their inherent limitations, enables the efficient utilization of these test modalities.

INTRODUCTION

The dizzy patient presents a formidable diagnostic challenge. Dizziness is one of the most common symptoms prompting clinical evaluation.[1] Afflicted patients experience poor quality of life, risk of falling with injury, and frequently require sick leave, job changes, or disability.[1–4] Clinicians must consider a wide range of benign to life-threatening etiologies within the time constraints of modern practice. The demands are compounded by the absence of a comprehensive clinical practice guideline for the dizziness diagnostic evaluation.

The admixture of distressed, at-risk patients, diagnostic uncertainty, and time pressure generates an explosion of test acquisition.[5–7] Vestibular tests consistently rank among the most billed office procedures associated with otolaryngologic practices in the United States,[8] and are also frequently obtained by other specialists and primary care clinicians.[9] However, there is no "standard practice," and vestibular test use varies markedly between geographic regions, medical specialties, and individual practices.[9–11]

Choosing Wisely Canada, a campaign to reduce unnecessary tests and treatments through the development of common-sense guidelines, specifically recommends, "[d]on't order specialized audiometric and vestibular neurodiagnostic tests in an attempt

Department of Otolaryngology—Head and Neck Surgery, University of Minnesota, 420 Delaware Street, MMC 396, Minneapolis, MN 55455, USA
* Corresponding author.
E-mail address: zunig085@umn.edu

Otolaryngol Clin N Am 54 (2021) 875–891
https://doi.org/10.1016/j.otc.2021.05.011
0030-6665/21/© 2021 Elsevier Inc. All rights reserved.

Abbreviations	
BPPV	Benign paroxysmal positional vertigo
cVEMP	Cervical VEMP
GEN	Gaze-evoked nystagmus
IVN	Inferior vestibular nerve
oVEMP	Ocular VEMP
PT	Physical therapy
SCDS	Superior semicircular canal dehiscence
SCV	Slow component velocity
SHA	Sinusoidal harmonic acceleration
SPV	Slow phase velocity
SVN	Superior vestibular nerve
VEMP	Vestibular evoked myogenic potential
VNG	Videonystagmography
VOR	Vestibulo-ocular reflex

to screen for peripheral vestibular disease."[12] Rather, the diagnosis should be guided by the presenting symptoms and office examination, and tests "should only be ordered if clinically indicated."[12] Accordingly, this article aims to help clinicians apply an accessible decision-making rubric to identify clinical scenarios that may and may not benefit from data derived from specific vestibular function tests.

MAKING WISE CHOICES

The etiology of dizziness can often be identified with a detailed history and focused physical examination without additional testing.[13–17] To illustrate, predictive accuracy of 78.5% for the final diagnosis was achieved by a previsit questionnaire that differentiated dizziness causes by episode description, symptoms (including auditory) characteristic of peripheral versus central etiologies, and general and emotional health.[18] Diagnostic criteria for common disorders, including Meniere's disease and benign paroxysmal positional vertigo (BPPV), do not include vestibular test data.[19,20] Best practices for using history and exam for dizziness diagnosis are presented elsewhere in this edition.

We also need to count the costs of our diagnostic approaches. Beyond the obvious monetary costs borne by patients, systems, and payors,[9,10] patients undergoing testing will experience morbidity and opportunity costs.[21] For example, videonystagmography (VNG) with caloric testing can induce nausea/vomiting, headaches, and other residual symptoms that preclude a return to work or activities of daily living for several days.[21] These tests may also require the involvement of additional family members (for the drive home) and finding child care alternatives, thus creating collateral social and financial burdens.

How then does a clinician determine if vestibular testing is clinically indicated? The decision-making checklist developed by Dr. William Follansbee[22] is particularly helpful in this regard. Prior to obtaining testing, a differential diagnosis is generated from the symptoms and exam. To determine what tests to order, *if any*, clinicians should: (1) define the specific question they are asking with the test; (2) determine if they truly need to know the answer because it will refine the diagnosis and/or affect patient management or outcomes; (3) identify the test that will best answer the specific question.

What Questions May Vestibular Tests Answer?

1. Site of Lesion. Vestibular tests may localize lesions to central versus peripheral vestibular pathways and by laterality and topography (eg, superior vs inferior vestibular nerve, otolithic organ vs semicircular canal).

2. Extent of Lesion. Vestibular tests may quantify the severity of vestibular hypofunction over the vestibulo-ocular reflex (VOR) frequency range, characterizing disease stage/progression to inform treatment decisions (eg, ablation).
3. Level of Compensation. Following acute vestibular loss, vestibular tests can assess compensation status to direct uncompensated individuals to vestibular physical therapy (PT)[23] and track progress over time.
4. Functional Integration of Sensory Inputs. A complex network of sensory inputs must be successfully integrated to maintain stance and gait. Tests including computerized dynamic posturography assess visual, vestibular, and postural contributions to balance.

What Questions May Vestibular Tests NOT Answer?

Vestibular tests offer more insight into vestibular physiology (eg, VOR function) than pathophysiology and do not typically provide a specific diagnosis (eg, Meniere's disease).[24] For example, VNG reveals nystagmus generated by asymmetric peripheral vestibular system stimulation, but supplementary information is required to elucidate the cause. Vestibular tests also do not determine the level of disability resulting from vestibular impairment. Patient-reported disability measures (eg, dizziness handicap inventory) and vestibular test results are poorly correlated,[25] potentially due to variations in physiologic and behavioral adaptation.

VESTIBULAR PHYSIOLOGY: KEY CONCEPTS FOR TEST SELECTION AND INTERPRETATION
Visual–Vestibular Interaction

Vestibular tests interrogate the function of the vestibular system largely through the measurement and interpretation of eye movements. A common goal of eye movements is to optimize visual acuity by directing and maintaining an object of interest on the fovea.[26] When the head is static and the object moves, central visual tracking systems are used. The *saccade* control system generates fast voluntary and involuntary eye movements that focus objects in the visual periphery on the fovea.[26] The *smooth pursuit* system maintains images of small, slowly moving objects on the fovea, driven by retinal slip from visual motion.[24] The peripherally-mediated VOR maintains fixation on a stable target during head movements by generating eye movements that are equal in velocity but opposite in direction to head movements (**Fig. 1**). During simultaneous movement of the head and visual surround, a complex interaction between vestibular and visual ocular control systems is necessary.

Nystagmus is generated by a combination of peripherally and centrally mediated eye movements.[26] The VOR holds images on the retina by producing reflexive compensatory eye movements during head rotations, but VOR-driven eye rotation is limited by anatomic constraints. As the eyes approach their orbital limit, central processes "reset" the position of the eyes, quickly moving them in the opposite direction and directing the gaze toward the oncoming visual scene. The slow phase of nystagmus is driven by tonic asymmetry in the neural activity of the vestibular system, and its velocity (degrees/s) is a common vestibular test outcome measure. The centrally generated fast phase movement is more discernible to observers and is used to name the direction of nystagmus (see **Fig. 1**).

Contributions from the Brainstem and Cerebellum

The VOR is maximally efficient and demonstrates nearly perfect gain (ie, eye velocity approximates head velocity) at frequencies between 0.05 and 6 Hz (**Fig. 2**).[27] VOR efficiency declines at higher and lower frequencies. Low-frequency transduction is

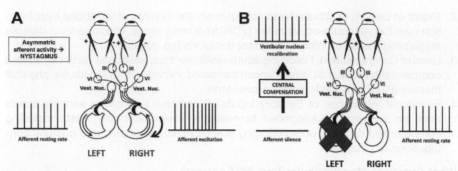

Fig. 1. Horizontal Vestibulo-ocular reflex (VOR). (*A*) While the head is at rest, vestibular afferents demonstrate an approximately symmetric baseline firing rate of 10 to 100 action potentials per second. This tonic neural activity affords bidirectional sensitivity to the system; excitatory head movements increase and inhibitory head movements decrease the firing rate, respectively.[24] The direction of cupular deflection determines whether action potential frequency increases or decreases with head motion, and the complementary arrangement of the canals ensures that an increase in firing rate for one results in a decrease in its coplanar mate. Stimulation of the horizontal semicircular canal produces eye movements in the plane of that canal (Ewald's first law) that are equal in velocity but opposite in direction to the associated head movement. In this case, sustained rightward head motion stimulates and inhibits the right and left horizontal canal afferents, respectively, resulting in leftward slow phase eye movement (*curved arrows*), and right beat (fast phase) nystagmus. (*B*) Acute left peripheral hypofunction creates a similar asymmetry in vestibular afferent firing rates with corresponding eye movements. Central static compensation occurs following an acute vestibular lesion and involves tonic rebalancing of the resting activity of the vestibular nuclei. This minimizes the tonic firing rate asymmetry in the second-order neurons originating in the vestibular nuclei.

improved by the perseveration of raw rotational signals by brainstem vestibular nuclei by the central *velocity storage* mechanism.[28] Velocity storage may be transiently diminished with acute unilateral vestibulopathy, leading to prerotary and postrotatory nystagmus (rotary chair) and head-shake nystagmus.

The *neural integrator* is a brainstem mechanism that allows the eyes to be held in an eccentric position for visual acuity instead of drifting back to neutral gaze position from elastic restoring forces of the orbit.[28] With acute unilateral vestibulopathy, the neural

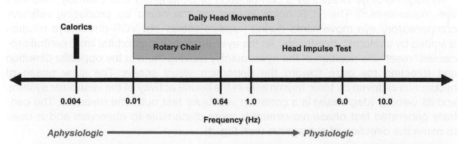

Fig. 2. Vestibulogram. In isolation, the VOR optimally functions between head rotation frequencies of 0.05 and 6 Hz, relying on supplementary central processing to improve function across its dynamic range (ie, velocity storage). Clinicians may assess the integrity of the horizontal VOR across its frequency range using caloric testing (low frequencies), rotary chair testing (low to middle frequencies), and head impulse testing (high frequencies).

integrator's ability to hold eccentric gaze is diminished (ie, unilaterally inhibited), and the eyes drift back to a central position. Corrective saccades are needed to maintain eye position, generating gaze-evoked nystagmus (GEN). The combination of GEN and VOR-driven nystagmus from a peripheral vestibular lesion results in increased nystagmus intensity when looking away from the lesion (ie, toward the nystagmus fast phase) and decreased intensity when looking toward the lesion. This nystagmus intensifies when visual fixation is denied. The effect is known as *Alexander's law* and is useful in distinguishing nystagmus of peripheral from central origin[29] and assessing for compensation.

Adjustment to asymmetries in peripheral vestibular input or compensation for insults within the central vestibular pathways relies on the adaptive plasticity of the cerebellum and brainstem nuclei.[30] Vestibular compensation occurs in 2 stages: (1) static compensation, which occurs in the absence of head movements and involves recalibration of the resting tonic activity of the vestibular nuclei; and (2) dynamic compensation, which is driven by persistent disequilibrium and motion-provoked vertigo.[24]

VIDEONYSTAGMOGRAPHY

VNG employs high-speed infrared cameras and sophisticated algorithms to record and measure eye movements in response to visual or vestibular stimuli. The VNG battery interrogates the oculomotor and vestibular systems and detects pathologic (spontaneous, gaze, positional, and positioning) nystagmus. VNG can be used to identify the site and extent of vestibular lesions and compensation status.

Oculomotor Testing (Central Lesions)

The oculomotor test battery interrogates central pathways responsible for generating voluntary and involuntary eye movements including saccades and smooth pursuit. The head is static during these tests permitting oculomotor system assessment *independent* of the peripheral vestibular system. The timing, speed, and accuracy of eye movements are compared with those of visual target stimuli. Abnormalities of saccades or smooth pursuit represent a dysfunction of neurologic substrates originating anywhere from supranuclear central control centers through the extraocular muscles.[26] Abnormalities of latency and velocity primarily result from dysfunction in the pontine reticular formation and brainstem structures[31]; abnormalities of accuracy often result from dysfunction of the vestibulocerebellum.[32] Oculomotor tests are influenced by age, alertness, medications/substances, and ophthalmologic pathology.[24] The reader is referred to Leigh and Zee[26] for a detailed analysis of neural pathways underlying oculomotor abnormalities.

Spontaneous Eye Movements (Central or Peripheral Lesions)

Eye movements are recorded during visual fixation on a static target and in darkness with eyes open, removing fixation, in midline gaze (primary position) and gazing 30° off midline in each direction (left, right, up, down).[33] Persistent nystagmus in place of steady gaze is considered to be abnormal. *Spontaneous nystagmus* may be observed while the patient looks straight ahead. Nystagmus unobserved in the primary position that appears with eccentric gaze is *GEN*. *End-gaze nystagmus* manifests as small-amplitude nystagmus when gazing more than 30° from midline and is seen in normal individuals.[33]

Nystagmus may be of central or peripheral origin. *Ewald's first law* describes the stereotypic eye movements resulting from semicircular canal stimulation. This canal-fixed frame of reference predicts the ocular movements the peripheral system is capable of producing (**Fig. 3**). Peripheral nystagmus typically has a horizontal component and is direction-fixed, while pure vertical, pure torsional, or direction-changing nystagmus is of central origin until proven otherwise. In contrast to central nystagmus, peripheral nystagmus intensifies when fixation is removed and should follow Alexander's law.[24] Bilateral superior canal dehiscence can result in simultaneous bilateral canal stimulation, representing a potential peripheral source of transient down-beat nystagmus.[30]

Gaze testing may also reveal abnormal eye movements with fixation that have equal velocity and amplitude in all directions, collectively referred to as saccadic intrusions and oscillations,[26] and implicate brainstem or cerebellar pathology.[24] Leigh and Zee (2015)[26] comprehensively review their pathogenesis.

Positional and Positioning Testing

Positional tests change labyrinthine orientation to gravity, uncovering imbalances in peripheral or central neural pathways. Nystagmus is recorded in static supine/precaloric, head right/left, and/or body right/left positions. Representing the most common VNG finding,[24] positional nystagmus is abnormal if it is present in more than half of the positions, direction changing, or average peak slow phase velocity (SPV) exceeds 4°/sec.[33] It may be localizing when considered with other VNG results (discussed below).

Dynamic positioning tests include tests for BPPV under video-oculography. The diagnosis of BPPV is clinical, based on history and positive Dix-Hallpike or roll tests, and does not require VNG.[34] VNG recordings may facilitate challenging diagnoses (eg, laterality of horizontal canalithiasis or cupulolithiasis). Vestibular testing is warranted when patients with positional vertigo have atypical nystagmus, another vestibular pathology is suspected, following frequent BPPV recurrences, or failure of repositioning maneuvers.[34]

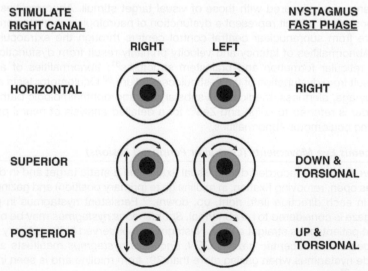

Fig. 3. Compensatory eye movements in response to canal stimulation (right ear). Arrows indicate slow phase compensatory eye movements. In considering whether nystagmus is of central or peripheral origin, it is important to consider whether the peripheral vestibular system is capable of producing the observed pattern of nystagmus.

Caloric Testing (Peripheral Lesions)

Bithermal caloric testing has long been the consensus standard for quantitative evaluation of peripheral vestibular function. Patients lie supine, head elevated 30°, placing the horizontal canal in the earth-vertical plane. Cool and warm irrigations of water or air are alternately delivered to each ear canal.[24] While preventing visual fixation, eye movements are recorded during and after each irrigation. Irrigations alternately stimulate (warm) or inhibit (cool) the horizontal canal VOR in an aphysiologic frequency range (0.003–0.008 Hz) (see **Fig. 2**).[35]

The peak SPV of caloric-induced nystagmus is used to generate the main outcome measures of the caloric test.[36] The *caloric weakness* is a comparison of responses between right and left ears. Responses are compared between ears because absolute responses to calorics are highly variable between individuals. The *directional preponderance* is a comparison of responses to irrigations yielding right versus left beat nystagmus and is analogous to the asymmetry outcome in rotary chair.

What do we learn from an abnormal caloric test? Caloric weaknesses result from lesions along the horizontal VOR pathway, including the horizontal semicircular canal, superior vestibular nerve, vestibulocochlear nerve root entry zone, and vestibular nucleus. Although exact localization is difficult, calorics isolate 1 vestibular periphery from the other,[35] defining laterality (sidedness) and quantifying the severity of vestibular hypofunction based on the percent weakness.

When unilateral weakness is identified, spontaneous and positional nystagmus tests help clinicians assess compensation status. On these tests, peripheral nystagmus follows Alexander's law and disappears with static compensation (**Figs. 4** and **5**). Persistent spontaneous nystagmus of greater than 2 to 3°/s suggests incomplete compensation[24] that may improve with therapy. Directional preponderance most often results from spontaneous nystagmus (eg, right beat nystagmus produces right DP), which characterizes acute uncompensated vestibular hypofunction or irritative lesions.[24]

Bilaterally reduced or absent horizontal VOR function is suggested when the total eye speed (ie, the sum of warm and cool caloric responses) per ear is less than 6°/sec.[37] However, rotary chair or vHIT is needed to determine whether there is a functionally significant residual function at higher physiologic frequencies.

What do we learn from a normal caloric test? Normal caloric results do not "rule out" vestibular disease. Calorics stimulate the horizontal canal VOR; lesions of the otolith organs, vertical canals, or other neural pathways (eg, superior semicircular canal dehiscence (SCDS), inferior vestibular neuritis) would not produce caloric asymmetry.[24] Further, peripheral disorders do not always cause canal hypofunction (eg, Meniere's disease).[38,39] Laboratories set cutoffs for unilateral weakness to avoid false positives, but the level of asymmetry sufficient to produce symptoms is unknown. A milder asymmetry may be significant in a symptomatic patient.[24]

ROTARY CHAIR TESTING

Rotary chair testing is a calibrated, midfrequency test of the horizontal VOR and its superior vestibular nerve (SVN) afferents (see **Fig. 2**). The common test paradigms are sinusoidal harmonic acceleration (SHA) and step testing. In SHA protocols, the chair rotates back and forth at frequencies 0.01 to 0.64 Hz at a set velocity.[24] Step testing consists of chair acceleration to sustained velocity followed by equal deceleration to a full stop[24]; the test is repeated in the opposite direction. Outcome measures are gain, phase or time constant (for SHA and step testing, respectively), and symmetry. Gain refers to the ratio of peak eye velocity to peak head velocity. Phase represents the

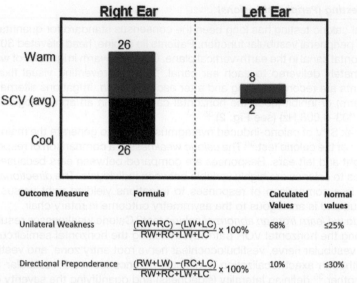

Outcome Measure	Formula	Calculated Values	Normal values
Unilateral Weakness	$\dfrac{(RW+RC)-(LW+LC)}{RW+RC+LW+LC} \times 100\%$	68%	≤25%
Directional Preponderance	$\dfrac{(RW+LW)-(RC+LC)}{RW+RC+LW+LC} \times 100\%$	10%	≤30%

Fig. 4. VNG results from a patient with persistent disequilibrium 3 months following acute vestibular syndrome, consistent with vestibular neuritis. Maximal slow component velocity (SCV) resulting from each caloric irrigation is presented (red, warm irrigation; blue, cool irrigation). Calculation of key outcome measures is illustrated, and normative values presented. Findings are consistent with left peripheral hypofunction. LC, left cool; LW, left warm; RC, right cool; RW, right warm; SCV, slow component velocity.

difference in time between the head and eyes reach peak velocity. Symmetry is a comparison of slow phase eye velocity during rightward versus leftward movements.

While some labs routinely employ rotary chair for vestibular deficit detection,[40] our decision-making rubric favors selective use. Rotational tests activate the VOR in a physiologic manner but, during rotation, the simultaneous push–pull (ie, excitation–inhibition) of semicircular canal pairs limits inferences about unilateral deficits and laterality. One intact labyrinth is sufficient to maintain normal VOR gain. Rotary chair is most useful for confirming and quantifying the severity of *bilateral* vestibular

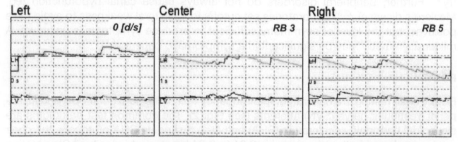

Fig. 5. Gaze testing in a patient with persistent disequilibrium 3 months following acute vestibular syndrome. Caloric testing revealed a 70% left caloric weakness. VNG tracings during gaze testing show spontaneous right beat nystagmus in center gaze (3 deg/s) that follows Alexander's law, intensifying to 5 deg/s when looking toward the fast phase (right). This is consistent with incomplete compensation. d/s = degrees/s; RB = Right Beat.

hypofunction. Bilateral loss of VOR function manifests as reduced VOR gain (<0.1 on SHA) and phase leads greater than 68° or time constant less than 5 seconds[37] (**Fig. 6**). Test results can reveal ototoxicity and direct PT, as verifying intact or reduced but viable VOR gain at high frequencies informs vestibular rehabilitation.[24] A secondary use of rotary chair is the assessment of compensation. Unilateral losses may manifest as borderline low gain and slight phase leads,[24] but these findings are not localizing. Rather, like spontaneous nystagmus on VNG, the asymmetry value reflects compensation, pointing to either the weaker side or an irritative lesion. Rotary chair is costly but may be used in populations poorly suited for calorics (eg, children) or vHIT (eg, limited neck range of motion).[37]

VIDEO HEAD IMPULSE TEST

The head impulse test is a bedside test of VOR integrity.[41] The patient is instructed to fixate on a stable visual target while the examiner applies small amplitude, high peak velocity head rotations in each of the paired semicircular canal planes. During vHIT, similar impulses are administered while patients wear tight-fitting video-oculography goggles outfitted to simultaneously measure eye and head velocity.[24]

The primary vHIT outcome parameters are gain (eye velocity/head velocity) and the response profile (saccades). Normal VOR function drives eye movement to keep up with head movement, producing a gain near 1.0. With VOR impairment, the eyes initially move *with* the head until the individual generates a refixation saccade to correct eye position back onto the target. This manifests as reduced gain and repeatable saccades after the impulse (overt) and/or during the impulse (covert) (**Fig. 7**).[42,43]

With its high-frequency physiologic stimulus (1-6 Hz) (see **Fig. 2**), vHIT affords repeatable, relatively quick, quantitative measures of VOR function for the 6 semicircular canals and their corresponding vestibular afferents, permitting more granular lesion localization.[44,45] The diagnostic accuracy of vHIT for detecting a VOR deficit (defined as a gain of <0.68) has been validated for horizontal[44] and vertical[45] semicircular canal hypofunction, with sensitivity and specificity (compared with a scleral search coil technique) as high as 100%.[46] Importantly, caloric testing may be abnormal while vHIT remains normal, a phenomenon commonly seen in Meniere's disease,[47] suggesting vHIT is complementary to calorics. vHIT assesses dynamic semicircular canal function at high frequencies (but does not reveal diagnoses),[48] and may serve as a first test of VOR function. Additional testing at lower frequencies may be indicated based on results (eg, normal vHIT despite symptoms). While the investigation is ongoing, vHIT may also assess compensation following vestibular loss, with better outcomes being noted for patients who demonstrate conversion from overt to covert saccades following a vestibular loss.[24,49,50]

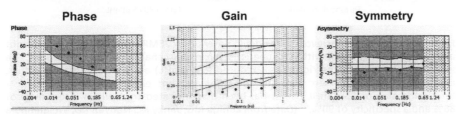

Fig. 6. Rotary chair results for a patient with imbalance and oscillopsia 6 weeks following therapy with intravenous gentamicin. There is a pronounced phase lead and low gain values across the frequency range, consistent with bilateral vestibular hypofunction.

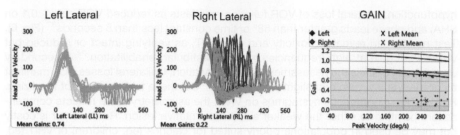

Fig. 7. vHIT response profile and gain measurements for the horizontal canal from a patient with episodic vertigo. On the right, eye movements (*green*) fail to keep up with head movements (*orange*), resulting in low gain (0.22) and corrective saccades (*red*) as the patient re-fixates on the target. The left ear demonstrates higher gain than the right (0.74) and no corrective saccades.

VESTIBULAR-EVOKED MYOGENIC POTENTIALS

VEMPs assess otolith function. Repetitive sound stimuli are sequentially applied to each ear. Resultant electromyographic (EMG) activity is recorded in target muscles. Cervical VEMP (cVEMP) measures relaxation potentials in the ipsilateral contracted sternocleidomastoid, generated primarily by the saccule and inferior vestibular nerve

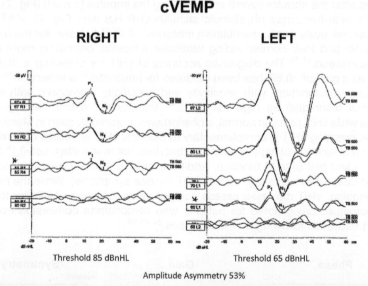

Fig. 8. Cervical vestibular evoked myogenic potential (cVEMP) response profile for right and left ears in a patient with left superior semicircular canal dehiscence syndrome. The stimulus threshold for the right ear is reduced (65 dBnHL) and an abnormal amplitude asymmetry (53%) is present between the right and left ears. Using a cVEMP cutoff threshold value of 85 dBnHL or less has been demonstrated to result in a sensitivity of 86% and a specificity of 90%.[61] (*Data from* Zuniga MG, Janky KL, Nguyen KD, Welgampola MS, Carey JP. Ocular Versus Cervical VEMPs in the Diagnosis of Superior Semicircular Canal Dehiscence Syndrome. *Otol Neurotol.* 2013;34(1):121-126. https://doi.org/10.1097/MAO.0b013e31827136b0.)

Table 1
Key tests, applications, and findings of common clinical questions from differential diagnosis

Clinical Scenarios	Sample Clinical Questions	Vestibular Function Tests and Pertinent Findings			
		VNG	Rotary Chair	vHIT	VEMP
Diagnostic refinement					
Acute vestibular syndrome	Is there a unilateral peripheral vestibular lesion?	**Caloric Asymmetry** **Spontaneous, gaze, or positional nystagmus obeys Alexander's law**	(+/−) Low gain Phase lead	**Reduced ipsilesional VOR gain** **Ipsilesional corrective saccades**	Absent/reduced oVEMP (SVN lesion) or cVEMP (IVN lesion)
	Has vestibular compensation occurred?[a]	**Spontaneous, gaze, positional, post head shake nystagmus**	Asymmetry	(+/−) Conversion of overt to covert saccades	NA
Episodic vestibular syndrome	Positional vertigo: BPPV vs central positional vertigo? Which canal is affected?	Positioning ± positional tests: nystagmus direction or duration (in) consistent with canal excitation	NA	NA	NA
	Is there a third window lesion?	NA	NA	NA	**Low thresholds, Amplitude asymmetry**
	Meniere's Disease: Which ear(s) are active? What is the level of hypofunction?	+/− **Caloric asymmetry** **Spontaneous, positional nystagmus (may point to irritative lesion or hypofunction)**	Asymmetry (may point to irritative lesion or hypofunction)	Gain may be normal even with caloric weakness	Asymmetric air conduction cVEMP (absent or reduced) and oVEMP (intact)
Chronic dizziness	Is there bilateral vestibular hypofunction?[b]	**Low total eye speed bilaterally** **Poor response to ice water caloric**	Low gain Phase lead	**Reduced VOR gain & saccades bilaterally**	(+/−)Absent/ reduced oVEMP (SVN), cVEMP (IVN)
	Is dizziness nonorganic or aphysiologic?	NA	NA	NA	NA

(continued on next page)

Table 1
(continued)

Clinical Scenarios	Sample Clinical Questions	Vestibular Function Tests and Pertinent Findings			
		VNG	Rotary Chair	vHIT	VEMP
Profound diagnostic uncertainty	What is happening?	NA	NA	NA	NA
Vestibular ablation: candidacy & efficacy assessment	How much vestibular function exists in each ear?	**Caloric asymmetry** **Total eye speed (to assess for bilateral weakness)**	Low gain if bilateral hypofunction	**VOR gain** **Corrective saccades**	oVEMP (SVN), cVEMP (IVN) response amplitude
Surgical Considerations[c]	Which ear has better vestibular function?	Caloric asymmetry	NA	**VOR gain** **Corrective saccades**	oVEMP (SVN), cVEMP (IVN) response amplitude
Clinical resources	Time to complete test in minutes (Mean [SD])[21,44]	71 [23]	26 [13]	10–15	~90 (estimate)
Billing – 2021 Medicare fee schedule	CPT Code(s) (Reimbursement Non-Facility/Facility)	92540 ($109.71/$112.01) 92537 ($42.59/$42.57)	92526 ($113.68/ $121.43)	No CPT code available	92517 ($87.23/ $43.97) 92518 ($81.30/ $43.97) 92519 ($135.39/ $65.95)

Denotes vestibular test modality with greatest potential to afford clinically meaningful results given the specific clinical scenario and question.

Abbreviations: BPPV, benign paroxysmal positional vertigo; CPT, current procedural terminology; cVEMP, cervical vestibular evoked myogenic potential; IVN, inferior vestibular nerve; NA, not applicable; oVEMP, ocular vestibular evoked myogenic potential; SVN, superior vestibular nerve; UVH, unilateral vestibular hypofunction; VEMP, vestibular evoked myogenic potential; vHIT, video head impulse test; VNG, videonystagmography; VOR, vestibulo-ocular reflex.

[a] Pertinent findings refer to evidence of an uncompensated lesion.

[b] Extent of frequency range involvement dependent on extent of lesion.

[c] Examples may include decisions regarding initial, bilateral, or contralateral cochlear implantation or stapes surgery, or postoperative assessments of symptomatic patients.

through the vestibulocollic reflex.[51] Ocular VEMP (oVEMP) measures excitation potentials in the contralateral inferior oblique, generated primarily by the utricle and superior vestibular nerve.[52] The outcome measures of cVEMP and oVEMP are their thresholds, peak-to-peak amplitudes, and latencies.

VEMP testing is most valuable for affirming the diagnosis of SCDS (**Fig. 8**).[53] In the presence of a third mobile window, otolith activation by sound is *enhanced*.[54] On the affected side(s), lower intensity sound stimuli induce the response (ie, lower VEMP threshold), and response amplitude may be abnormally increased (ie, amplitude asymmetry).[53] For the diagnosis of SCDS, the reported sensitivity and specificity of cVEMP are 42% to 91% and 90% to 100%, respectively, and of oVEMP are 62% to 100% and 73% to 100%, respectively.[55,56] VEMPs also detect *loss* of otolith function, manifesting as absent, reduced, or asymmetric cVEMP and/or oVEMP responses. While the clinical utility of loss-of-function applications is incompletely defined,[53] VEMPs may characterize vestibular nerve division(s) affected by vestibular neuritis or schwannoma,[54] ears with Meniere's disease,[57] and residual function after surgery/ablation.

SELECTING A VESTIBULAR TEST BATTERY

While clinical history is the cornerstone of vestibular investigation, vestibular function tests have clinically significant implications for diagnosis and management in specific scenarios. **Table 1** summarizes key tests, applications, and findings organized by common clinical questions that arise after clinicians craft a differential diagnosis. When diagnostic criteria are satisfied on clinical grounds (eg, BPPV, Meniere's), vestibular tests provide little additional information to bolster diagnostic confidence. However, as outlined, there are scenarios for which tests provide insight into lesion sites, severity, and compensation status, aiding in diagnostic refinement and management selection. The degree of vestibular impairment in unilateral pathology and the functional capacity of the contralateral vestibular system impacts management decisions, particularly regarding ablative therapies. Tests also inform decisions regarding initial or sequential otologic surgeries that risk vestibular loss (eg cochlear implantation, stapedectomy). Patients reporting vestibular symptoms before or after surgery may benefit from quantitative vestibular assessment, as documented hypofunction may contraindicate contralateral procedures. The majority of vestibular lesions initially impact the lower frequencies with preservation of the mid to high frequencies.[24] Patients with presumed bilateral vestibular areflexia require vestibular testing for diagnostic confirmation and quantification of injury extent. Determination of partial or complete vestibular loss across the frequency range informs the optimal treatment strategy (ie vestibular rehabilitation vs vestibular substitution for partial or complete loss, respectively).

SUMMARY

Despite the prevalence of dizziness and ample availability of diagnostic modalities, many affected individuals do not receive the prompt or accurate diagnoses needed to facilitate proper clinical management.[58–60] While most vestibular disorders may be diagnosed and managed based on data derived from history and exams, there are clinical scenarios in which vestibular function tests prove useful for diagnostic refinement and management decisions. An understanding of the insights that may be provided by vestibular tests and the limitations of the modalities facilitates efficient utilization.

CLINICS CARE POINTS

- The majority of vestibular disorders may be diagnosed based on history and physical exam findings.

- Vestibular function testing does not typically reveal the diagnosis but may provide insights that allow for diagnostic refinement and may inform management decisions.

- After formulating a differential diagnosis, tests should be selected to answer specific clinical questions rather than to "screen" for vestibular disease.

- Vestibular tests provide information about vestibular lesion localization, severity, compensation, and functional status.

- VNG and calorics provide data regarding laterality and severity of vestibular hypofunction and compensation status.

- Rotary chair may diagnose and/or confirm bilateral vestibular hypofunction and compensation status.

- vHIT provides an accessible means of assessing the function of all 6 semicircular canals and both superior and inferior vestibular nerve divisions.

- VEMP affords adjunctive data primarily efficacious in confirming the diagnosis of third window lesions including superior canal dehiscence.

- An understanding of vestibular physiology and the benefits and limitations of vestibular testing is requisite to the efficient use of this technology.

DISCLOSURE

The authors have no conflicts of interest to disclose. This work was supported by NIDCD R21DC016359 (M.E. Adams).

REFERENCES

1. Agrawal Y, Carey JP, Della Santina CC, et al. Disorders of balance and vestibular function in US adults: Data from the National Health and Nutrition Examination Survey, 2001-2004. Arch Intern Med 2009;169(10):938–44.

2. Lin HW, Bhattacharyya N. Balance disorders in the elderly: Epidemiology and functional impact. Laryngoscope 2012;122(8):1858–61.

3. Lin HW, Bhattacharyya N. Otologic diagnoses in the elderly: Current utilization and predicted workload increase. Laryngoscope 2011;121(7): 1504–7.

4. Lin HW, Bhattacharyya N. Impact of dizziness and obesity on the prevalence of falls and fall-related injuries. Laryngoscope 2014;124(12): 2797–801.

5. Saber Tehrani A, Coughlan D, Hsieh Y-H, et al. Rising Annual Costs of Dizziness Presentations to US Emergency Departments (P06.002). Neurology 2013;80(7 Supplement):689–96.

6. Kim AS, Sidney S, Klingman JG, et al. Practice variation in neuroimaging to evaluate dizziness in the ED. Am J Emerg Med 2012;30(5):665–72.

7. Newman-Toker DE, McDonald KM, Meltzer DO. How much diagnostic safety can we afford, and how should we decide? A health economics perspective. BMJ Qual Saf 2013;22(SUPPL.2):ii11–20.

8. American Academy of Otolaryngology - Head and Neck Surgery. Top 100 ENT CPT codes for 2015. Available at: https://www.entnet.org/wp-content/uploads/2021/06/non-facility-2021.pdf.

9. Adams ME, Yueh B, Marmor S. Clinician Use and Payments by Medical Specialty for Audiometric and Vestibular Testing among US Medicare Beneficiaries. JAMA Otolaryngol Head Neck Surg 2019;146(2):143–9.

10. Adams ME, Marmor S, Yueh B, et al. Geographic Variation in Use of Vestibular Testing among Medicare Beneficiaries. Otolaryngol Head Neck Surg 2017; 156(2):312–20.

11. Piker EG, Schulz K, Parham K, et al. Variation in the Use of Vestibular Diagnostic Testing for Patients Presenting to Otolaryngology Clinics with Dizziness. Otolaryngol Head Neck Surg 2016;155(1):42–7.

12. Canadian Society of Otolaryngology - Head & neck Surgery. Choosing Wisely Canada. 2020. Available at: https://choosingwiselycanada.org/otolaryngology/%0D%0A.

13. Phillips JS, Mallinson AI, Hamid MA. Cost-effective evaluation of the vestibular patient. Curr Opin Otolaryngol Head Neck Surg 2011;19(5):403–9.

14. Phillips JS, Fitzgerald JE, Bath AP. The role of the vestibular assessment. J Laryngol Otol 2009. https://doi.org/10.1017/S0022215109005611.

15. Grill E, Strupp M, Müller M, et al. Health services utilization of patients with vertigo in primary care: A retrospective cohort study. J Neurol 2014;261(8):1492–8.

16. Zhao JG, Piccirillo JF, Spitznagel EL, et al. Predictive capability of historical data for diagnosis of dizziness. Otol Neurotol 2011;32(2):284–90.

17. Jaynstein D. HINTS for differentiating peripheral from central causes of vertigo. J Am Acad Physician Assist 2016;29(10):56–7.

18. Roland LT, Kallogjeri D, Sinks BC, et al. Utility of an abbreviated dizziness questionnaire to differentiate between causes of vertigo and guide appropriate referral: A multicenter prospective blinded study. Otol Neurotol 2015;36(10): 1687–94.

19. Von Brevern M, Bertholon P, Brandt T, et al. Benign paroxysmal positional vertigo: Diagnostic criteria. J Vestib Res Equilib Orientat 2015;25(3–4):105–17.

20. Lopez-Escamez JA, Carey J, Chung WH, et al. Diagnostic criteria for Menière's disease. J Vestib Res Equilib Orientat 2015;25(1):1–7.

21. Kelly EA, Stocker C, Kempton CM, et al. Vestibular testing: Patient perceptions, morbidity, and opportunity costs. Otol Neurotol 2018;39(10):1222–8.

22. Follansbee WP. Diagnostic Decision Making: Time to Take Two Steps Back. Available at: http://ddmchecklist.upmc.com/.

23. Hall CD, Herdman SJ, Whitney SL, et al. Vestibular rehabilitation for peripheral vestibular hypofunction: An evidence-based clinical practice guideline: From the American physical therapy association neurology section. J Neurol Phys Ther 2016;40(2):124–55.

24. Jacobson GP, Shepard NT, Barin K, et al. Balance function assessment and management. In: Jacobson GP, Shepard NT, Barin K, et al, editors. Rotational Vestibular Assessment. 3rd edition. San Diego (CA): Plural Publishing; 2021. p. 283–332.

25. Yip CW, Strupp M. The Dizziness Handicap Inventory does not correlate with vestibular function tests: a prospective study. J Neurol 2018;265(5):1210–8.

26. Leigh RJ, Zee DS. The neurology of eye movements. In: Zee DS, editor. Diagnosis of Nystagmus and Saccadic Intrusions. 5th edition. New York: Oxford University Press; 2015. p. 658–768.

27. Goldberg JM, Wilson VJ, Cullen KE, et al. The vestibular system: a Sixth sense. New York: Oxford University Press; 2012. https://doi.org/10.1093/acprof:oso/9780195167085.001.0001.

28. Jellinger KA. The Neurology of Eye Movements 4th edn. Eur J Neurol 2009;16(7): e132.

29. Robinson DA, Zee DS, Hain TC, et al. Alexander's law: Its behavior and origin in the human vestibulo-ocular reflex. Ann Neurol 1984;16(6):714–22.

30. Curthoys IS, Michael Halmagyi G. Vestibular compensation: A review of the oculomotor, neural, and clinical consequences of unilateral vestibular loss. J Vestib Res 1995;5(2):67–107.

31. Walton MMG, Mustari MJ. Abnormal tuning of saccade-related cells in pontine reticular formation of strabismic monkeys. J Neurophysiol 2015;114(2):857–68.

32. Quaia C, Lefèvre P, Optican LM. Model of the control of saccades by superior colliculus and cerebellum. J Neurophysiol 1999;82(2):999–1018.

33. Shepard NT. Practical management of the balance disorder patient. In: Telian SA, editor. San Diego (CA): Singular Pub. Group; 1996.

34. Bhattacharyya N, Gubbels SP, Schwartz SR, et al. Clinical Practice Guideline: Benign Paroxysmal Positional Vertigo (Update). Otolaryngol Head Neck Surg 2017;156(3_suppl):S1–47.

35. Shepard N, Jacobson G. The caloric irrigation test. Handb Clin Neurol 2016;137: 119–31.

36. JONGKEES LB, MAAS JP, PHILIPSZOON AJ. Clinical nystagmography. A detailed study of electro-nystagmography in 341 patients with vertigo. Pract Otorhinolaryngol (Basel) 1962;24:65–93.

37. Strupp M, Kim JS, Murofushi T, et al. Bilateral vestibulopathy: Diagnostic criteria consensus document of the classification committee of the barany society. J Vestib Res Equilib Orientat 2017;27(4):177–89.

38. Palomar-Asenjo V, Boleas-Aguirre MS. S??nchez-Ferr??ndiz N, Perez Fernandez N. Caloric and Rotatory Chair Test Results in Patients with M??ni??re's Disease. Otol Neurotol 2006;27(7):945–50.

39. Yacovino DA, Hain TC, Musazzi M. Fluctuating vestibulo-ocular reflex in ménière's disease. Otol Neurotol 2017;38(2):244–7.

40. Arriaga MA, Chen DA, Cenci KA. Rotational chair (ROTO) instead of electronystagmography (ENG) as the primary vestibular test. Otolaryngol Head Neck Surg 2005;133(3):329–33.

41. Halmagyi GM, Curthoys IS. A Clinical Sign of Canal Paresis. Arch Neurol 1988; 45(7):737–9.

42. Weber KP, Aw ST, Todd MJ, et al. Head impulse test in unilateral vestibular loss: vestibulo-ocular reflex and catch-up saccades. Neurology 2008;70(6):454–63.

43. Halmagyi GM, Curthoys IS, Cremer PD, et al. The human horizontal vestibulo-ocular reflex in response to high-acceleration stimulation before and after unilateral vestibular neurectomy. Exp Brain Res 1990;81(3):479–90.

44. MacDougall HG, Weber KP, McGarvie LA, et al. The video head impulse test: Diagnostic accuracy in peripheral vestibulopathy. Neurology 2009;73(14): 1134–41.

45. MacDougall HG, McGarvie LA, Halmagyi GM, et al. The Video Head Impulse Test (vHIT) Detects Vertical Semicircular Canal Dysfunction. PLoS One 2013;8(4): e61488.

46. Curthoys IS, Manzari L. Clinical application of the head impulse test of semicircular canal function. Hearing, Balance and Communication 2017;15(3):113–26. https://doi.org/10.1080/21695717.2017.1353774.

47. Kaci B, Nooristani M, Mijovic T, et al. Usefulness of video head impulse test results in the identification of meniere's disease. Front Neurol 2020;11:581527.

48. Curthoys IS, Halmagyi GM. What does head impulse testing really test? JAMA Otolaryngol Head Neck Surg 2019;145(11):1080.

49. Sjögren J, Fransson P-A, Karlberg M, et al. Functional Head Impulse Testing Might Be Useful for Assessing Vestibular Compensation After Unilateral Vestibular Loss. Front Neurol 2018;9(NOV):979.

50. MacDougall HG, Curthoys IS. Plasticity during vestibular compensation: The role of saccades. Front Neurol 2012. https://doi.org/10.3389/fneur.2012.00021.

51. Colebatch JG, Halmagyi GM, Skuse NF. Myogenic potentials generated by a click-evoked vestibulocollic reflex. J Neurol Neurosurg Psychiatry 1994;57(2): 190–7.

52. Todd NPMA, Rosengren SM, Aw ST, et al. Ocular vestibular evoked myogenic potentials (OVEMPs) produced by air- and bone-conducted sound. Clin Neurophysiol 2007;118(2):381–90.

53. Fife TD, Colebatch JG, Kerber KA, et al. Practice guideline: Cervical and ocular vestibular evokedmyogenic potential testing: Report of the guideline development, dissemination, and implementation subcommittee of the American Academy of Neurology. Neurology 2017;89(22):2288–96.

54. Rosengren SM, Colebatch JG, Young AS, et al. Vestibular evoked myogenic potentials in practice: Methods, pitfalls and clinical applications. Clin Neurophysiol Pract 2019;4:47–68.

55. Noij KS, Rauch SD. Vestibular Evoked Myogenic Potential (VEMP) Testing for Diagnosis of Superior Semicircular Canal Dehiscence. Front Neurol 2020;11:695.

56. Fife TD, Satya-Murti S, Burkard RF, et al. Vestibular evoked myogenic potential testing Payment policy review for clinicians and payers. Neurol Clin Pract 2018; 8(2):129–34.

57. Taylor RL, Wijewardene AA, Gibson WPR, et al. The vestibular evoked-potential profile of Ménière's disease. Clin Neurophysiol 2011;122(6):1256–63.

58. To-Alemanji J, Ryan C, Schubert MC. Experiences Engaging Healthcare When Dizzy. Otol Neurotol 2016;37(8):1122–7.

59. Fife D, Fitzgerald JE. Do patients with benign paroxysmal positional vertigo receive prompt treatment? Analysis of waiting times and human and financial costs associated with current practice. Int J Audiol 2005;44(1):50–7.

60. Bhattacharyya N, Baugh RF, Orvidas L, et al. Clinical practice guideline: Benign paroxysmal positional vertigo. Otolaryngol Head Neck Surg 2008;139(5 SUPPL. 4). https://doi.org/10.1016/j.otohns.2008.08.022.

61. Zuniga MG, Janky KL, Nguyen KD, et al. Ocular Versus Cervical VEMPs in the Diagnosis of Superior Semicircular Canal Dehiscence Syndrome. Otol Neurotol 2013;34(1):121–6.

Neuroimaging of Dizziness and Vertigo

Wassim Malak, MD, Mari Hagiwara, MD, Vinh Nguyen, MD*

KEYWORDS

• Dizziness • Vertigo • Central • Peripheral • CT scan • MRI

KEY POINTS

- Vertigo and dizziness are symptoms of a broad scope of diseases affecting the peripheral and central vestibular system.
- Neuroimaging is particularly valuable for patients with neurologic signs or symptoms, and can be diagnostic when utilized appropriately.
- Frequent overlap in symptomatology necessitates a multidisciplinary approach toward diagnosis, image interpretation, and management of these patients.

INTRODUCTION

Dizziness and vertigo are symptoms that are often associated with each other, although the terms are sometimes used interchangeably. Dizziness refers to a general sensation of disturbed or impaired spatial orientation without a false sense of motion. Causes of dizziness are broad and include neurologic, metabolic, cardiovascular, and psychiatric etiologies. Vertigo, separate from dizziness, specifically refers to a false sensation of spinning, often believed to be of vestibular etiology.[1]

In this article, we discuss the role of imaging modalities used in the diagnostic workup and management of patients with dizziness, vertigo, or both. The clinical presentation, differential diagnoses, anatomy, and imaging findings are reviewed. Peripheral etiologies are more common and are due to disease processes involving the eighth cranial nerve or inner ear structures. Conversely, central pathologies are less common and typically owing to pathologies involving the brain parenchyma, more specifically, affecting the vestibular nuclei within the pons and medulla.

PROTOCOLS

The determination of an appropriate imaging study for a patient with dizziness and/or vertigo is based on whether the disease process is suspected to be peripheral or

Department of Radiology, NYU Langone Health, 222 East 41st Street, 5th Floor Radiology, New York, NY 10017, USA
* Corresponding author.
E-mail address: Vinh.Nguyen@nyulangone.org

Otolaryngol Clin N Am 54 (2021) 893–911
https://doi.org/10.1016/j.otc.2021.06.001

central in origin. Once the hypothesized site of pathology is established, an appropriate disease- and anatomy-targeted imaging study can be performed.

Computed Tomography Scans

A temporal bone computed tomography (CT) scan is the most appropriate imaging modality when certain peripheral processes are suspected owing to its high spatial resolution allowing visualization of the fine anatomic structures of the middle and inner ear. This imaging allows for the optimal evaluation in disease processes such as fracture, semicircular canal dehiscence, bony changes from infection or malignancy, and postsurgical follow-up. The use of ionizing radiation has been considered a major disadvantage of a temporal bone CT scan, although there has been considerable progress in decreasing exposure using deconvolution techniques and iterative reconstruction.[2]

A routine noncontrast head CT scan is not beneficial in assessing peripheral causes of dizziness and vertigo because it does not provide sufficient detail of the inner ear. However, a noncontrast head CT scan may be beneficial in the initial workup of central causes of dizziness and vertigo, especially to rule out urgent causes such as hemorrhage, infarct and herniation.[3] A contrast-enhanced head CT scan may be useful if malignancy or infection is suspected.

MRI

An MRI of the brain and internal auditory canals (IACs) are usually performed concurrently in the workup of dizziness and vertigo, for both peripheral and central causes.

When evaluating peripheral causes, high-resolution fluid-weighted images (including constructive interference in steady state, fast imaging employing steady-state acquisition, and T2 sampling perfection with application-optimized contrasts using different flip angle evolution sequences) best depict the normal anatomy and pathology of the fluid filled inner ear structures and cranial nerve VIII.[4,5] Postcontrast T1-weighted images are used to assess infectious processes such as labyrinthitis and neoplastic processes such as schwannomas.

When assessing for central causes, noncontrast whole brain MRI sequences are used to evaluate for infarct, demyelination, or structural abnormalities such as Chiari malformations. Postcontrast images are adjunctively useful in evaluating neoplasms.

Vascular Imaging

Vascular imaging such as a CT angiogram (CTA) and MR angiogram (MRA) are often not useful when assessing for peripheral causes of dizziness and vertigo. However, these studies are useful in assessing for central causes such as vertebrobasilar insufficiency, which may occur in up to 25% of elderly patients presenting with dizziness, possibly owing to high prevalence of atherosclerotic disease.[6] CTA and MRA are most useful in defining the degree of arterial stenoses supplying the posterior circulation.

DIFFERENTIAL DIAGNOSES
Peripheral Etiologies

Peripheral etiologies of dizziness and vertigo make up about 80% of cases and are limited to cranial nerve VIII and all distal structures of the vestibular system, including the 3 semicircular canals (posterior, superior, and lateral) and otolithic organs (saccule and utricle).[3]

Neoplastic

A vestibular schwannoma (**Fig. 1**) is a benign tumor of the Schwann cells arising from the vestibular nerve, most commonly from the inferior division.[7] These tumors

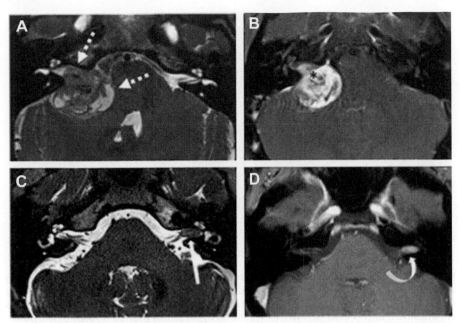

Fig. 1. Schwannoma. Axial fast imaging employing steady-state acquisition (*A*) imaging shows a heterogeneous solid and cystic mass (*dotted arrows*) in the internal auditory canal and cerebellopontine angle, which indents the brainstem. Postcontrast T1 image (*B*) demonstrates heterogeneous enhancement and widening of the porus acousticus (*asterisk*). A smaller schwannoma is seen on constructive interference in steady state (*C*) imaging as a filling defect in the left internal auditory canal (*arrow*). Enhancement (*D*) of the filling defect is present following contrast administration (*curved arrow*).

comprise approximately 80% of cerebellopontine angle (CPA) masses. Most are sporadic, but bilateral vestibular schwannomas can be found in neurofibromatosis type 2.[8] These tumors tend to arise near the porus acousticus of the IAC where there is a transition point between the glial and Schwann cells. Common symptomatology include hearing loss (80%), although ataxia and vertigo have also been reported (4% and 3%, respectively).[9] MRI of the brain and IAC with and without contrast allows for tumor characterization, surgical planning, and post-treatment evaluation, as well as to rule out other posterior fossa tumors. Vestibular schwannomas most commonly have an intracanalicular component widening the porus acousticus, called the trumpet sign. Extracanalicular extension from the IAC toward the CPA can display the ice cream cone sign, where the CPA portion is the ice cream and the intracanalicular portion is the cone. There is also a cystic variant that presents as a heterogeneously enhancing tumor with rapid and unpredictable growth.[10]

Meningiomas (**Fig. 2**) are the most common intracranial tumor, with approximately 1% of all intracranial meningiomas occurring in the CPA, and are the second most common CPA mass.[11] These usually occur in the fifth decade of life, with a female predominance. Meningiomas can extend into the IAC, or more rarely originate from the IAC itself.[12] When there is involvement of cranial nerve VIII, patients experience hearing loss, but up to 60% of patients can also have vertigo or imbalance.[13] In contrast with vestibular schwannomas, meningiomas grow as dural-based masses and do not expand the porus acousticus, best evaluated with an MRI of the brain and IAC

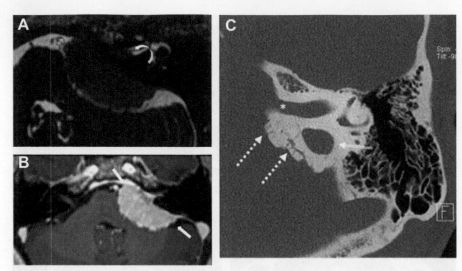

Fig. 2. Meningioma. Axial fast imaging employing steady-state acquisition (A) imaging shows a dural based mass in the CPA indenting the brainstem and overlying and extending into the internal auditory canal (*curved arrow*). The postcontrast T1 image (B) demonstrates enhancement of this mass (*arrows*). CT (C) shows hyperostosis (*dotted arrows*) of the posterior petrous ridge at the base of the mass with narrowing the porus acousticus (*asterisk*). Note is made of a high riding jugular bulb (*double lined arrow*).

with and without contrast. CT scans frequently demonstrate hyperostosis of the underlying bone.[14]

Glomus tumors (paragangliomas) are rare neuroendocrine tumors arising from paraganglia, which are neural crest derivatives. In the skull base, these neoplasms can arise from glomus bodies along the inferior tympanic nerve (Jacobson's nerve) of cranial nerve IX, overlying the cochlear promontory, giving rise to glomus tympanicum. Glomus bodies within the jugular foramen along the auricular branch of cranial nerve X (Arnold's nerve) or also Jacobson's nerve give rise to glomus jugulare.[15] Glomus jugulotympanicum refers to tumor involving both the jugular foramen and middle ear. The most common presenting symptom is pulsatile tinnitus, which may be accompanied by conductive hearing loss. Vertigo is a rare symptom, but can occur if the tumor erodes into the bony labyrinth.[16] Glomus tympanicum on imaging (**Fig. 3**) appears as a round enhancing mass on the cochlear promontory projecting into the mesotympanum. Glomus jugulare appears as a bony destructive, aggressive, enhancing lesion in the jugular foramen. T1-weighted images may show a salt and pepper appearance, with the salt corresponding with high-intensity T1 foci representing hemorrhage and pepper corresponding with the flow voids.[17]

Metastatic disease, most commonly from lung cancer, makes up about 3% of all temporal bone masses, usually occurring in the seventh decade of life.[18] Patients usually present with hearing loss and facial palsy, although dizziness has also been reported.[19]

Vascular

Jugular bulb diverticulum is an irregular outpouching of the jugular bulb in the temporal bone. Symptoms include hearing loss and pulsatile tinnitus associated with extension to the middle ear cavity, and vertigo associated with extension to the inner ear or the IAC.[20] CT scans demonstrate a smooth focal outpouching of the pars vascularis of the jugular foramen.[21]

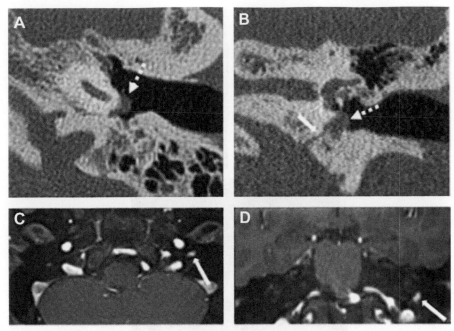

Fig. 3. Glomus tympanicum. Axial (*A*) and coronal (*B*) CT imaging of the left temporal bone show a soft tissue lesion on the cochlear promontory (*dashed arrows*). Extension into and widening of the inferior tympanic canaliculus (*solid arrow* in *B*) is seen as these tumors arise from the tympanic branch of the glossopharyngeal nerve. Contrast enhanced MR imaging shows avid enhancement of this lesion (*solid arrows*) on the axial (*C*) and coronal (*D*) views.

Infectious or inflammatory

In labyrinthitis, there is inflammation of the membranous labyrinth as well as vestibular and cochlear divisions of cranial nerve VIII.[3] These patients present with symptoms of vestibular neuritis and sensorineural hearing loss.[22] Illness usually begins with a viral upper respiratory tract infection. Spread can occur directly from bacterial meningitis or otitis media.[23,24] Imaging findings depend on the stage of disease. Acute labyrinthitis demonstrates enhancement of the membranous labyrinth on postcontrast MRI (**Fig. 4**). Chronic labyrinthitis will show resolution of enhancement but loss of normal fluid signal within the membranous labyrinth. In the ossifying stage (labyrinthitis ossificans), a CT scan shows an osseous matrix filling the membranous labyrinth.[25]

Cholesteatomas (**Fig. 5**) are benign collections of keratinized squamous epithelium within the middle ear. The congenital subtype occurs behind an intact tympanic membrane without a history of trauma or infection, whereas the acquired subtype is due to tympanic membrane retraction.[26] Common symptoms are conductive hearing loss and painless otorrhea.[27] Vertigo can indicate erosion into the inner ear and possibly a perilymphatic fistula.[28] A CT scan is used to detect or confirm disease, assess extension, and evaluate for complications. The CT scan will show a soft tissue mass, classically originating in Prussak's space, eroding surrounding osseous structures. MRI is most often used to evaluate for residual or recurrent disease and will demonstrate a nonenhancing, diffusion-restricted mass.[29]

Traumatic

Temporal bone fractures often result from high-energy blunt head injuries.[30] Temporal bone fractures are divided into otic capsule–sparing and otic capsule–violating

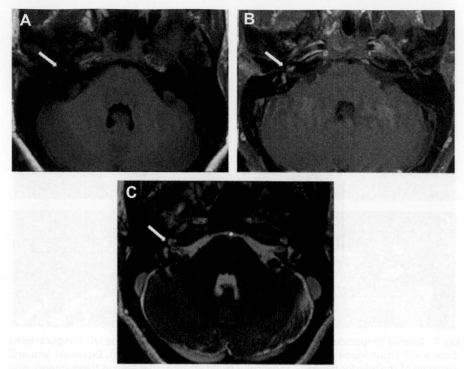

Fig. 4. Labyrinthitis. Axial T1 precontrast image (*A*) shows patchy high intense signal within the right inner ear structures, representing proteinaceous and/or hemorrhagic debris with superimposed diffuse enhancement on post contrast T1 (*B*) imaging (*arrows*). Axial high-resolution T2-weighted image (*C*) shows preservation of normal fluid signal within the labyrinth (*arrow*).

fractures. When the otic capsule is violated, presenting symptoms include facial nerve paresis, cerebrospinal fluid leakage, hearing loss, and dizziness and disequilibrium.[31] A CT scan of the temporal bone is the study of choice and allows for the visualization of the fracture line and involvement of the otic capsule.[32]

Perilymphatic fistula is a rare abnormal connection between the inner ear and sur-rounding structures, usually via the round or oval window. This is usually due to trauma (**Fig. 6**), but can also be due to cholesteatoma or be iatrogenic.[33] Free air within the membranous labyrinth disrupts the propagation of sound waves and causes irritation within the inner ear, resulting in hearing loss and rotational vertigo.[34] A CT scan of the temporal bone may show pneumolabyrinth, disorientation of the stapedial footplate (if the perilymphatic fistula is via the oval window), or effusion of the round window niche (if the perilymphatic fistula is via the round window).[34]

Degenerative or progressive
Meniere disease (**Fig. 7**), also known as idiopathic endolymphatic hydrops, is a disor-der of the inner ear resulting in vertigo, tinnitus, sensorineural hearing loss, and aural fullness.[35] Conventional MRI may be performed to exclude an underlying inner ear or retrocochlear lesion. Recent advances allow evaluation for endolymphatic hydrops using MRI 4 hours after the intravenous or intratympanic injection of gadolinium contrast; delayed preferential enhancement of the perilymphatic space allows for the detection of an enlarged nonenhanced endolymphatic space.[36]

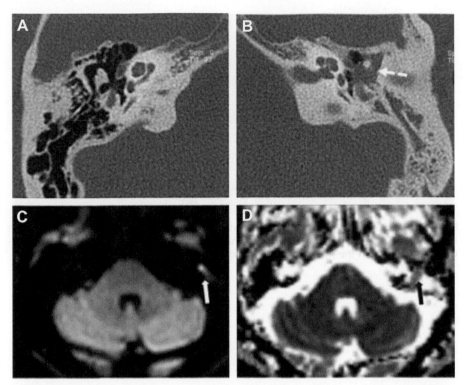

Fig. 5. Cholesteatoma. Using the normal right side (*A*) for comparison, abnormal soft tissue is seen in the left tympanic cavity (*B*) eroding the incus (*dashed arrow*). Diffusion-weighted imaging (*C*) demonstrates corresponding hyperintense signal with signal drop out on the apparent diffusion coefficient map (*D*), indicating diffusion restriction (*arrows*).

Otosclerosis is osteodystrophy of the otic capsule that results in progressive conductive hearing loss owing to fixation of the stapedial footplate along its anterior annulus.[37] This disease is more common in Caucasians and females, with a reported overall prevalence of 0.1% to 1.0%.[38] Otosclerosis is divided into 2 types: fenestral (**Fig. 8**) and retrofenestral otosclerosis. On temporal bone CT scans, fenestral otosclerosis appears as focal bony osseous demineralization limited to the fissula ante fenestram located anterior to the oval window. These patients present with progressive conductive hearing loss. Retrofenestral otosclerosis is the less common subtype and appears as bony demineralization involving the remainder of the otic capsule. These patients typically present with progressive sensorineural or mixed hearing loss. However, dizziness and/or vertigo may ensue if the osteodystrophy involves the vestibular structures.[39]

Anatomic
Superior semicircular canal dehiscence (**Fig. 9**) is a vestibular disorder caused by a pathologic third window into the labyrinth, creating altered pressure gradients. Classically, presentation is Tulio's phenomenon, which is vertigo or nystagmus in response to loud noises.[40] Additional common symptoms are autophony, or hyperacusis to bone-conducted sound as well as conductive hearing loss. A CT scan of the temporal bone with special oblique reformatted images parallel or orthogonal to the plane of the superior semicircular canal, termed Poschl's and Stenver's views, respectively, is the

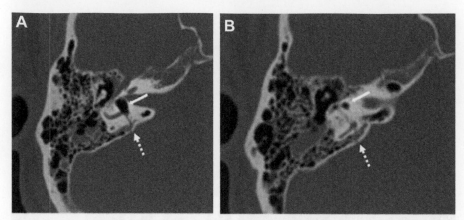

Fig. 6. Perilymphatic fistula. Axial high-resolution CT imaging demonstrates free air within the vestibule (*A*) and superior semicircular canal (*B*) (*solid arrows*) owing to an otic capsule-violating fracture in the posterior right temporal bone (*dashed arrows*).

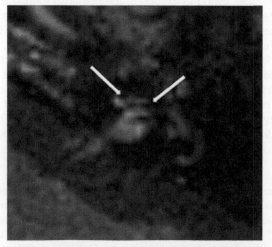

Fig. 7. Meniere disease. Axial 3D fluid-attenuated inversion recovery image of the left vestibulocochlear complex 4 hours after the intravenous injection of contrast demonstrates marked enlargement of the unenhanced endolymphatic space (*arrows*).

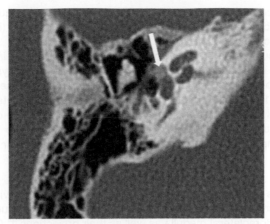

Fig. 8. Otosclerosis. Lucency and bony demineralization of the fissula ante fenestram, located anterior to the oval window (*arrow*).

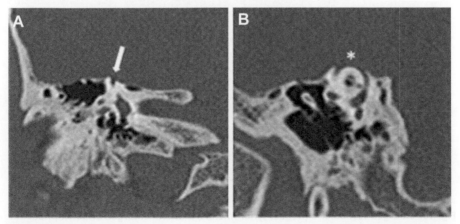

Fig. 9. Superior semicircular canal dehiscence. (*A*) A coronal CT scan shows a bony defect in the arcuate eminence (*arrow*). (*B*) Poschl reformat shows loss of bony integrity over the superior semicircular canal (*asterisk*).

modality of choice owing to the high spatial resolution and exquisite bony detail display. Imaging demonstrates a defect in the arcuate eminence (bony covering of the superior semicircular canal).[41]

Enlarged vestibular aqueduct syndrome (**Fig. 10**) is a congenital inner ear anomaly characterized by sensorineural hearing loss and/or vertiginous symptoms.[42] A CT scan of the temporal bone demonstrates a widened diameter of the vestibular aqueduct greater than 1.5 mm at its midpoint, and greater than the diameter of the posterior semicircular canal. There is also a strong association with absence of the bony modiolus. High resolution fluid-weighted MRI sequences may also demonstrate an enlarged endolymphatic sac and duct, housed within the vestibular aqueduct.[43]

Central

Central vertigo is the false sensation of motion or spinning owing to pathology involving the central vestibular structures, namely, the vestibular nuclei in the caudal pons and rostral dorsolateral medulla as well as their projections.[44] Central etiologies

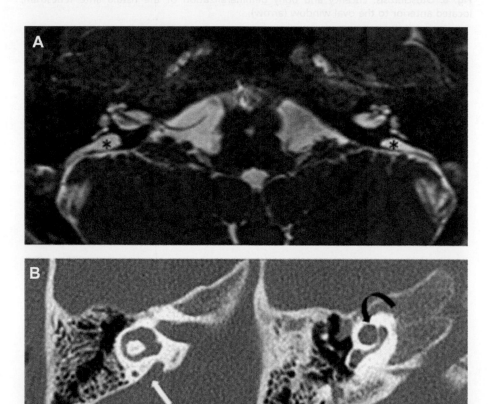

Fig. 10. Enlarged vestibular aqueduct syndrome. (*A*) Bilateral enlarged endolymphatic sacs (*asterisks*) on axial constructive interference in steady state imaging. (*B*) The vestibular aqueduct diameter is larger than the posterior semicircular canal (*arrow*). (*C*) An absent modiolus is seen (*curved arrow*).

account for approximately 20% of vertigo presentations.[45] These etiologies may be subdivided into vascular, neoplastic, anatomic, infectious or inflammatory, and miscellaneous.

Vascular

Approximately 20% of intracranial infarcts are in the posterior (vertebrobasilar) circulation, with dizziness and vertigo presenting as the most common symptoms.[46] Patients may also present with falling toward the side of the infarction, diplopia, multidirectional nystagmus, ipsilateral Horner, and contralateral loss of pain and temperature sensation.[47]

A noncontrast head CT is typically the initial study of choice to look for infarct (loss of gray–white differentiation, focal hypodensity, sulcal effacement), hemorrhage, or brain herniation. However, owing to the low sensitivity of CT scans for the evaluation of posterior fossa infarcts, MRI is the imaging modality of choice for evaluation of infarct in patients with dizziness.[48] Either CTA or MRA may be used to look for large vessel occlusion.

Vertebrobasilar insufficiency indicates inadequate blood flow through the posterior circulation and may be due to cardiogenic pathology, medications, or vascular compromise.[6] The most common symptoms are vertigo and dizziness. Cranial nerve palsies and ataxic symptoms can be seen in brainstem and cerebellar infarcts, respectively. CTA and MRA are the studies of choice to assess for vascular stenosis or large vessel occlusion, seen as luminal narrowing or loss of contrast or flow-related enhancement.

Anatomic

A Chiari 1 malformation is characterized by downward descent of the cerebellar tonsils through the foramen magnum.[49] Patients usually complain of headaches, and less commonly dizziness and vertigo.[50] MRI is the imaging modality of choice and demonstrates peg-like cerebellar tonsils extending more than 5 mm below the level of the foramen magnum (**Fig. 11**). An MRI of the cervical spine may also be considered to evaluate for syrinx, a common associated complication.[51]

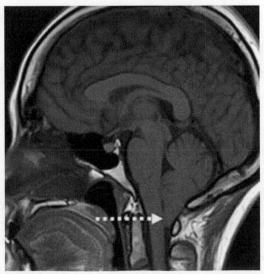

Fig. 11. Chiari 1 Malformation. Sagittal T1-weighted image demonstrates 0.9 cm of downward herniation of the cerebellar tonsils (*arrow*), crowding the foramen magnum.

Neoplastic

Posterior fossa tumors are an uncommon yet potential cause for vertigo and dizziness from compression of central vestibular structures. Common pediatric tumors include astrocytoma (usually pilocytic astrocytoma), medulloblastoma (**Fig. 12**), and ependymoma,[52] whereas common adult tumors are metastases and hemangioblastoma.[53] An MRI of the brain with and without contrast is the study of choice.

Infectious or inflammatory

Multiple sclerosis is a chronic autoimmune inflammatory disease of the cranial central nervous system resulting in demyelination, gliosis, and neuronal loss.[54] It affects approximately 400,000 people in the United States with a 3-fold higher incidence in

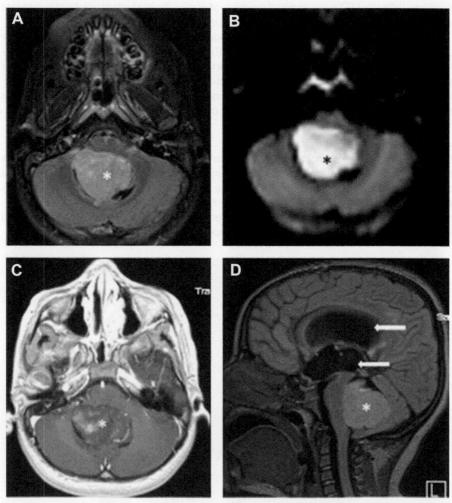

Fig. 12. Medulloblastoma. Axial fluid-attenuated inversion recovery (*A*), diffusion-weighted imaging (*B*), axial postcontrast, (*C*) and sagittal fluid-attenuated inversion recovery (*D*) images demonstrates a diffusion-restricted, heterogeneously enhancing mass within the fourth ventricle (*asterisks*) resulting in obstructive hydrocephalus (*arrows*).

females.[55] Presentation depends on the burden and location of these plaques. When there are insults to the brainstem, patients can present with vertigo, dysarthria, diplopia, and facial sensory loss.[56] MRI of the brain is the imaging of choice. The fluid-attenuated inversion recovery sequence is sensitive for disease identification. Enhancement or diffusion restriction of a plaque suggests active disease.

Cerebrospinal fluid homeostasis

Intracranial hypertension and hypotension refer to abnormally increased or decreased pressure of the cerebrospinal fluid within the cranial vault, respectively. The most common presentation for both entities is headache. However, vertigo/dizziness was found in up to 75% of patients presenting with intracranial hypertension[57] and 30% of patients with intracranial hypotension.[58]

The etiologies of intracranial hypertension can be divided into primary or intracranial (eg, trauma, tumor, hydrocephalus, idiopathic) and secondary or extracranial (eg, hypoventilation, hypertension, metabolic, seizures).[59] In cases of idiopathic intracranial hypertension, an MRI of the brain demonstrates slit-like ventricles, prominence of the optic nerve sheaths, flattening of the posterior globes, enlarged arachnoid

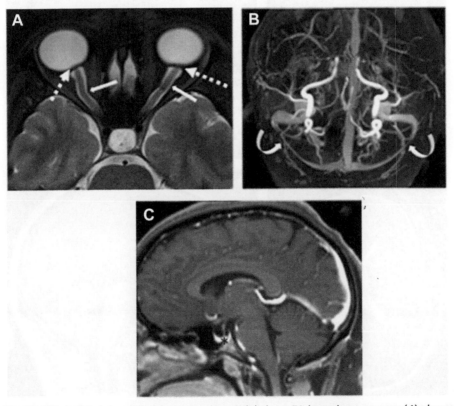

Fig. 13. Idiopathic intracranial hypertension. Axial short T1 inversion recovery (*A*) shows prominence of the distal optic nerve sheaths (*solid arrow*) and indentation and flattening of the optic discs (*dashed arrows*). Severe stenosis of the distal transverse sinuses (*curved arrows*) is seen on the postcontrast maximum intensity projection MR venogram of the brain (*B*). Sagittal T1 postcontrast (*C*) demonstrates a partially empty sella (*asterisk*).

outpouchings, venous sinus stenosis or thrombosis (usually lateral aspects of the transverse sinuses), and acquired cerebellar tonsillar ectopia[60] (**Fig. 13**).

Intracranial hypotension occurs when there is cerebrospinal fluid leak, which may be iatrogenic (usually after a lumbar puncture) or spontaneous owing to dural tear related to minor trauma, connective tissue disorders, or idiopathic.[61] The classic imaging triad of intracranial hypotension on MRI is pachymeningeal thickening or enhancement, brain sagging, and subdural hematomas and/or hygromas. Other imaging signs include inferior cerebellar tonsillar ectopia, distended venous sinuses, and an engorged pituitary gland[62] (**Fig. 14**).

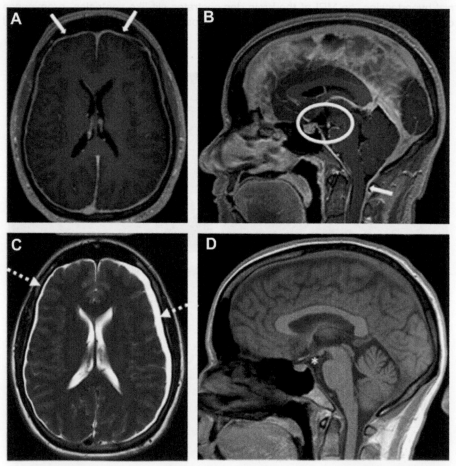

Fig. 14. Intracranial hypotension. Axial (*A*) and sagittal (*B*) postcontrast T1 images show diffuse pachymeningeal enhancement extending to upper cervical spine (*solid arrows*), a sagging midbrain and decreased mamillopontine distance (*oval*). Axial T2 image (*C*) shows bilateral subdural hygromas (*dashed arrows*). Following epidural blood patch, there has been resolution of crowding at the suprasellar cistern (*asterisk*) on sagittal T1 imaging (*D*).

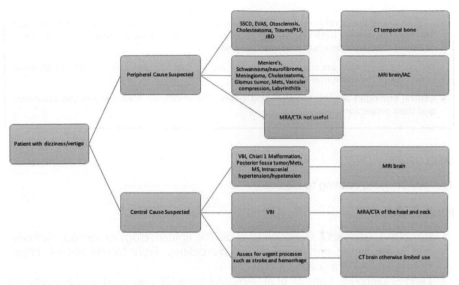

Fig. 15. Imaging decision algorithm. A simplified model to aid in deciding which imaging modality to order based on whether a peripheral or central etiology for the dizziness/vertigo is suspected. Each imaging modality is accompanied with differential diagnoses it is most apt at evaluating. CTA, computed tomography angiography; EVAS, enlarged vestibular aqueduct syndrome; JBD, jugular bulb diverticulum; MRA, MR angiography; PLF, perilymphatic fistula; SSCD, superior semicircular canal dehiscence; VBI, vertebrobasilar insufficiency.

SUMMARY

There is a wide range of pathophysiologic processes that can contribute to a patient's symptoms of dizziness and vertigo. When deciding which imaging modality to perform, it is beneficial to first establish whether the disease process is most likely peripheral or central. Generally, if a peripheral pathology is suspected, a CT scan of the temporal bone is the initial study of choice to evaluate the inner ear structures, otic capsule, and bony vascular foramina. A major exception is a CPA tumor, for which MRI of the IAC with and without contrast is recommended. If a central pathology is suspected, MRI of the brain and IAC with and without contrast is the preferred imaging modality because it is best for evaluating the brainstem, cerebellum, cranial nerve VIII, and IACs. CTA or MRA may be performed to evaluate for central vertebrobasilar insufficiency. A robust history should accompany requested imaging studies to aid the radiologist in addressing suspected pathologies as well as correlate imaging findings to patient symptomatology. This process is summarized in **Fig. 15**.

Patient presentations may not fit exactly within the peripheral or central category. Complicated histories and differential diagnoses requiring diagnostic imaging investigation would benefit from consultation with the radiologist. CT and MRI studies may play complimentary roles in the diagnostic workup for many cases.

CLINICS CARE POINTS

- Dizziness refers to a general sensation of disturbed or impaired spatial orientation, whereas vertigo specifically refers to a false sense of motion.

- CT scan of the temporal bone is used to assess for peripheral etiologies of vertigo, whereas MRI may be used for both central and peripheral etiologies. CTA and MRA are useful for assessing for central etiologies of vascular origin.

- Peripheral etiologies are more common and are limited to cranial nerve VIII and all distal structures of the vestibular system.

- Central etiologies are less common and involve the vestibular nuclei within the brainstem and their projections.

DISCLOSURE

The authors have nothing to disclose.

REFERENCES

1. Bisdorff A, Bosser G, Gueguen R, et al. The epidemiology of vertigo, dizziness, and unsteadiness and its links to co-morbidities. Front Neurol 2013;4. https://doi.org/10.3389/fneur.2013.00029.
2. Leng S, Diehn FE, Lane JI, et al. Temporal bone CT: improved image quality and potential for decreased radiation dose using an ultra-high-resolution scan mode with an iterative reconstruction algorithm. AJNR Am J Neuroradiol 2015;36(9): 1599–603.
3. Thompson TL, Amedee R. Vertigo: a review of common peripheral and central vestibular disorders. Ochsner J 2009;9(1):20–6.
4. Conte G, Lo Russo FM, Calloni SF, et al. MR imaging of endolymphatic hydrops in Ménière's disease: not all that glitters is gold. Acta Otorhinolaryngol Ital 2018; 38(4):369–76.
5. van Steekelenburg JM, van Weijnen A, de Pont LMH, et al. Value of endolymphatic hydrops and perilymph signal intensity in suspected Ménière disease. AJNR Am J Neuroradiol 2020;41(3):529–34.
6. Lima Neto AC, Bittar R, Gattas GS, et al. Pathophysiology and diagnosis of vertebrobasilar insufficiency: a review of the literature. Int Arch Otorhinolaryngol 2017;21(3):302–7.
7. DeLong M, Kirkpatrick J, Cummings T, et al. Vestibular schwannomas: lessons for the neurosurgeon part ii: molecular biology and histology. Contemp Neurosurg 2011;33(21):1–3.
8. Meola A, Chang SD. Bilateral vestibular schwannomas in neurofibromatosis type 2. N Engl J Med 2018;379(15):1463.
9. Foley RW, Shirazi S, Maweni RM, et al. Signs and symptoms of acoustic neuroma at initial presentation: an exploratory analysis. Cureus. 2017; 9(11): e1846.
10. Nguyen D, de Kanztow L. Vestibular schwannomas: a review. Appl Radiol 2019; 48(3): 22–27.
11. Bonneville F, Savatovsky J, Chiras J. Imaging of cerebellopontine angle lesions: an update. Part 1: enhancing extra-axial lesions. Eur Radiol 2007;17(10): 2472–82.
12. Gao K, Ma H, Cui Y, et al. Meningiomas of the cerebellopontine angle: radiological differences in tumors with internal auditory canal involvement and their influence on surgical outcome. PLoS One 2015;10(4): e0122949.
13. Granick MS, Martuza RL, Parker SW, et al. Cerebellopontine angle meningiomas: clinical manifestations and diagnosis. Ann Otol Rhinol Laryngol 1985;94(1 Pt 1):34–8.

14. Smirniotopoulos JG, Yue NC, Rushing EJ. Cerebellopontine angle masses: radio-logic-pathologic correlation. Radiographics 1993; 13(5): 1131–47.
15. Lee KY, Oh YW, Noh JH, et al. Extraadrenal paragangliomas of the body: imaging features. AJR 2006;187:492–504.
16. Gjuric M, Gleeson M. Consensus statement and guidelines on the management of paragangliomas of the head and neck. Skull Base 2009;19(1):109–16.
17. Bozek P, Kluczewska E, Lisowska G, et al. [Imaging and assessment of glomus jugulare in MRI and CT techniques]. Otolaryngol Pol 2011;65(3):218–27.
18. Gloria-Cruz TI, Schachern PA, Paparella MM, et al. Metastases to temporal bones from primary nonsystemic malignant neoplasms. Arch Otolaryngol Head Neck Surg 2000;126(2):209.
19. Song K, Park K-W, Heo J-H, et al. Clinical characteristics of temporal bone me-tastases. Clin Exp Otorhinolaryngol 2019;12(1):27–32.
20. Park JH, Son SB, Hong HP, et al. A case of jugular bulb diverticulum invading the internal auditory canal. Korean J Audiol 2012;16(1):39–42.
21. Iaccarino I, Bozzetti F, Bacciu A, Falcioni M. Imaging case of the month: jugular bulb diverticulum uncovering the internal auditory canal. J Case Rep Clin Images 2019;2(1):1015.
22. Tarnutzer AA, Berkowitz AL, Robinson KA, et al. Does my dizzy patient have a stroke? A systematic review of bedside diagnosis in acute vestibular syndrome. CMAJ 2011;183(9):E571–92.
23. Hearing loss as a sequela of meningitis - Nadol - 1978 - The laryngoscope - Wiley Online Library. Available at: https://onlinelibrary.wiley.com/doi/abs/10.1002/lary.1978.88.5.739. Accessed November 15, 2020.
24. Wu JF, Jin Z, Yang JM, Liu YH, Duan ML. Extracranial and intracranial complica-tions of otitis media: 22-year clinical experience and analysis. Acta Otolaryngol 2012;132(3):261–5.
25. Themes UFO. Labyrinthitis. Radiology key. 2019. Available at: https://radiologykey.com/labyrinthitis-2/. Accessed November 15, 2020.
26. Castle JT. Cholesteatoma pearls: practical points and update. Head Neck Pathol 2018;12(3):419–29.
27. Pusalkar AG. Cholesteatoma and its management. Indian J Otolaryngol Head Neck Surg 2015;67(3):201–4.
28. Agrup C, Gleeson M, Rudge P. The inner ear and the neurologist. J Neurol Neuro-surg Psychiatry 2007;78(2):114–22.
29. Baráth K, Huber AM, Stämpfli P, et al. Neuroradiology of cholesteatomas. AJNR Am J Neuroradiol 2011;32(2):221–9.
30. Patel A, Groppo E. Management of temporal bone trauma. Craniomaxillofac Trauma Reconstr 2010;3(2):105–13.
31. Little SC, Kesser BW. Radiographic classification of temporal bone fractures: clin-ical predictability using a new system. Arch Otolaryngol Head Neck Surg 2006; 132(12):1300.
32. Saraiya PV, Aygun N. Temporal bone fractures. Emerg Radiol 2009;16(4):255–65.
33. Hornibrook J. Perilymph fistula: fifty years of controversy. ISRN Otolaryngol 2012; 281248:9.
34. Sarna B, Abouzari M, Merna C, et al. Perilymphatic fistula: a review of classifica-tion, etiology, diagnosis, and treatment. Front Neurol 2020;11:1046.
35. Beasley NJ, Jones NS. Menière's disease: evolution of a definition. J Laryngol Otol 1996;110(12):1107–13.
36. Bernaerts A, De Foer B. Imaging of Ménière disease. Neuroimaging Clin N Am 2019;29(1):19–28.

37. Chole RA, McKenna M. Pathophysiology of otosclerosis. Otol Neurotol 2001; 22(2):249–57.
38. Crompton M, Cadge BA, Ziff JL, et al. The epidemiology of otosclerosis in a British cohort. Otol Neurotol 2019;40(1):22–30.
39. Purohit B, Hermans R, Op de beeck K. Imaging in otosclerosis: a pictorial review. Insights Imaging 2014;5(2):245–52.
40. Steenerson KK, Crane BT, Minor LB. Superior semicircular canal dehiscence syndrome. Semin Neurol 2020;40(01):151–9.
41. Gartrell BC, Gentry LR, Kennedy TA, et al. Radiographic features of superior semicircular canal dehiscence in the setting of chronic ear disease. Otol Neurotol 2014;35(1):91–6.
42. Ralli M, Nola G, Sparvoli L, et al. Unilateral enlarged vestibular aqueduct syndrome and bilateral endolymphatic hydrops. Case Rep Otolaryngol 2017;2017.
43. Okamoto K, Ito J, Furusawa T, et al. Large vestibular aqueduct syndrome with high CT density and high MR signal intensity. Am J Neuroradiol 1997; 18(3): 482–4.
44. Renga V. Clinical evaluation of patients with vestibular dysfunction. Neurol Res Int 2019;3931548:8.
45. Huon L-K, Wang T-C, Fang T-Y, et al. Vertigo and stroke: a national database survey. Otol Neurotol 2012;33(7):1131–5.
46. Savitz SI, Caplan LR. Vertebrobasilar disease. N Engl J Med 2005; 352(25): 2618–26.
47. Nouh A, Remke J, Ruland S. Ischemic posterior circulation stroke: a review of anatomy, clinical presentations, diagnosis, and current management. Front Neurol 2014;5:30.
48. Hwang DY, Silva GS, Furie KL, et al. Comparative sensitivity of computed tomography vs. magnetic resonance imaging for detecting acute posterior fossa infarct. J Emerg Med 2012;42(5):559–65.
49. Bejjani GK. Definition of the adult Chiari malformation: a brief historical overview. Neurosurg Focus 2001;11(1):1–8.
50. Greenlee JDW, Donovan KA, Hasan DM, et al. Chiari I malformation in the very young child: the spectrum of presentations and experience in 31 children under age 6 years. Pediatrics 2002;110(6):1212–9.
51. Chiapparini L, Saletti V, Solero CL, et al. Neuroradiological diagnosis of Chiari malformations. Neurol Sci 2011;32(3):283–6.
52. Prasad KSV, Ravi D, Pallikonda V, et al. Clinicopathological study of pediatric posterior fossa tumors. J Pediatr Neurosci 2017;12(3):245–50.
53. Chalal RA, Kessaci F, Mansouri B. Posterior fossa tumors in adults: MR imaging. ECR 2017 EPOS. 2017. Available at: https://epos.myesr.org/poster/esr/ecr2017/C-2241. Accessed November 21, 2020.
54. Ghasemi N, Razavi S, Nikzad E. Multiple sclerosis: pathogenesis, symptoms, diagnoses and cell-based therapy. Cell J 2017;19(1):1–10.
55. Dilokthornsakul P, Valuck RJ, Nair KV, et al. Multiple sclerosis prevalence in the United States commercially insured population. Neurology 2016;86(11):1014–21.
56. Ford H. Clinical presentation and diagnosis of multiple sclerosis. Clin Med (Lond) 2020;20(4):380–3.
57. Digre KB, Nakamoto BK, Warner JEA, et al. A comparison of idiopathic intracranial hypertension with and without papilledema. Headache 2009;49(2):185–93.
58. Chen S, Hagiwara M, Roehm PC. Spontaneous intracranial hypotension presenting with severe sensorineural hearing loss and headache. Otol Neurotol 2012; 33(8):e65–6.

59. Biousse V, Bruce BB, Newman NJ. Update on the pathophysiology and management of idiopathic intracranial hypertension. J Neurol Neurosurg Psychiatry 2012; 83(5):488–94.
60. Suzuki H, Takanashi J, Kobayashi K, et al. MR imaging of idiopathic intracranial hypertension. AJNR Am J Neuroradiol 2001;22(1):196–9.
61. Lin J, Zhang S, He F, et al. The status of diagnosis and treatment to intracranial hypotension, including SIH. J Headache Pain 2017;18(1).
62. Shah LM, McLean LA, Heilbrun ME, et al. Intracranial hypotension: improved MRI detection with diagnostic intracranial angles. AJR Am J Roentgenol 2013;200(2): 400–7.

Positional Vertigo

Ilana Yellin, MD*, Maja Svrakic, MD, MSEd

KEYWORDS

- Benign paroxysmal positional vertigo • Central paroxysmal positional vertigo
- Cervical vertigo • Persistent postural perceptual vertigo • Positional vertigo
- Vertebrobasilar insufficiency

KEY POINTS

- Positional vertigo can be both functional and structural in origin, and structural lesions may be peripherally or centrally located.
- A thorough history and physical exam is essential in identifying key features to distinguish the disorders on the differential diagnosis for a patient with positional vertigo.
- Benign paroxysmal positional vertigo (BPPV) is the most common cause of positional vertigo and is treated with repositioning maneuvers.
- Patients presenting with positional vertigo and a negative Dix–Hallpike, atypical nystagmus on Dix–Hallpike, or other neurologic symptoms should be further evaluated for alternative causes of positional vertigo, including central lesions and functional disorders.

INTRODUCTION

Positional vertigo refers to a spinning sensation produced by changes in head position relative to gravity.[1] BPPV is the most common form of positional vertigo and is the primary diagnosis for 17% to 42% of patients complaining of vertigo.[1] Given its high prevalence, BPPV has become synonymous with positional vertigo to many practitioners who do not often encounter other forms of positional vertigo. While there are many schemes by which vertigo may be classified, the presence or absence of positional vertigo itself is not a commonly used approach to understanding etiologies of vertigo, and thus the literature lacks a well-developed differential diagnosis for this common complaint. There is a common misconception that worsening dizziness with head motion implies a peripheral cause of vertigo when in fact, positional vertigo may be either structural or functional, or peripheral or central, in origin.[2] This chapter aims to explore the various causes of positional vertigo, including BPPV, central paroxysmal positional vertigo (CPPV), cervical vertigo and vertebrobasilar insufficiency, and persistent postural perceptual dizziness (PPPD). While this classification

Department of Otolaryngology, Zucker School of Medicine at Hofstra/Northwell, 430 Lakeville Road, New Hyde Park, NY 10040, USA
* Corresponding author.
E-mail address: iyellin@northwell.edu

Otolaryngol Clin N Am 54 (2021) 913–924
https://doi.org/10.1016/j.otc.2021.05.012
0030-6665/21/© 2021 Elsevier Inc. All rights reserved.

oto.theclinics.com

Abbreviations

BPPV	Benign paroxysmal positional vertigo
CBT	Cognitive behavioral therapy
CPPV	Central paroxysmal positional vertigo
CSD	Chronic subjective dizziness
DSA	Digital subtraction angiography
PPPD	Persistent postural perceptual dizziness
PPV	Phobic postural vertigo
VV	Visual vertigo

schema is not usually encountered in literature, it is quite relevant and practical in clinical settings.

EVALUATION OF PATIENTS WITH POSITIONAL VERTIGO

Positional vertigo can be either functional or structural in origin, and structural lesions can be either peripherally or centrally located. The first step in evaluating a patient with positional vertigo is to elicit a detailed history consistent with a triggered, episodic syndrome.[2] This allows for the distinction from syndromes of spontaneous and acute onset such as vestibular neuritis and viral labyrinthitis, both of which are characterized by dizziness at rest and are exacerbated by head motion.[2] Additional features such as the degree of imbalance or nausea, and the presence of auditory or neurologic symptoms, may help distinguish central from peripheral etiologies, but most often, the differential is narrowed by the structured physical exam.[3]

The physical exam focuses on the Dix–Hallpike and supine rolls tests, the evaluation of nystagmus, orthostatic vitals, and the neurologic exam. Orthostatic hypotension is distinguished from peripheral causes of positional vertigo by a negative Dix–Hallpike and a significant change in vitals with changes in position.[2] In functional disorders such as PPPD, there are no associated test findings, and the diagnosis is made based on the history that fulfills strict diagnostic criteria.[4]

Conversely, structural disorders of central and peripheral origin may be distinguished by patterns of observed nystagmus.[2,5,6] On the Dix–Hallpike and supine roll tests, patients with peripheral disorders such as BPPV will exhibit characteristic nystagmus that corresponds to the stimulated canal plane, while patients who exhibit upbeat, downbeat, or purely torsional nystagmus should be further evaluated for central disorders such as CPPV or vertebrobasilar insufficiency.[5] These patients require neuroimaging including CT/MRI, which may reveal CNS lesions or neck pathology, and angiography to assess the vertebral artery if vertebrobasilar insufficiency is suspected.

BENIGN PAROXYSMAL POSITIONAL VERTIGO
Prevalence and Pathophysiology

BPPV is defined as a disorder of the inner ear characterized by repeated episodes of positional vertigo, and it is the most common form of peripheral vertigo.[1] The estimated prevalence ranges from 10.7 to 140 per 100,000 with a lifetime prevalence of 2.4%.[1] Women are affected more commonly than men, with a female-to-male ratio in the range of 2:1 to 3:1. The peak age of onset is between the fifth and seventh decades of life.[1,6]

The 2 variants of BPPV include that of the posterior semicircular canal, which accounts for 85% to 95% of cases, and that of the lateral semicircular canal. The pathogenesis of each variant is related to either canalithiasis or cupulolithiasis. In canalithiasis, free-floating otoconia move from the utricle and collect near the cupula, causing an abnormal influence on the vestibular system, while in cupulolithiasis, the otoconia are attached to the cupula and have a similar effect.[1]

Presentation and Physical Exam

The key to diagnosis in BPPV is to establish a history consistent with a triggered episodic vestibular syndrome. The typical patient with BPPV caused by canalithiasis of either the posterior or the lateral semicircular canal will describe attacks of vertigo induced by changes in head position relative to gravity. The attacks appear after a short latency, last less than 1 minute, and decrease in intensity when the change in head position is repeated.[7] The episodes are not associated with hearing loss, tinnitus, aural fullness, or focal neurologic deficits. In patients whose BPPV is caused by cupulolithiasis, vertigo appears without latency and lasts for more than 1 minute without a decrease in intensity.[7]

The Dix–Hallpike (**Fig. 1**) and supine roll test (**Fig. 2**) are useful maneuvers in differentiating the variants of BPPV from one another and from other disorders of positional vertigo. In BPPV of the posterior canal, the Dix–Hallpike induces an upbeat-torsional nystagmus that develops after a brief latency of 5 to 20 seconds, lasts less than 1 minute, and diminishes on repeat testing.[1,6] When the etiology is cupulolithiasis of the posterior canal, the nystagmus may be induced without latency and lasts greater than 1 minute.[7] If the induced nystagmus varies from this pattern, the diagnosis of

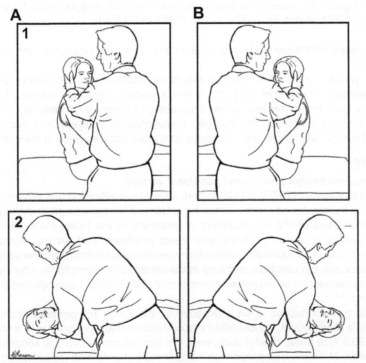

Fig. 1. Dix–Hallpike maneuver. In Dix–Hallpike to the right (*A*), the patient begins in the seated position (1) and is lowered to the supine position with the neck extended (2). Dix–Hallpike to the left (*B*). (*From* Fife TD, von Brevern M. Benign Paroxysmal Positional Vertigo in the Acute Care Setting. Neurol Clin. 2015 Aug;33(3):601-17, viii-ix. doi: 10.1016/j.ncl.2015.04.003. Epub 2015 Jun 12. PMID: 26231274.)

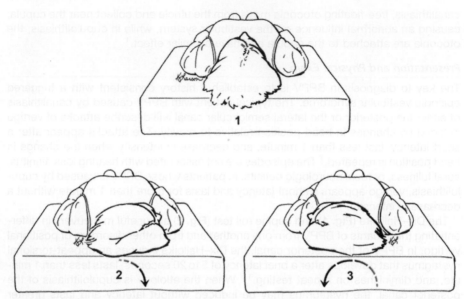

Fig. 2. Supine roll test. The patient is in the supine position (1), and the head is turned 90° to the right (2) and 90° to the left (3). (*From* Fife TD, von Brevern M. Benign Paroxysmal Positional Vertigo in the Acute Care Setting. Neurol Clin. 2015 Aug;33(3):601-17, viii-ix. doi: 10.1016/j.ncl.2015.04.003. Epub 2015 Jun 12. PMID: 26231274.)

posterior canal BPPV cannot be made, and other causes of positional vertigo must be explored.

When the etiology BPPV is canalithiasis of the lateral canal, the supine roll test induces geotropic positional nystagmus that appears with short latency, lasts less than 1 minute, and increases before decreasing in intensity.[7] In lateral canal BPPV caused by cupulolithiasis, the induced nystagmus is apogeotropic and appears without latency, lasts more than 1 minute, and does not decrease in intensity.

Treatment

Posterior canal benign paroxysmal positional vertigo

Once the diagnosis of BPPV is established, several repositioning maneuvers aimed at redirecting the displaced otoconia may be employed for symptomatic management.[6] In posterior canal BPPV, the mainstay of treatment is the Epley maneuver (**Fig. 3**), which involves a series of body and head positions that evoke characteristic nystagmus. These sequential movements move otoconial debris from the semicircular canals back into the vestibule and lead to the resolution of symptoms when successful. The maneuver has an estimated success rate of 80% after 1 attempt and 92% after 4 attempts.[6,8]

The Semont maneuver is an alternative to the Epley for posterior canal BPPV (**Fig. 4**). In a randomized, double-blind trial comparing this maneuver with a sham procedure, 86.8% of patients who underwent the Semont maneuver had recovered from vertigo after 24 hours, compared with none of the patients who underwent the sham procedure.[9]

Lateral canal benign paroxysmal positional vertigo

Lateral canal BPPV is treated with various maneuvers that target otoconia in the lateral canals. In the barbecue roll maneuver, the patient begins supine and rotates the body

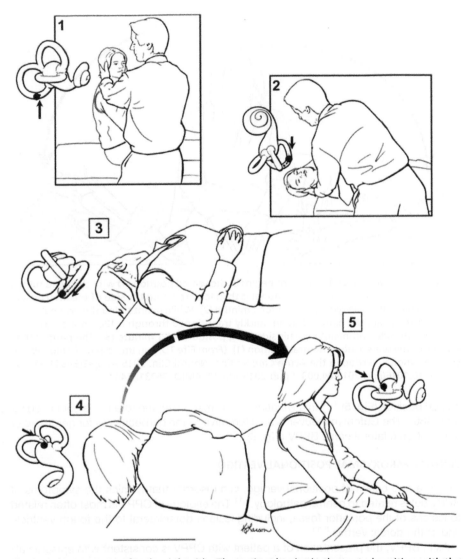

Fig. 3. Epley maneuver for the right side. The patient begins in the seated position with the head rotated 45° toward the affected ear (1). The patient is then lowered to the supine position with the head kept at 45° and the neck extended slightly below the horizontal plane (2). The patient is kept in this position until the evoked nystagmus disappears, at which point the head is turned 90° toward the unaffected ear and again kept in this position until the evoked nystagmus disappears (3). The patient's body is then rotated 90° toward the unaffected side while the head is rotated another 45° and kept in this position until any evoked nystagmus disappears (4). Finally, the patient is returned to the seated, head-neutral position (5). (*From* Fife TD, von Brevern M. Benign Paroxysmal Positional Vertigo in the Acute Care Setting. Neurol Clin. 2015 Aug;33(3):601-17, viii-ix. doi: 10.1016/j.ncl.2015.04.003. Epub 2015 Jun 12. PMID: 26231274.)

90° onto the affected side. After 30 seconds, the patient rotates back to the supine position. The patient then rotates the body in the same direction in increments of 90° until the body has been rotated 270°, at which point the patient returns to the upright,

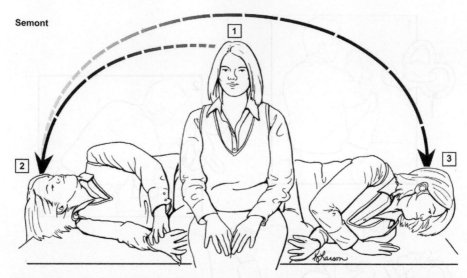

Fig. 4. Semont maneuver. The patient begins in the seated position (1) with the head turned 45° toward the unaffected ear. The patient is then lowered onto the side of the affected ear and remains in the side-lying position for 1 minute (2). While maintaining the original orientation of the head, the patient is then quickly transitioned through a 180° motion to lie on the opposite side and maintains this side-lying position for 1 minute (3). The patient then returns to the seated, head-neutral position (1). (*From* Fife TD, von Brevern M. Benign Paroxysmal Positional Vertigo in the Acute Care Setting. Neurol Clin. 2015 Aug;33(3):601-17, viii-ix. doi: 10.1016/j.ncl.2015.04.003. Epub 2015 Jun 12. PMID: 26231274.)

seated position (**Fig. 5**).[1,10] In a variation of this maneuver, the rotation is continued for a full 360°. The Gufoni maneuver is an alternative to the barbecue roll for geotropic or apogeotropic lateral canal BPPV (**Fig. 6**).[1,10]

CENTRAL PAROXYSMAL POSITIONAL VERTIGO

CPPV, a rare cause of positional vertigo, is a disorder that mimics the symptoms of BPPV but is related to central pathology.[5,11] The etiology of CPPV is most often related to lesions of the posterior fossa, including lesions dorsolateral to the fourth ventricle and of the dorsal vermis.[5,11]

As in BPPV, the presentation of a patient with CPPV is consistent with episodic attacks of positional vertigo. While the attack duration is typically shorter than those of BPPV, the greatest distinction between the disorders is in the observed nystagmus.[5] In contrast to BPPV, the nystagmus of CPPV does not correspond to the stimulated canal plane and is typically purely vertical, with downbeat nystagmus being most common, or purely torsional.[5] It appears with either no latency or a short latency of up to 5 seconds, does not exhibit the characteristic crescendo-decrescendo nature or fatigability of the nystagmus in BPPV, and is not inhibited by fixation.[5,12] In addition to this characteristic nystagmus, patients with CPPV often present with cerebellar and other neurologic signs, including cerebellar dysmetria and periodic alternating and gaze-evoked nystagmus.[11,13] However, it is possible for the distinctive history and nystagmus of CPPV to occur in the absence of any other neurologic signs, despite the presence of CNS pathology.[11]

Unlike benign causes of positional vertigo that do not require further workup beyond the history and physical exam, further workup including imaging is indicated in the

Lempert Roll Maneuver

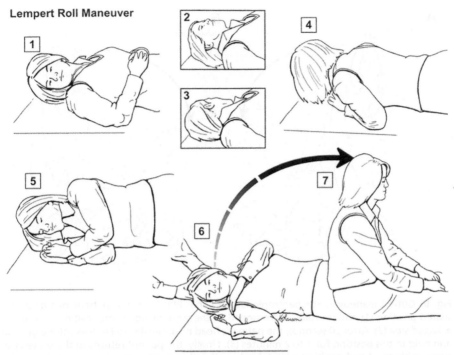

Fig. 5. Barbecue roll maneuver. Numbers 1 to 7 illustrate the sequential rotations of the body in the maneuver. (*From* Fife TD, von Brevern M. Benign Paroxysmal Positional Vertigo in the Acute Care Setting. Neurol Clin. 2015 Aug;33(3):601-17, viii-ix. doi: 10.1016/j.ncl.2015.04.003. Epub 2015 Jun 12. PMID: 26231274.)

case of positional vertigo with an atypical nystagmus pattern, whether or not any additional neurologic signs are present. In their series of patients, Lee and colleagues[11] describe 4 patients with positional vertigo who underwent MRI and were found to have cerebellar lesions of both primary CNS and metastatic origin, including hemangioblastoma, high-grade glioma, and metastatic lung and colon cancer. These patients with suspected central causes of positional vertigo should be referred for neurology consultation and neurosurgical consultation depending on imaging findings.

CERVICAL VERTIGO AND VERTEBROBASILAR INSUFFICIENCY
Cervical Vertigo

Cervical vertigo is characterized by dizziness related to the position of the cervical spine in patients with neck pathology.[14] The disease entity is poorly understood, and no consensus expert opinion defines it.[15] Thomson-Harvey and colleagues[15] define cervical vertigo as dizziness combined with a neck disorder when reasonable alternatives have been ruled out, while Wrisley and colleagues[16] stipulate that neck pain is required to make the diagnosis. Given this lack of consensus defining cervical vertigo, neither epidemiologic data nor population studies describe the disease.[17]

There are multiple proposed mechanisms for the pathophysiology of cervical vertigo, including proprioceptive and posttraumatic cervical vertigo, and cervical vertigo related to vertebrobasilar insufficiency.[17] The neck contains mechanisms involved in

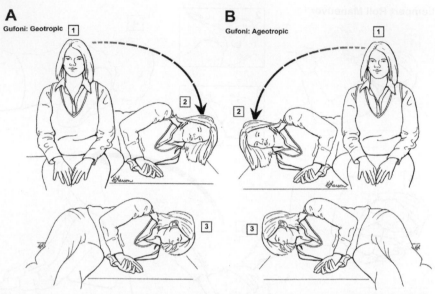

Fig. 6. Gufoni maneuver. For geotropic lateral canal BPPV (*A*), the patient begins in the seated position (1) and is rapidly transitioned to the straight side-lying position on the unaffected side (2). After 30 seconds, the patient's head is turned 45° to 60° toward the ground and held in this position for 1 to 2 minutes (3). Finally, the patient returns to the seated position with the head position maintained until fully upright, at which point it may be straightened. In the case of apogeotropic lateral canal BPPV (*B*), the patient is brought to the straight side-lying position on the affected side (2), and the head is turned 45° to 60° either toward the floor (3) if the otoconial debris is thought to be on the utricular side of the cupula, or toward the ceiling if the debris is thought to be on the canal side of the cupula. (*From* Fife TD, von Brevern M. Benign Paroxysmal Positional Vertigo in the Acute Care Setting. Neurol Clin. 2015 Aug;33(3):601-17, viii-ix. doi: 10.1016/j.ncl.2015.04.003. Epub 2015 Jun 12. PMID: 26231274.)

balance control, including proprioceptors and joint receptors, and thus it is reasonable that injury to the neck may be associated with the sensation of dizziness.[16] Ryan and Cope[18] postulate that cervical vertigo is due to abnormal afferent input to the vestibular nucleus caused by damaged joint receptors in the upper cervical region. This type of cervical vertigo is most often associated with flexion-extension injuries such as whiplash but is also reported in patients with severe cervical arthritis and herniated discs.[16]

Cervical vertigo is a diagnosis of exclusion based on the correlation of dizziness symptoms with head and neck movements, with or without neck pain, and the exclusion of peripheral vestibular disease in a patient with neck injury.[16] Episodes of dizziness may last minutes to hours, and symptoms may occur suddenly or days to years following injury.[16] On physical exam, vestibular disease is excluded with a negative Dix–Hallpike and normal vestibular testing. Imaging such as CT or MRI may be useful in detecting structural injury to the neck but does not definitively rule in cervical vertigo.[17]

When cervical vertigo is proprioceptive or posttraumatic, treatment focuses on manual therapy and vestibular rehab.[16] Manual therapy decreases irritation on cervical proprioceptors from muscle spasms and trigger points, while vestibular rehab improves dizziness symptoms.[16]

Vertebrobasilar Insufficiency

Cervical vertigo may also present as symptomatic vertebrobasilar insufficiency resulting from mechanical occlusion or stenosis of the vertebral artery during head and neck rotation or extension.[19] These cases are referred to as rotational vertebral artery occlusion syndrome. As the vertebral artery ascends the neck, it passes through the transverse foramina of C2–C6, where it is susceptible to dynamic compression by abnormal bony structures such as osteophytes, disc herniation, and tumors.[19,20]

Symptoms of this syndrome are related to ischemia from the resulting vertebrobasilar insufficiency and include vertigo, syncope, diplopia, dysarthria, and nausea. On physical exam, patients may exhibit sensory or motor deficits with head rotation and a central pattern of nystagmus.[19,20] These patients should undergo routine imaging including CT/CTA and MRI/MRA to detect abnormal bony strictures, stenotic arteries, or infarction.[19] The gold standard for diagnosis is digital subtraction angiography (DSA), which shows patent arteries in the neutral position and stenotic arteries in the head-rotated position.[19,21]

Treatment options for vertebrobasilar insufficiency resulting from rotational vertebral artery occlusion syndrome include conservative management, surgical decompression, and endovascular intervention. Conservative management involves avoiding head and neck rotation with the use of a cervical collar as well as antiplatelet or anticoagulation therapy.[19,21] Surgical intervention has an estimated success rate of 85% and involves decompression of the vertebral artery.[20,22] Finally, endovascular repair involves coil embolization or angioplasty with stenting, both of which preserve neck range of motion and are minimally invasive.[19]

PERSISTENT POSTURAL PERCEPTUAL DIZZINESS

PPPD is best understood as a chronic, functional vestibular disorder characterized by vertigo exacerbated by upright posture and exposure to complex visual stimuli.[4,23] The disease process results from maladaptive behavior, usually following peripheral vestibular disorders such as BPPV or vestibular neuritis, or central disorders such as vestibular migraine or traumatic brain injury.[23] In normal dizziness response, patients activate high-risk postural control strategies, including adopting a stiffened stance and shorter strides and increasing reliance on visual rather than vestibular input.[23] However, these adaptations are meant to be abandoned when the threat to postural stability is resolved. In PPPD, these patients have a high level of anxiety regarding vestibular and balance sensations and develop an excessive degree of self-observation that ultimately results in the persistent dependence on visual rather than vestibular input for spatial orientation.[4,23] While PPPD is considered a functional rather than psychiatric disorder, patients with existing psychiatric disorders such as generalized anxiety disorder are at higher risk for developing PPPD following vestibular insult.[4,24]

The incidence and prevalence of PPPD are based on years of research on chronic subjective dizziness (CSD), phobic postural vertigo (PPV), and visual vertigo (VV), the well-documented precursors to this newly termed disorder.[23] Among patients with vestibular symptoms, the prevalence of CSD or PPV is an estimated 15% to 20%.[4] The incidence of PPPD among patients followed for vestibular neuritis, BPPV, vestibular migraine, and Meniere's disease is further estimated to be 25%, with an average duration of illness of 4.5 years.[4]

The diagnosis in PPPD is based on eliciting a history that sufficiently fulfills the diagnostic criteria established by the Barany Society; it is not a diagnosis of exclusion.[23]

The criteria include 1 or more symptoms of dizziness, unsteadiness, or nonspinning vertigo present for most days for 3 or more months that occur without provocation but are exacerbated by upright posture, active or passive motion, or exposure to moving visual stimuli. These symptoms cause significant distress or functional impairment and are not better explained by another disease. Finally, the disorder is precipitated by acute, episodic, or chronic vestibular syndromes.[4]

In a statistical analysis of clinical aspects of patients with PPPD, the main trigger in the onset of dizziness symptoms in 52% of patients was body movements.[24] Other chronic vestibular disorders such as bilateral vestibulopathy and neurodegenerative disorders are best distinguished from PPPD by physical exam findings. As the name "perceptual dizziness" implies, PPPD has no associated test findings. In contrast, bilateral vestibulopathy may exhibit bilateral positive head thrust and diminished responses on head impulse, testing, caloric irrigation, or sinusoidal stimulation in the rotary chair.[4]

The mainstay of treatment in PPPD includes vestibular rehabilitation, medication, and cognitive behavior therapy (CBT).[23] Vestibular rehab aims to promote habituation by focusing on techniques that help fatigue the abnormal reflexive responses to movement and reduce sensitivity to visual stimuli.[23] The use of medication focuses on SSRIs and SNRIs that have been effective in treating CSD.[23–25] Finally, the role of CBT is to reduce anxiety and self-monitoring of vestibular symptoms and has been shown to reduce disability and dizziness symptoms on the Dizziness Handicap Inventory and Dizziness Symptoms Inventory, respectively, after 3 weekly treatment sessions.[26]

While they may not meet the criteria for a diagnosis of PPPD, patients with anxiety or exaggerated stress responses to vestibular stimuli may develop a fear with positioning maneuvers. Reporting of nausea during a Dix–Hallpike exam is commonly seen in patients with motion sickness and vestibular migraines. Patients fearful of such positioning may exhibit a sympathetic response with visible sweating, hyperventilating, and tachycardia. In turn, they feel lightheaded and may even refuse the exam. While such responses are not classified as symptoms synonymous with positional vertigo, they offer a clue into the diagnosis and contributing and exacerbating factors. As with PPPD, behavioral therapy, habituation therapy, and even medication can be helpful in this population.

SUMMARY

Positional vertigo refers to a spinning sensation produced by changes in head position relative to gravity. It can be a symptom of a functional disorder or structural disorders of central or peripheral origin. The first step in evaluating patients presenting with positional vertigo is the comprehensive history and physical exam to identify key features that distinguish the disorders on the differential diagnosis. BPPV is the most common cause of positional vertigo and is diagnosed by eliciting the characteristic upbeat-torsional or horizontal nystagmus on Dix–Hallpike. Patients presenting with positional vertigo and a negative Dix–Hallpike, atypical nystagmus on Dix–Hallpike, or other neurologic symptoms should undergo further evaluation, including neuroimaging to rule out structural lesions of central origin.

CLINICS CARE POINTS

- Positional vertigo can be both functional and structural in origin, and structural lesions may be either peripherally or centrally located.

- A thorough history and physical exam are essential in identifying key features to distinguish the disorders on the differential diagnosis for a patient with positional vertigo.
- BPPV is the most common cause of positional vertigo and is treated with repositioning maneuvers.
- Patients presenting with positional vertigo and a negative Dix–Hallpike, atypical nystagmus on Dix–Hallpike, or other neurologic symptoms should be further evaluated for alternative causes of positional vertigo, including central lesions and functional disorders.

DISCLOSURE

None.

REFERENCES

1. Bhattacharyya N, Gubbels SP, Schwartz SR, et al. Clinical practice guideline: benign paroxysmal positional vertigo (update). Otolaryngol Head Neck Surg 2017;156(3_suppl):S1–47.
2. Newman-Toker DE, Edlow JA. TiTrATE: a novel, evidence-based approach to diagnosing acute dizziness and vertigo. Neurol Clin 2015;33(3):577–99, viii.
3. Baloh RW. Differentiating between peripheral and central causes of vertigo. Otolaryngol Head Neck Surg 1998;119(1):55–9.
4. Staab JP, Eckhardt-Henn A, Horii A, et al. Diagnostic criteria for persistent postural-perceptual dizziness (PPPD): Consensus document of the committee for the Classification of Vestibular Disorders of the Bárány Society. J Vestib Res 2017;27(4):191–208.
5. Büttner U, Helmchen C, Brandt T. Diagnostic criteria for central versus peripheral positioning nystagmus and vertigo: a review. Acta Otolaryngol 1999;119(1):1–5.
6. Kim JS, Zee DS. Clinical practice. Benign paroxysmal positional vertigo. N Engl J Med 2014;370(12):1138–47.
7. Cho EI, White JA. Positional vertigo: as occurs across all age groups. Oto Clin North Am 2011;44:347–60.
8. Hunt WT, Zimmermann EF, Hilton MP. Modifications of the Epley (canalith repositioning) manoeuvre for posterior canal benign paroxysmal positional vertigo (BPPV). Cochrane Database Syst Rev 2012;(4):2012. :CD008675.
9. Mandalà M, Santoro GP, Asprella Libonati G, et al. Double-blind randomized trial on short-term efficacy of the Semont maneuver for the treatment of posterior canal benign paroxysmal positional vertigo. J Neurol 2012;259(5):882–5.
10. Oron Y, Cohen-Atsmoni S, Len A, et al. Treatment of horizontal canal BPPV: pathophysiology, available maneuvers, and recommended treatment. Laryngoscope 2015;125(8):1959–64.
11. Lee HJ, Kim ES, Kim M, et al. Isolated horizontal positional nystagmus from a posterior fossa lesion. Ann Neurol 2014;76(6):905–10.
12. Maire R, Duvoisin B. Localization of static positional nystagmus with the ocular fixation test. Laryngoscope 1999;109(4):606–12.
13. Bassani R, Della Torre S. Positional nystagmus reversing from geotropic to apogeotropic: a new central vestibular syndrome. J Neurol 2011;258(2):313–5.
14. Yenigun A, Ustun ME, Tugrul S, et al. Classification of vertebral artery loop formation and association with cervicogenic dizziness. J Laryngol Otol 2016;130(12):1115–9.

15. Thompson-Harvey A, Hain TC. Symptoms in cervical vertigo. Laryngoscope Investig Otolaryngol 2018;4(1):109–15.
16. Wrisley DM, Sparto PJ, Whitney SL, et al. Cervicogenic dizziness: a review of diagnosis and treatment. J Orthop Sports Phys Ther 2000;30(12):755–66.
17. Yacovino DA, Hain TC. Clinical characteristics of cervicogenic-related dizziness and vertigo. Semin Neurol 2013;33(3):244–55.
18. Ryan GM, Cope S. Cervical vertigo. Lancet 1955;269(6905):1355–8.
19. Duan G, Xu J, Shi J, et al. Advances in the pathogenesis, diagnosis and treatment of bow hunter's syndrome: a comprehensive review of the literature. Interv Neurol 2016;5(1–2):29–38.
20. Kuether TA, Nesbit GM, Clark WM, et al. Rotational vertebral artery occlusion: a mechanism of vertebrobasilar insufficiency. Neurosurgery 1997;41:427–32.
21. Bergl PA. Provoked dizziness from bow hunter's syndrome. Am J Med 2017; 130(9):e375–8.
22. Lu DC, Zador Z, Mummaneni PV, et al. Rotational vertebral artery occlusion-series of 9 cases. Neurosurgery 2010;67(4):1066–72 [discussion 1072].
23. Popkirov S, Staab JP, Stone J. Persistent postural-perceptual dizziness (PPPD): a common, characteristic and treatable cause of chronic dizziness. Pract Neurol 2018;18(1):5–13.
24. Bittar RS, Lins EM. Clinical characteristics of patients with persistent postural-perceptual dizziness. Braz J Otorhinolaryngol 2015;81(3):276–82.
25. Staab JP, Ruckenstein MJ, Amsterdam JD. A prospective trial of sertraline for chronic subjective dizziness. Laryngoscope 2004;114(9):1637–41.
26. Edelman S, Mahoney AE, Cremer PD. Cognitive behavior therapy for chronic subjective dizziness: a randomized, controlled trial. Am J Otolaryngol 2012; 33(4):395–401.

Acute Vestibular Syndrome and ER Presentations of Dizziness

Richard Baron, MD[a], Kristen K. Steenerson, MD[a,b], Jennifer Alyono, MD, MS[b,*]

KEYWORDS

- Acute vestibular syndrome • Dizzy • Emergency • HINTS Plus • Stroke • TiTrATE
- Vestibular neuritis

KEY POINTS

- Acute vestibular syndrome (AVS) describes severe, continuous dizziness typically associated with nausea, unsteadiness, head-motion intolerance, and nystagmus that develops suddenly and persists for more than 24 hours.
- History can identify provoking factors like medication changes or trauma as well as new neurologic symptoms or risk factors for stroke.
- The HINTS Plus exam is the best clinical tool to differentiate between central versus peripheral causes of AVS and guide imaging decisions.
- Vestibular neuritis (VN) is the most common cause of AVS; it is self-limited, and treatment relies on vestibular therapy with only a limited role for vestibular suppressants.
- Posterior circulation strokes can present with symptoms indistinguishable from other types of AVS and are frequent and primary causes of AVS.

INTRODUCTION

Acute vestibular syndrome (AVS) is a term first introduced by Hotson and Baloh in 1998[1] to describe severe, continuous dizziness (vertigo, lightheadedness, disequilibrium) that develops rapidly (over seconds to hours) but persists longer than 24 hours and is associated with nausea, vomiting, gait unsteadiness, head-motion intolerance, and nystagmus. AVS is usually monophasic and reaches its symptomatic peak during the first week, followed by gradual recovery over weeks to months with residual symptoms in a minority of patients.[2]

[a] Department of Neurology and Neurological Sciences, Stanford University School of Medicine, 801 Welch Road, Stanford, CA 94305, USA; [b] Department of Otolaryngology–Head & Neck Surgery, Stanford University School of Medicine, 801 Welch Road, Stanford, CA 94305, USA
* Corresponding author.
E-mail address: jalyono@stanford.edu

Otolaryngol Clin N Am 54 (2021) 925–938
https://doi.org/10.1016/j.otc.2021.05.013
oto.theclinics.com

Abbreviations	
AVS	Acute vestibular syndrome (expansion retained twice, as the second use is referential)
BPPV	Benign paroxysmal positional vertigo
CN	Cranial nerve
CT	Computed tomography
ED	Emergency department
EVS	Episodic vestibular syndrome
VN	Vestibular neuritis
VOR	Vestibulo-ocular reflex

AVS stands in contrast to episodic vestibular syndrome (EVS), in which patients are symptomatic in recurrent, stereotyped paroxysms. Attacks may last seconds to minutes and are strictly triggered by a specific head motion or position change, as is classically seen in benign paroxysmal positional vertigo (BPPV), or attacks may be spontaneous with symptoms that can last for minutes to hours, such as in vestibular migraine or Ménière's disease.

A thorough clinical evaluation of dizziness is particularly important in the emergency department (ED) context to properly identify posterior circulation strokes. While stroke is responsible for only 3% to 5% of all ED presentations for dizziness, up to 25% of patients presenting with Acute Vestibular Syndrome specifically have been found to have a stroke. (3) In 2011, there were 2.5 million ED visits for dizziness, an estimated 10% to 20% of which were for symptoms consistent with AVS (250,000 - 500,000). Therefore we can estimate that about 70,000 to 100,000 stroke patients per year present to the ED with dizziness.[3]

The key to the differentiation between AVS, EVS, and the variety of their central and peripheral etiologies lies in a careful history focusing on timing, triggers, and exposures, and a targeted bedside examination as described in the TiTrATE model[2] (*Ti*ming, *Tr*iggers, *A*nd *T*argeted *Ex*am).

ACUTE VESTIBULAR SYNDROME ETIOLOGIES
Spontaneous

Vestibular neuritis
VN is the most common cause of AVS (approximately 60% of cases[3]) and is the third most common cause of peripheral vertigo among all dizzy patients (following BPPV and Ménière's[4]).

Vestibular neuritis etiology. The vestibular ganglion lies in the internal auditory canal; these bipolar afferent neurons receive input from the vestibular hair cells and relay these signals to the brainstem. The vestibular nerve has a superior division (innervating the utricle, superior and horizontal semicircular canals) and an inferior division (innervating the saccule and posterior semicircular canal) that together form a central trunk. Both superior and inferior divisions are usually affected in VN (55%), although some patients will have only superior division involvement (42%). Isolated inferior division involvement is rare (2%).[5] This may be explained by the double innervation of the posterior canal by the accessory singular nerve and the fact that the bony canal around the superior division is longer (~2 mm vs 0.3 mm) and more spiculated[6] and thereby more susceptible to inflammatory injury.

VN is traditionally thought to be a viral or postviral reactivation analogous to Bell's Palsy. Latent HSV-1 has been detected in about 60% of otherwise asymptomatic vestibular ganglia in human autopsy studies,[7,8] similar to the trigeminal ganglion. In addition, VN can be induced in mice models by inoculation with HSV.[9]

Epidemiologic studies have noted that the risk of VN increases with age, vascular risk factors,[10] and is associated with the presence of carotid plaques,[11] which has raised the possibility of a vascular etiology for VN. However, increased microglial activity on [18]GE180 PET[12] studies and contrast enhancement and FLAIR abnormalities on research MRI protocols[13] have shifted focus back to an inflammatory peri-viral process. Of note, dizziness is the most common neurologic symptom among patients with COVID-19 (present in 16.8% of hospitalized COVID patients in Wuhan[14]). Severe dizziness consistent with AVS as a presenting symptom of COVID has been reported in at least 3 case reports as of September 2020.[15]

Vestibular neuritis natural history. Symptoms from VN are typically most severe in the first 1 to 3 days, with significant recovery after 5 to 7 days when spontaneous nystagmus will be mostly suppressible with fixation. Most patients have minimal symptoms within 6 weeks,[4] but complete vestibular recovery on caloric testing occurs in only 50% to 70% of patients.[16] Recurrence occurs in only 2%[17]–10%[18] of patients, but 30% to 50% of patients will have persistent symptoms at long-term follow-up.[19] Of note, long-term prognosis in VN patients is linked more strongly to anxiety, personality, and somatization traits than to objective vestibular deficits[20]– especially fear of bodily sensations, catastrophic thoughts, and dependent personality.[21]

Labyrinthitis

Labyrinthitis traditionally refers to cochleovestibular neuritis—a VN-like condition that also involves hearing loss, suggesting inflammatory involvement of the whole labyrinth (vestibular + auditory structures). This condition is thought to be benign and viral/postviral, similar to VN, but acute bacterial otitis media, temporal bone trauma, hemorrhage, and tumors can infrequently cause inflammation in the labyrinth as well. In rare cases, the membranous labyrinth will ossify in response to the inflammation, resulting in labyrinthitis ossificans with changes visible on CT and MRI.

Newman Toker and colleagues[2] suggest that a diagnosis of labyrinthitis should be looked upon with suspicion, as the presence of AVS with hearing loss is also a common presentation for stroke.[22,23]

Stroke

Posterior circulation strokes are a less common but important cause of AVS. While stroke comprises only 3% to 5% of all patients who present to the ED with dizziness, stroke occurs in about 25% of patients presenting with symptoms consistent with AVS, and among patients with AVS and greater than 1 stroke risk factor, the rate of stroke is as high as 55% to 60%.[24,25] They are often missed by physicians and can be challenging to identify clinically.[26] Missed diagnosis of stroke occurs more frequently in those presenting with dizziness (35%) than those with motor deficits (4%).[27] Routine tools like the NIH Stroke Scale are not sensitive to posterior circulation strokes and can mislead clinicians.[28]

Stroke Localization

One study of 240 isolated cerebellar infarcts noted that only 10% presented with isolated dizziness; 90% of patients had other focal neurologic findings or concerning symptoms.[29] Of note, virtually all infarcts causing isolated dizziness occurred in the medial branch of the PICA. Other cohorts have shown a 3:1 preponderance of PICA to AICA strokes.[30] Strokes of the AICA, which supplies the internal auditory artery in 90% of people,[31] sometimes presents as dizziness with hearing loss,[32] though larger territory infarcts can affect the pons, thus causing more prominent sensorimotor deficits. About 25% of stroke patients are younger than age 50, with those strokes most commonly due to vertebral dissection.[3]

Other
There have been many case reports of AVS due to demyelinating lesions in multiple sclerosis.[33,34] In 1 cohort, demyelination accounted for approximately 4% of all cases of AVS. Causal lesions were scattered throughout the brainstem.[35] All patients had central oculomotor signs (upbeat nystagmus, internuclear ophthalmoplegia, seesaw nystagmus, skew deviation, direction-changing, gaze-evoked horizontal nystagmus) or a normal head impulse test. Isolated cranial nerve (CN) involvement occurs in 10% of multiple sclerosis cases.[36] The trigeminal (CN V) and facial (CN VII) nerves were most commonly involved, and vestibulocochlear nerve involvement was quite rare (4% of isolated CN palsy)[36] despite the vestibulocochlear nerve being highly myelinated.[37]

Although uncommon, AVS can also be a presenting symptom in patients with thiamine deficiency. Wernicke encephalopathy classically presents as a triad of ophthalmoplegia, ataxia, and encephalopathy in a malnourished patient.[38] Encephalopathy is present in 90% of patients diagnosed, but in a case series of nonencephalopathic thiamine deficiency, several patients presented with clinical AVS with peripheral vestibular findings (horizontal, bilateral gaze-evoked nystagmus, and bilaterally abnormal head impulse tests), most of whom improved if not resolved with thiamine repletion.[39]

Patients with brainstem encephalitis or cerebellitis can present with vertigo, nausea/vomiting, and nystagmus, but the onset of symptoms is typically subacute, and patients may have additional symptoms such as headaches, fevers, altered mentation, or ataxia.[40]

Neoplasms will typically have a gradual onset of symptoms or grow slowly enough that the central nervous system can compensate; however, there have been reported cases of vestibular schwannoma mimicking labyrinthitis,[41,42] particularly in aggressive schwannomas with p27 loss-of-function mutations[43].

Postexposure
AVS can occur as a result of drug or toxin exposure or due to head trauma. Antiepileptic drugs are a particularly common cause of dizziness, even at therapeutic doses.[44,45] Aminoglycosides (particularly gentamicin) can cause profound, often permanent loss of vestibular function. Such a loss can be seen in as many as 3% of patients treated with gentamicin[46] and occurs rather idiosyncratically without correlation to serum drug level or total drug exposure.[47] Patients typically present with prominent gait unsteadiness and oscillopsia with head movement; hearing is typically spared. Dizziness is common, but room-spinning vertigo is rare, thought to be due to the underlying symmetric bilateral nature of the vestibulopathy.

Head trauma can cause AVS if there is direct vestibular nerve injury or labyrinthine concussion, and has been described in cases of blunt force head trauma,[48] blast injuries,[49] whiplash,[50] and barotrauma.[51] Dizziness is the most common postconcussive symptom in the first 2 weeks post TBI[52] and can persist as a component of postconcussive syndrome (dizziness, headaches, fatigue, and mild cognitive impairment), especially in vestibular subtype postconcussive syndrome.

Assessment of patients with acute vestibular syndrome
The TiTrATE model has been proposed as a systematic method to differentiate various etiologies for dizziness.[2] A differential diagnosis is first narrowed by history taking,

dividing *Ti*ming into episodic, acute, or chronic in duration. *Tri*ggers for the underlying pathology are reviewed, including positional triggers, toxins, medications, and trauma. *Ta*rgeted bedside examination, including differentiating central from peripheral signs of vertigo, helps guide whether other workups, such as imaging, may be indicated (**Fig. 1**).

History

Taking a history is critical in developing a differential diagnosis for dizziness. The onset and duration of symptoms, associated symptoms, demographics, and past medical history help establish pretest probabilities of the cause.

Headache can suggest an intracranial mass or bleed, and in combination with fever, raise suspicion for meningitis and encephalitis. New neurologic symptoms such as weakness, sensory loss, dysphagia, dysarthria, or extraocular movement abnormalities may be signs of a stroke, demyelinating lesion, or mass. Sudden severe neck pain can signify vertebral dissection (though pain is absent in 25% of dissections),[53] and hearing loss, as previously discussed, is common in both AICA strokes and labyrinthitis.

If dizziness is the main or only symptom, consider whether the timeline and persistence of symptoms are more consistent with AVS (persistent, classically lasting >24 hours) or EVS (intermittent, short-lived symptoms, possibly with trigger). The circumstances surrounding the onset of symptoms may help assess exposures: trauma, malnutrition, and alcoholism (Wernicke), drug exposure (especially aminoglycosides or antiepileptics), recent otologic surgery, or immune suppression (encephalitis).

Demographics and past medical history can be useful for risk stratifying patients. Although patients who are older and have more vascular risk factors are more likely to have a stroke, age is a risk factor for *both* VN and stroke, and patients with VN often have underlying vascular risk factors.

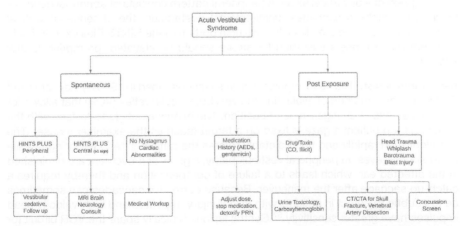

Fig. 1. Acute Vestibular Diagnostic Pathway. AEDs, antiepileptic drugs; CO, carbon monoxide; HINTS, Head Impulse Test, Nystagmus, Test of Skew. (*Adapted from* Newman-Toker DE, Edlow JA. TiTrATE: A Novel, Evidence-Based Approach to Diagnosing Acute Dizziness and Vertigo. Neurol Clin. 2015 Aug;33(3):577-99, viii. https://doi.org/10.1016/j.ncl.2015.04.011. PMID: 26231273; PMCID: PMC4522574.)

Exam

General neurologic and ENT exam

Patients with AVS often appear uncomfortable and in distress. In patients who are actively nauseated or vomiting and appear in extremis, it is important to remember ABCs (airway, breathing, circulation) and obtain vital signs, an electrocardiogram, and cardiac exam to rule out arrhythmia, acute coronary syndrome, or severe hypotension.

A routine head and neck examination should be performed on all patients. Particular attention should be given to the cranial nerves to evaluate the integrity of the brainstem and cerebellar-pontine angle and an otoscopic exam to evaluate for acute otitis media, which in rare cases may lead to bacterial labyrinthitis. A neurologic exam should include extremity motor and sensory testing—pronator drift and finger tapping are particularly sensitive tests for even mild weakness.[54] An ataxic gait may be observed, characterized by a wide base, truncal swaying, and inability to tandem. Truncal ataxia can graded as Grade 1 (able to walk independently despite imbalance), Grade 2 (requires support to ambulate), or Grade 3 (unable to remain upright or unable to ambulate). Appendicular ataxia can be assessed with finger–nose–finger, heel–shin slide, or rapid pronation–supination of the arms. Abnormalities on the coordination exam that are out of proportion to the degree of dizziness typically reflect central etiologies. Grade 3 truncal ataxia, in particular, is strongly associated with primary causes of AVS (100% sensitivity and 61% specificity in 1 cohort[30]), whereas appendicular ataxia is only present in 60% of patients with cerebellar strokes.[55] In all patients, a HINTS Plus exam (Head Impulse, Nystagmus, Test of Skew, hearing loss) should always be performed given its very high accuracy for differentiating central and peripheral lesions.

HINTS plus exam

The HINTS Plus exam consists of head impulse testing, characterization of nystagmus, a test of skew, and evaluating for acute hearing loss. A central pattern consists of a normal head impulse test, vertical or direction-changing nystagmus, and the presence of vertical skew. A peripheral pattern consists of abnormal head impulse with catch-up saccades, unidirectional nystagmus, the absence of vertical skew, and no acute hearing loss. If any single portion of the HINTS Plus exam reflects a central pattern, one's suspicion for stroke should be elevated, prompting further evaluation.

Head impulse test. The head impulse test was first described in 1998 by Halmagyi and Curthoys[56] as a method of evaluating the vestibulo-ocular reflex (VOR) that allows for fixed gaze despite changes in head position. The examiner sits face-to-face with the patient as the patient's gaze is fixed on a target (such as the examiner's nose). The examiner then rapidly and unpredictably rotates the patient's head left or right while observing the eyes. In peripheral vestibulopathy, signals of movement are diminished in the affected ear, which leads to a failure of compensation and thereby requires a catch-up saccade after the maneuver. Because corrective saccades can sometimes be too subtle to detect in patients with milder injury, repeated and high-velocity head impulses have greater sensitivity.[57] Central lesions typically spare the VOR circuit (or else cause frank extraocular movement impairment).[58]

Nystagmus. Nystagmus should be assessed with the patient sitting in a neutral position, first observing for spontaneous movement then screening for gaze-evoked nystagmus in all cardinal directions. Peripheral nystagmus is caused by an imbalance of vestibular tone between the 2 sides that leads to spontaneous eye movement in a slow phase toward the side of vestibular deficit, with quick saccadic eye movements in the opposite direction. Peripheral nystagmus is horizontal and unidirectional, intensifying when looking toward the fast phase direction and improving when looking toward the slow phase. Central nystagmus involves vertical, purely torsional, or direction-changing nystagmus. There are rare cases of isolated inferior division VN affecting the posterior canals that cause downbeat nystagmus.[5] In contrast with central causes, peripheral nystagmus can generally be suppressed with visual fixation.

Test of skew. The cover–uncover test for vertical skew looks for evidence of vertical misalignment due to an impaired otolith-ocular reflex. This impairment is caused by central lesions, usually on the same side as the lower eye; pontine lesions are most common, followed by midbrain and medulla.[59] To perform the test, the examiner alternates between covering one and then the other eye of the patient. In a healthy patient, the eyes remain motionless. The test is positive, or abnormal, when the eye has a vertical refixation saccade after the cover is moved, indicating ocular misalignment (**Table 1**).

Plus. Since AICA strokes can cause ischemia to CN VIII or the labyrinth itself,[31] these patients can paradoxically demonstrate peripheral catch-up saccades on head impulse testing.[22] These patients will exhibit hearing loss, however, so the inclusion of "Plus hearing" as a central sign improves the sensitivity of the HINTS exam.[58] Formal audiology testing is usually not possible in the ED, but simple bedside screening can be performed. The 2 ears can be compared using finger rub or tuning fork testing. Additionally, multiple smartphone-based hearing tests are available but vary in quality, and most have not been validated.[60]

Computed tomography

Neuroimaging is a powerful diagnostic tool in the workup of dizziness in the ED. However, with rising healthcare costs largely due to trends toward more imaging,[61] it is important that imaging is used in the appropriate context.

While CTs are commonly performed for dizziness,[62] they are rarely clinically significant. In 1 study where CTs were obtained in 48% of 1681 patients, only 0.74% changed management.[63] Another study evaluating 228 CT/CTAs performed in dizzy patients had a yield of 2.2%.[64] In an earlier study of 200 consecutive patients presenting with isolated dizziness, a noncontrast head CT provided a diagnostic explanation in 0 patients.[65]

This low yield is likely explained by the fact that the pathologies that CT is useful in detecting (large masses, hemorrhage, bony abnormalities) are relatively rare causes of isolated dizziness.[66] There is a role for CT in patients with a history of trauma, suspected vertebral artery dissection (associated head/neck pain and visual loss), or suspected canal dehiscence (autophony, pulsatile tinnitus). However, the sensitivity of CT in posterior fossa stroke is low. Even when looking retrospectively at patients who were confirmed to have had a stroke on MRI, attending neuroradiologists were able to find CT changes in only 40%.[67]

MRI

MRI is the preferred diagnostic imaging modality in the evaluation of patients with AVS. MRI in dizzy patients is useful primarily in ruling out stroke,[66] though it can also be helpful to evaluate for multiple sclerosis, masses, and intralabyrinthine hemorrhages and can demonstrate enhancement in labyrinthitis. MRIs in patients with VN, unlike Bell's palsy, are typically normal.

Table 1
Peripheral versus central oculomotor abnormalities

	Peripheral	Central
Nystagmus Direction	Unidirectional	Direction may change with gaze position
Spontaneous Nystagmus	Horizontal or torsional; suppressed by gaze fixation	Pure vertical, horizontal, or torsional; not suppressed by gaze fixation
Head Impulse Test	Impaired with catch up saccades	Intact, able to maintain fixed gaze
Test of Skew	No correction	Vertical correction

MRI should be performed in patients with AVS if there are accompanying neurologic findings (ex. cranial neuropathy, visual changes, motor/sensory weakness, ataxia), or if the patient demonstrates any components of a central pattern on a HINTS Plus exam: if the head impulse test is normal, nystagmus is direction-changing or vertical, skew deviation is present, or hearing loss is present.

Studies have shown that a HINTS exam outperforms MRI in detecting strokes in the ED with a sensitivity and specificity greater than 95% in most studies.[24,68] The few patients in whom strokes are missed by an initial HINTS exam are usually captured by adding sensorineural hearing loss as a central sign, for a so-called composite HINTS Plus exam.[58] The accuracy of HINTS, however, decreases to a sensitivity of 83% and specificity of 44%, when performed by physicians of mixed training rather than just neurologists/otologists.[69]

While the presence of diffusion restriction on MRI is the gold standard for diagnosing stroke, lesions that are smaller than 1 cm in size (15% of posterior circulation strokes) are often missed by MRI during the first 48 hours, with a sensitivity of only 50%.[24] This leads to the previously discussed superiority of a well-performed HINTS Plus exam on initial evaluation and suggestions of obtaining an MRI after 72 hours from symptom onset if a patient is thought to be at high risk for stroke.

Treatment

Pharmacologic
Symptomatic management of nausea and vertigo can include several classes of medications including antihistamines (promethazine, meclizine, diphenhydramine), 5-HT3 serotonin receptor antagonists (ondansetron, granisetron, and metoclopramide at higher doses), dopamine receptor 2 antagonists (droperidol, haloperidol, metoclopramide at lower doses), M1 anticholinergics (scopolamine), benzodiazepines (lorazepam, diazepam), and glucocorticoids (prednisone).

Histamine and M1 acetylcholine are thought to be the receptors most active in the vestibular pathway for dizziness, but 5-HT3 and D2 are also expressed more centrally. Comparison studies have generally suggested the superiority of antihistamines like promethazine over 5HT-3 antagonists like ondansetron (51% vs 37% reduction in vertigo symptoms[70]) or benzodiazepines like diazepam (95% excellent improvement vs 17% good improvement[71]) and lorazepam (66% vs 38% reduction[72]). However, 1 study suggested that 5HT-3 antagonists like ondansetron are more effective in treating nausea/vomiting and cause greater symptomatic relief, whereas an antihistamine like promethazine more strongly improves the sense of motion and shows decreased rates of readmission, though it is associated with a higher rate of side effects,[70] primarily sedation. Other side effects include sedation or delirium in antihistamines and benzodiazepines, QTC prolongation and torsades de pointes or serotonin syndrome in 5HT-3 antagonists, and extrapyramidal side effects or neuroleptic malignant syndrome in antidopaminergics.

None of these medications should be used longer than 72 hours, as prolonged use may interfere with central compensation and long-term recovery.[73]

Vestibular therapy

Vestibular therapy is the mainstay of treatment for AVS. Vestibular therapy is primarily aimed at desensitizing the vestibular system and teaching compensatory techniques (ie, fixation) and has been shown to improve gaze stabilization[74] and reduce symptom severity.[75]

Vestibular neuritis treatment

In patients with sudden sensorineural hearing loss accompanying their acute vertigo (ie, labyrinthitis), steroids remain the standard of care. In isolated VN, treatment paradigms are less clear.

Early results established no benefit to the use of antiviral medications,[76] but the use of steroids has remained controversial. The most recent Cochrane Review from 2011[77] and multiple meta-analyses in the early 2010s[78,79] did not find sufficient evidence to support the use of corticosteroids in the treatment of VN. Since then, prospective placebo-controlled trials comparing corticosteroids with vestibular therapy did not show clinical improvement.[80,81] However, steroids remain the standard of care in some institutions,[82] and it is reasonable to consider whether a patient has comorbidities that would be aggravated by steroid side effects (eg, diabetes, hypertension, dementia).

Given the strong association between long-term recovery and psychological factors,[20,21] it is prudent to identify patients at risk and address underlying psychiatric comorbidities. A simple screen can be performed in the ED with the PHQ-2 for depression[83] (Little interest or pleasure in doing things? Feeling down depressed or hopeless? on a 0–3 frequency scale) or the GAD-2 for anxiety[84] (Feeling nervous, anxious or on edge? Not being able to stop or control worrying? 0–3 frequency scale). There is evidence that cognitive behavioral therapy and psychotherapy are both effective in promoting recovery after VN,[85] and they may help prevent long-term morbidity and development of persistent postural perceptual dizziness.[86]

Stroke

The detection of stroke is a high priority, and patients with a central pattern HINTS exam should have an MRI and a neurology consult. Posterior fossa strokes, particularly vertebral or basilar artery occlusions, may be sufficiently disabling to warrant thrombolytic therapy or thrombectomy. Posterior fossa infarctions may become complicated by edema or hemorrhage, which can lead to acute hydrocephalus, herniation, and even death. Patients with critical stenoses in the posterior circulation may exhibit pressure-dependent brain perfusion, requiring ICU admission for pressure support. In all patients with strokes, etiology should be assessed (small vessel disease vs intracranial atherosclerosis, vs artery to artery embolism, vs cardioembolic, vs hypercoagulability), and treatment will involve management of risk factors for secondary prevention, including LDL, A1c, and hypertensive management as well as possible anticoagulation.

SUMMARY

AVS is defined by the acute onset of severe, continuous dizziness that persists for more than 24 hours and is associated with nausea, vomiting, gait unsteadiness, head-motion intolerance, and nystagmus. Evaluation can differentiate peripheral from central causes and should follow the TiTrATE approach to assess the timing of symptoms, possible triggers, prior exposures, and a targeted bedside examination.[2] While VN is the most common cause of AVS in all patients, ruling out stroke is important. The HINTS Plus exam is the most sensitive and specific tool to detect central causes of AVS and should be performed on every patient. Vestibular therapy is a mainstay of treatment, and care should be taken to ensure that patients do not use vestibular suppressants for more than 72 hours.

CLINICS CARE POINTS

- Use the TiTrATE model (*Ti*ming, *Tr*iggers, *A*nd *T*argeted *Ex*am) to evaluate causes of AVS.[2]
- Stroke is responsible for 4% of all patients presenting to the ED with dizziness but 25% of patients with AVS and up to 60% of patients with AVS and more than 1 stroke risk factor.[24,25]
- HINTS Plus (Head Impulse, Nystagmus, Test of Skew, plus hearing loss) should be used in examining patients with AVS.
- CT scans are very low yield in patients with dizziness[63] and should be reserved for patients with a history of trauma, suspected vertebral artery dissection, or suspected canal dehiscence.
- MRI is the preferred diagnostic imaging modality in evaluating patients with AVS, though it may miss small strokes of less than 1 cm and is not as sensitive or specific as a HINTS Plus exam.
- Vestibular suppressants should not be used for more than 72 hours, as this can interfere with central compensation and is associated with poorer outcomes.[73]
- There is no role for antiviral medication in the treatment of VN[76]; there is insufficient evidence to recommend steroids,[77] but they are still frequently used in clinical practice and reasonable to employ when there is a low risk of side effects.

DISCLOSURE

"The authors have nothing to disclose."

REFERENCES

1. Hotson JR, Baloh RW. Acute vestibular syndrome. N Engl J Med 1998;339(10): 680–5.
2. Newman-Toker DE, Edlow JA. TiTrATE: a novel, evidence-based approach to diagnosing acute dizziness and vertigo. Neurol Clin 2015;33(3):577–99, viii.
3. Tarnutzer AA, Berkowitz AL, Robinson KA, et al. Does my dizzy patient have a stroke? A systematic review of bedside diagnosis in acute vestibular syndrome. CMAJ 2011;183(9):E571–92.
4. Strupp M, Brandt T. Vestibular neuritis. Semin Neurol 2009;29(5):509–19.
5. Taylor RL, McGarvie LA, Reid N, et al. Vestibular neuritis affects both superior and inferior vestibular nerves. Neurology 2016;87(16):1704–12.
6. Gianoli G, Goebel J, Mowry S, et al. Anatomic differences in the lateral vestibular nerve channels and their implications in vestibular neuritis. Otol Neurotol 2005; 26(3):489–94.
7. Furuta Y, Takasu T, Fukuda S, et al. Latent herpes simplex virus type 1 in human vestibular ganglia. Acta Otolaryngol (Stockh) 1993;113(sup503):85–9.

8. Arbusow V, Schulz P, Strupp M, et al. Distribution of herpes simplex virus type 1 in human geniculate and vestibular ganglia: implications for vestibular neuritis. Ann Neurol 1999;46(3):416–9.

9. Hirata Y, Gyo K, Yanagihara N. Herpetic vestibular neuritis: an experimental study. Acta Otolaryngol Suppl 1995;519:93–6.

10. Oron Y, Shemesh S, Shushan S, et al. Cardiovascular risk factors among patients with vestibular neuritis. Ann Otol Rhinol Laryngol 2017;126(8):597–601.

11. Wada M, Takeshima T, Nakamura Y, et al. Carotid plaque is a new risk factor for peripheral vestibular disorder: a retrospective cohort study. Medicine (Baltimore) 2016;95(31):e4510.

12. Becker-Bense S, Zwergal A, Unterrainer M, et al. Imaging neuroinflammation along the vestibular nerve and nucleus in acute unilateral vestibulopathy by [18F]GE180-PET. Eur J Neurol 2018;25(S 2):561.

13. Venkatasamy A, Huynh TT, Wohlhuter N, et al. Superior vestibular neuritis: improved detection using FLAIR sequence with delayed enhancement (1 h). Eur Arch Otorhinolaryngol 2019;276(12):3309–16.

14. Mao L, Jin H, Wang M, et al. Neurologic manifestations of hospitalized patients with coronavirus disease 2019 in Wuhan, China. JAMA Neurol 2020;77(6):683.

15. Saniasiaya J, Kulasegarah J. Dizziness and COVID-19. Ear Nose Throat J 2021; 100(1):29–30.

16. Ohbayashi S, Oda M, Yamamoto M, et al. Recovery of the vestibular function after vestibular neuronitis. Acta Otolaryngol Suppl 1993;503:31–4.

17. Mandalà M, Santoro GP, Awrey J, et al. Vestibular neuritis: recurrence and incidence of secondary benign paroxysmal positional vertigo. Acta Otolaryngol (Stockh) 2010;130(5):565–7.

18. Kim YH, Kim K-S, Kim KJ, et al. Recurrence of vertigo in patients with vestibular neuritis. Acta Otolaryngol (Stockh) 2011;131(11):1172–7.

19. Okinaka Y, Sekitani T, Okazaki H, et al. Progress of caloric response of vestibular neuronitis. Acta Otolaryngol Suppl 1993;503:18–22.

20. Godemann F, Siefert K, Hantschke-Brüggemann M, et al. What accounts for vertigo one year after neuritis vestibularis - anxiety or a dysfunctional vestibular organ? J Psychiatr Res 2005;39(5):529–34.

21. Heinrichs N, Edler C, Eskens S, et al. Predicting continued dizziness after an acute peripheral vestibular disorder. Psychosom Med 2007;69(7):700–7.

22. Lee H. Audiovestibular loss in anterior inferior cerebellar artery territory infarction: a window to early detection? J Neurol Sci 2012;313(1–2):153–9.

23. Lin HC, Pin Zhir C, Lee HC. Sudden sensorineural hearing loss increases the risk of stroke. Stroke 2008;39(10):2744–8.

24. Saber Tehrani AS, Kattah JC, Mantokoudis G, et al. Small strokes causing severe vertigo. Neurology 2014;83(2):169–73.

25. Newman-Toker DE, Kerber KA, Hsieh Y-H, et al. HINTS outperforms ABCD2 to screen for stroke in acute continuous vertigo and dizziness. Acad Emerg Med 2013;20(10):986–96.

26. Kuruvilla A, Bhattacharya P, Rajamani K, et al. Factors associated with misdiagnosis of acute stroke in young adults. J Stroke Cerebrovasc Dis 2011;20(6): 523–7.

27. Newman-Toker DE, Moy E, Valente E, et al. Missed diagnosis of stroke in the emergency department: a cross-sectional analysis of a large population-based sample. Diagn Berl Ger 2014;1(2):155–66.

28. Schneck Michael J. Current stroke scales may be partly responsible for worse outcomes in posterior circulation stroke. Stroke 2018;49(11):2565–6.

29. Lee H, Sohn S-I, Cho Y-W, et al. Cerebellar infarction presenting isolated vertigo: frequency and vascular topographical patterns. Neurology 2006;67(7):1178–83.
30. Carmona S, Martínez C, Zalazar G, et al. The diagnostic accuracy of truncal ataxia and HINTS as cardinal signs for acute vestibular syndrome. Front Neurol 2016;7:125.
31. Delion M, Dinomais M, Mercier P. Arteries and veins of the cerebellum. Cerebellum 2017;16(5–6):880–912.
32. Lee H, Sohn S-I, Jung D-K, et al. Sudden deafness and anterior inferior cerebellar artery infarction. Stroke 2002;33(12):2807–12.
33. Surmeli R, Surmeli M, Yalcin AD, et al. Multiple sclerosis attack case presenting with pseudo-vestibular neuritis. Int J Neurosci 2020;1–5.
34. Valente P, Pinto I, Aguiar C, et al. Acute vestibular syndrome and hearing loss mimicking labyrinthitis as initial presentation of multiple sclerosis. Int J Pediatr Otorhinolaryngol 2020;134:110048.
35. Pula J, Kattah J, Newman-Toker D. Acute Vestibular Syndrome from Demyelinating Lesions (P02.247). Neurology 2012;78(1 Supplement). P02.247-P02.247.
36. Zadro I, Barun B, Habek M, et al. Isolated cranial nerve palsies in multiple sclerosis. Clin Neurol Neurosurg 2008;110(9):886–8.
37. Silverstein H, Norrell H. Histologic study of the vestibulocochlear nerve. Ann Otol Rhinol Laryngol 1986;95(5 Pt 1):545–6.
38. Victor M, Adams RD, Collins GH. The Wernicke-Korsakoff syndrome. A clinical and pathological study of 245 patients, 82 with post-mortem examinations. Contemp Neurol Ser 1971;7:1–206.
39. Kattah JC, Dhanani SS, Pula JH, et al. Vestibular signs of thiamine deficiency during the early phase of suspected Wernicke encephalopathy. Neurol Clin Pract 2013;3(6):460–8.
40. Van Samkar A, Poulsen MNF, Bienfait HP, et al. Acute cerebellitis in adults: a case report and review of the literature. BMC Res Notes 2017;10:610.
41. Lee JD, Lee BD, Hwang SC. Vestibular schwannoma in patients with sudden sensorineural hearing loss. Skull Base 2011;21(2):75–8.
42. Han DY, Jang WI, Lee JD. A case of vestibular schwannoma mimicking acute labyrinthitis. Res Vestib Sci 2009;8(2):164–7.
43. Seol HJ, Jung H-W, Park S-H, et al. Aggressive vestibular schwannomas showing postoperative rapid growth - their association with decreased p27 expression. J Neurooncol 2005;75(2):203–7.
44. Kattah JC, Talkad AV, Wang DZ, et al. HINTS to diagnose stroke in the acute vestibular syndrome: three-step bedside oculomotor examination more sensitive than early MRI diffusion-weighted imaging. Stroke 2009;40(11):3504–10.
45. St. Louis E. Minimizing AED adverse effects: improving quality of life in the interictal state in epilepsy care. Curr Neuropharmacol 2009;7(2):106–14. https://doi.org/10.2174/157015909788848857.
46. Kahlmeter G, Dahlager JI. Aminoglycoside toxicity - a review of clinical studies published between 1975 and 1982. J Antimicrob Chemother 1984;13(Suppl A):9–22.
47. Ahmed RM, Hannigan IP, MacDougall HG, et al. Gentamicin ototoxicity: a 23-year selected case series of 103 patients. Med J Aust 2012;196(11):701–4.
48. Davies RA, Luxon LM. Dizziness following head injury: a neuro-otological study. J Neurol 1995;242(4):222–30.
49. Hoffer ME, Balaban C, Gottshall K, et al. Blast exposure: vestibular consequences and associated characteristics. Otol Neurotol 2010;31(2):232–6.

50. Vibert D, Häusler R. Acute peripheral vestibular deficits after whiplash injuries. Ann Otol Rhinol Laryngol 2003;112(3):246–51.
51. Klingmann C, Praetorius M, Baumann I, et al. Barotrauma and decompression illness of the inner ear: 46 cases during treatment and follow-up. Otol Neurotol 2007;28(4):447–54.
52. Yang C-C, Tu Y-K, Hua M-S, et al. The association between the postconcussion symptoms and clinical outcomes for patients with mild traumatic brain injury. J Trauma 2007;62(3):657–63.
53. Gottesman RF, Sharma P, Robinson KA, et al. Imaging characteristics of symptomatic vertebral artery dissection: a systematic review. Neurologist 2012;18(5): 255–60.
54. Teitelbaum JS, Eliasziw M, Garner M. Tests of motor function in patients suspected of having mild unilateral cerebral lesions. Can J Neurol Sci J Can Sci Neurol 2002;29(4):337–44.
55. Edlow JA, Newman-Toker DE, Savitz SI. Diagnosis and initial management of cerebellar infarction. Lancet Neurol 2008;7(10):951–64.
56. Halmagyi GM, Curthoys IS. A clinical sign of canal paresis. Arch Neurol 1988; 45(7):737–9.
57. Weber KP, Aw ST, Todd MJ, et al. Head impulse test in unilateral vestibular loss: vestibulo-ocular reflex and catch-up saccades. Neurology 2008;70(6):454–63.
58. Kattah JC. Update on HINTS plus, with discussion of pitfalls and pearls. J Neurol Phys Ther 2019;43:S42.
59. Keane JR. Ocular skew deviation. Analysis of 100 cases. Arch Neurol 1975;32(3): 185–90.
60. Bright T, Pallawela D. Validated smartphone-based apps for ear and hearing assessments: a review. JMIR Rehabil Assist Technol 2016;3(2):e13.
61. Tehrani ASS, Coughlan D, Hsieh YH, et al. Rising annual costs of dizziness presentations to U.S. emergency departments. Acad Emerg Med 2013;20(7): 689–96.
62. Kim AS, Sidney S, Klingman JG, et al. Practice variation in neuroimaging to evaluate dizziness in the ED. Am J Emerg Med 2012;30(5):665–72.
63. Ahsan SF, Syamal MN, Yaremchuk K, et al. The costs and utility of imaging in evaluating dizzy patients in the emergency room. Laryngoscope 2013;123(9): 2250–3.
64. Fakhran S, Alhilali L, Branstetter BF. Yield of CT angiography and contrast-enhanced MR imaging in patients with dizziness. AJNR Am J Neuroradiol 2013;34(5):1077–81.
65. Wasay M, Dubey N, Bakshi R. Dizziness and yield of emergency head CT scan: Is it cost effective? Emerg Med J 2005;22(4):312.
66. Newman-Toker DE, Hsieh Y-H, Camargo CA, et al. Spectrum of dizziness visits to US emergency departments: cross-sectional analysis from a nationally representative sample. Mayo Clin Proc Mayo Clin 2008;83(7):765–75.
67. Hwang DY, Silva GS, Furie KL, et al. Comparative sensitivity of computed tomography vs. magnetic resonance imaging for detecting acute posterior fossa infarct. J Emerg Med 2012;42(5):559–65.
68. Jorns-Häderli M, Straumann D, Palla A. Accuracy of the bedside head impulse test in detecting vestibular hypofunction. J Neurol Neurosurg Psychiatry 2007; 78(10):1113–8.
69. Ohle R, Montpellier R-A, Marchadier V, et al. Can emergency physicians accurately rule out a central cause of vertigo using the HINTS examination? A systematic review and meta-analysis. Acad Emerg Med 2020;27(9):887–96.

70. Saberi A, Pourshafie SH, Kazemnejad-Leili E, et al. Ondansetron or promethazine: which one is better for the treatment of acute peripheral vertigo? Am J Otolaryngol 2019;40(1):10–5.

71. Shafipour L, Khatir IG, Shafipour V, et al. Intravenous promethazine versus diazepam for treatment of peripheral vertigo in emergency department. J Mazandaran Univ Med Sci 2017;27(149):88–98.

72. Amini A, Heidari K, Asadollahi S, et al. Intravenous promethazine versus lorazepam for the treatment of peripheral vertigo in the emergency department: a double blind, randomized clinical trial of efficacy and safety. J Vestib Res Equilib Orientat 2014;24(1):39–47.

73. Walker MF. Treatment of vestibular neuritis. Curr Treat Options Neurol 2009; 11(1):41–5.

74. Hall CD, Herdman SJ, Whitney SL, et al. Vestibular rehabilitation for peripheral vestibular hypofunction: an evidence-based clinical practice guideline: From the American Physical Therapy Association Neurology Section. J Neurol Phys Ther JNPT 2016;40(2):124–55.

75. Teggi R, Caldirola D, Fabiano B, et al. Rehabilitation after acute vestibular disorders. J Laryngol Otol 2009;123(4):397–402.

76. Strupp M, Zingler VC, Arbusow V, et al. Methylprednisolone, valacyclovir, or the combination for vestibular neuritis. N Engl J Med 2004;351(4):354–61.

77. Fishman JM, Burgess C, Waddell A. Corticosteroids for the treatment of idiopathic acute vestibular dysfunction (vestibular neuritis). Cochrane Database Syst Rev 2011;5:CD008607.

78. Goudakos JK, Markou KD, Franco-Vidal V, et al. Corticosteroids in the treatment of vestibular neuritis: a systematic review and meta-analysis. Otol Neurotol 2010; 31(2):183–9.

79. Wegner I, van Benthem PPG, Aarts MCJ, et al. Insufficient evidence for the effect of corticosteroid treatment on recovery of vestibular neuritis. Otolaryngol Head Neck Surg 2012;147(5):826–31.

80. Goudakos JK, Markou KD, Psillas G, et al. Corticosteroids and Vestibular Exercises in Vestibular Neuritis: Single-blind Randomized Clinical Trial. JAMA Otolaryngol Neck Surg 2014;140(5):434.

81. Yoo MH, Yang CJ, Kim SA, et al. Efficacy of steroid therapy based on symptomatic and functional improvement in patients with vestibular neuritis: a prospective randomized controlled trial. Eur Arch Otorhinolaryngol 2017;274(6):2443–51.

82. Sjögren J, Magnusson M, Tjernström F, et al. Steroids for acute vestibular neuronitis—the earlier the treatment, the better the outcome? Otol Neurotol 2019;40(3): 372–4.

83. Arroll B, Goodyear-Smith F, Crengle S, et al. Validation of PHQ-2 and PHQ-9 to screen for major depression in the primary care population. Ann Fam Med 2010;8(4):348.

84. Sapra A, Bhandari P, Sharma S, et al. Using generalized anxiety disorder-2 (GAD-2) and GAD-7 in a primary care setting. Cureus 2020;12(5):e8224.

85. Schmid G, Henningsen P, Dieterich M, et al. Psychotherapy in dizziness: a systematic review. J Neurol Neurosurg Psychiatry 2011;82(6):601–6.

86. Staab JP, Eckhardt-Henn A, Horii A, et al. Diagnostic criteria for persistent postural-perceptual dizziness (PPPD): consensus document of the committee for the Classification of Vestibular Disorders of the Bárány Society. J Vestib Res Equilib Orientat 2017;27(4):191–208.

Chronic Central Vestibulopathies for the Otolaryngologist

Bibhuti Mishra, MD[a,b,*], Neeraj Singh, MD[a,c]

KEYWORDS

- Central vestibulopathy • Vestibular migraine • Vertigo • Nystagmus • Balance

KEY POINTS

- Central and peripheral vestibulopathies can have similar presenting symptoms and signs but can be distinguished with careful neurologic examination and appropriate testing.
- Central vestibulopathies can include vestibular migraines, which can result from abnormal neuroanatomy or neuronal signaling.
- The etiologies for some central vestibulopathies still are not understood fully.

INTRODUCTION

Central vestibulopathies refer to disorders of the central nervous system that can contribute to symptoms and signs affecting balance, including dizziness, vertigo, and nystagmus. The components of the central nervous system that typically are affected in central vestibulopathies include the rostral cerebellum and brainstem, in particular the medulla oblongata. This is in contrast to peripheral vestibulopathies, in which problems affecting balance originate from outside the central nervous system, most often the inner ear.

A typical case example of a central nervous system lesion that leads to dizziness is that of a middle-aged man presenting to an emergency department for persistent vertigo lasting a few days, independent of position, and not responding to meclizine, with findings of horizontal nystagmus and dysmetria with left finger-to-nose test. In this case, a subacute cerebellar stroke can be diagnosed with neuroimaging. Features telling of a central disorder of the vestibular system are persistence of symptoms, independence of position, and poor response to medication trials meant for peripheral lesions.

[a] LIJ Forest Hills Hospital, Northwell Health, NY 11375, USA; [b] George Washington University, Washington, DC, USA; [c] Zucker School of Medicine at Hofstra/Northwell
* Corresponding author.
E-mail address: BMishra1@northwell.edu

Otolaryngol Clin N Am 54 (2021) 939–948
https://doi.org/10.1016/j.otc.2021.06.004
0030-6665/21/© 2021 Elsevier Inc. All rights reserved.

DEFINITION

Dizziness is a common reason for visiting an acute care center (4% of emergency room visits). Its causes and treatments vary, depending on the kind of dizziness and the different etiologies of each kind of dizziness.[1] Chronic central vestibulopathies can be divided into those arising from vestibular migraine and those with other causes of pathology. Diagnosis of vestibular migraine in the dizzy patient only recently has been formalized.[2] For further information on the specifics of diagnosis of vestibular migraine, see Ashley Zaleski-King and Ashkan Monfared's article, "Vestibular Migraine and its Comorbidities," in this issue.

NEUROPHYSIOLOGY

Understanding of the anatomy of the systems that produce a sensation of dizziness and pain in migraine has improved significantly with the availability of functional magnetic resonance imaging (fMRI)-based brain imaging to investigate brain networks during attacks of migraine and animal models of migraine.

Comparative anatomy of primate brain, electrical stimulation of the human brain, or lesion localization in humans points to widely distributed cortical areas that are involved in balance and movement perception. Particular concentrations of cortical vestibular representations are found in the parietal operculum and posterior and posterior insula and the retroinsular cortex. Anterior cingulate cortex, hippocampus, and parahippocampus also show significant connections with the vestibular network.[3]

Using brain oxygen level–dependent signals in resting state brain fMRI of healthy controls and in bilateral vestibulopathy, a reciprocal inhibitory connection between the visual and vestibular cortex is observed. Such a reciprocal inhibitory connection between the vestibular cortex and other sensory modalities might be important for the perception of equilibrium. For example, loss of coherence between visual and vestibular inputs produces changes in signals in these areas and correlates with symptoms of oscillopsia or vertigo.[4]

The importance of the corpus callosum in this network is to connect and balance the information arriving in the vestibular cortex of one hemisphere with the opposite side and between bilateral visual hemispheric systems for the cognitive establishment of the body's reference to a 3-dimensional surrounding spatial frame.

Most afferent connections from the vestibular nuclei transit through the medial longitudinal fasciculus and relay in the thalamus. There also is an ipsilateral direct connection from the vestibular nucleus to the posterior insular cortex. There are 2 pathways that relay in the posterolateral thalamic nuclei or in the midline (centromedian, intralaminar) nuclei. The posterolateral vestibular thalamocortical relay is believed to be involved in maintenance of a sense of position during joint active and passive motion. A right-sided vestibular dominance in right-handed individuals and a similar left-sided vestibular dominance is expected in left-handed individuals are explained by the balance of connectivity measures.[5,6] The vestibular dominance is opposite to handedness, which refers to somatosensory and motor dominance. This difference in anatomy is proposed as the reason right hemispheric neglect is more prominent for the hemispace and left hemispherical neglect more categorical.

Vestibular Migraine: Mechanisms Underlying the Sensation of Dizziness, Pain, and Anxiety

One of the characteristics of the physiology of the vestibular system in the interictal period of those who suffer migraine is a heightened vestibular ocular reflex threshold and vestibular motion perceptual threshold for self-motion. This is heightened further by whole-field motion perception and is a unique interictal feature of vestibular migraine.[7] Descending modulatory pathways from the periaqueductal gray, rostral ventromedial nuclei hypothalamus may be the process by which increased network gain is produced.

Magnetic resonance images (MRIs) demonstrate that several distinct parts of the cortex—bilateral central sulcus, left medial frontal, left precuneus, and right occipital–temporal gyrus—are thinner in those who suffered migraine (138 subjects) compared with healthy controls (115 subjects) after adjustment for age gender and type of MRI. Duration of migraine and severity as well as presence or absence of aura appeared to make a difference in the location and degree of thinning. More recent fMRI study of regions of interest or resting state fMRI connectivity as well as diffusion tensor imaging and tractography during migraine attacks and in the interictal period have amassed a significant amount of human data that appear to corroborate data from studies of mice bearing mutated genes that cause human familial hemiplegic migraine.[8,9]

Many studies have confirmed connections between paraventricular and posterior hypothalamic nuclei and brainstem centers, such as the periaqueductal gray, locus coeruleus, and raphe nuclei, as well as the activation of these areas in animal and fMRI studies by pain in spontaneous or induced pain in dural structures.[10]

Interplay Between Migraine Headache and the Vestibular System

Vestibular afferents from the vestibular nuclei signal posterior and ventral thalamic nuclei via the glutamate neurotransmitter system as well as the intralaminar nuclei, mediated by γ-aminobutyric acid (GABA). Trigeminocervical somatic sensory afferents synapse in the same regions of the thalamus.

Thalamic circuits increase or decrease electrical activity and gain in the sensory relay cells of the thalamus resulting in reduced habituation of vestibular signals. This increases a perception of imbalance or vertigo. The process is bidirectional, so that the loss of dampening or loss of habituation could occur in the trigeminovascular reflex system, resulting in headache pain. Direct and indirect reciprocal collaterals of both systems to the median raphe (serotonergic/nonserotonergic), locus coeruleus (noradrenergic), brachium pontis nuclei (cholinergic and serotonergic), hypothalamus (dopaminergic), amygdala (dopaminergic, serotonergic, and GABA), pedunculopontine nuclei (cholinergic), mediate inattention, anxiety, stress response, and autonomic symptoms (sympathetic and parasympathetic)[11]

Long-term potentiation and recruitment of efferents that modulate pain and autonomic and vestibular input (periaqueductal gray, rostral ventromedial nuclei, and superior salivatory nucleus) may be the mechanisms of sustained activation of the network gain that have been described in animal models.[10] A similar mechanism could be relevant in humans.

Other Disorders of Tilt and Motion

Even in the absence of migraine, central vestibulopathies can affect sensory perception of position, leading to difficulty with balance. The mechanism by which a sensory awareness of position and motion occurs is incompletely understood. Head angular velocity is coded in the lower brainstem, which is integrated with the head direction coding networks in the rostral brainstem and a place system that creates a sensation of location in the 3-dimensional plane distributed in the anterior thalamus and hippocampus. The center that integrates these velocity inputs with visual clues to create a sense of stable motion is not yet known. The posterior hypothalamus and the cerebellum are contenders for this role of the creator of sensation of orientation and position in space during motion. Currently, the areas of the cortex that respond to vestibular stimulation also show activity in response to visual and proprioceptive sensation. The medial superior temporal gyrus is more responsive to visual motion judged by responses to motion in darkness. The vestibular insular cortex is more responsive to vestibular stimulation in light and darkness.

Table 1 summarizes other central vestibulopathies that can mimic vestibular migraine and thus are of interest to the otolaryngologist.

Table 1
Central vestibulopathies that mimic vestibular migraine

Vestibular Injury	Characteristic Symptoms	Mechanism	Reference
Stroke	Lateropulsion, pusher syndrome	Ischemic stroke of thalamus insular cortex: more commonly right hemispheric	Perennou et al,[12] 2008
Stroke	Ipsilateral hemiataxia, nausea vomiting, vertigo and ipsilateral (partial) Horner syndrome	Lateral medullary infarction due to vertebral artery or posterior inferior cerebellar artery thrombosis or dissection	Dorobisz et al,[13] 2020
Vertebral artery or carotid artery stenosis	Dizziness, balance disorder, nystagmus. Abnormal VEMP and VNG	Ischemia of vestibular and trigeminal nuclei and their connections	Venhovens et al,[14] 2016
Concussive trauma	Headache, benign paroxysmal positional vertigo, nystagmus, abnormalities on tandem gait, vestibular agnosia	Physical disruption of vestibular pathways and connections of cerebellum to the vestibular nucleus. Altered resting state network	Marcus et al,[15] 2019
Anxiety and depression	Dizziness, functional decline, subjective handicaps without objective findings	Altered connectivity with vestibular nuclei, cerebellum, thalamus during interictal state and during an attack	Balaban,[16] 2002

Using voxel-wise lesion behavior mapping in subjects who suffered ischemic strokes of the thalamus, the relationship of thalamic nuclei to contraversive or ipsiversive tilts of the subjective visual vertical (SVV) axis have been localized to different nuclei of the thalamus. Contraversive tilts occur with lesions of the superomedial and posterior thalamus, whereas ipsiversive tilts occur with lesions of the inferior perifascicular nuclei, the red nucleus, nuclei near the brachium conjunctivum, and related thalamic nuclei.[5]

Cerebral hemispheric infarctions limited to the parietoinsular vestibular cortex do not necessarily cause vestibular symptoms but unilateral, more commonly right hemispheric, lesions restricted to the areas of the vestibular cortical network may cause vertigo or disorder of coordination with or without nausea and vomiting.[17]

CENTRAL VESTIBULAR DISORDERS

Multiple well-defined neurologic disorders cause dizziness and vertigo, such as stroke, trauma, concussion, neoplasms, and demyelinating diseases, such as multiple sclerosis. Conditions that can cause skew deviation with or without headache include right superior cerebellar arteriovenous malformations,[25] lithium dose increase,[26] and late-onset cerebellar ataxia and sensory neuronopathy with vestibular areflexia syndrome.[27] Specific central vestibulopathies that may be of particular interest to otolaryngologists are described.

Epilepsy

Vertigo is an uncommon symptom of epilepsy and usually occurs in association with other sensory symptoms, most commonly auditory hallucinations and changes in vision or olfaction.[28] Furthermore, among those who have epilepsy and vertigo, only 4% to 5% appear to develop vertigo during an epileptic seizure.[29,30] In these cases, patients experience a room-spinning sensation that typically lasts for under 30 seconds at a time, without loss of consciousness[31] Even more rarely, vertigo symptoms that persist or worsen appear to be a manifestation of nonconvulsive focal epilepsy emanating from the frontal or temporal region.[32] In these cases, an electroencephalogram (EEG) is necessary to help distinguish between an epileptic seizure and a cerebrovascular syndrome, such as a posterior circulation stroke or vertebrobasilar insufficiency. Unfortunately, the EEG is equivocal in peripheral and central vestibular disorders.

Central Nervous System Infections

Rhombencephalitis (caused by Listeria monocytogenes), cysticercosis, and cerebellar abscesses are well known causes of headache and vertigo. Recently, severe acute respiratory syndrome coronavirus 2, or COVID-19, has resulted in an increase in the prevalence and incidence of headache, vertigo, and balance disorders. Both acute infection and a virus-negative postinfection phase are periods of risk for these symptoms.

Neurodegenerative Disorders

Parkinson disease (PD) and related disorders, including Lewy body disorder, progressive supranuclear palsy (PSP), and multisystem atrophy, have in common an elevated risk of falls, as does Alzheimer disease. Although being dizzy is a common complaint, most patients do not endorse vertigo but do admit to a disorder of balance and complain of unsteadiness. Vestibular abnormalities are confirmed in these individuals by tests, such as vestibular evoked myogenic potentials (VEMPs) and VNG.[33] VEMP abnormality reportedly has a high sensitivity for predicting those who fall in this group.[34]

PSP can present with loss of balance while walking, often in association with slow or restricted eye movements and poor control over eyelid movements. Increased sway on posturography correlates with reduced cerebral glucose metabolism in the thalamus and caudate nucleus, as visualized by PET, consistent with loss of neurons in these areas. In PSP, as opposed to PD, the earliest loss of neurons occurs in the pedunculopontine nucleus of the mesencephalon and the intralaminar nuclei of the thalamus.[35] These are cholinergic projections to the thalamus, correlating with reduced cholinergic activity in the thalamus of patients with PSP in contrast to PD, which is marked by reduced dopaminergic activity in the caudate.

Concussion

Vestibular agnosia is a term coined to describe the loss of subjective sensation of a vestibular disorder in the presence of objective vestibulopathy and is common after mild to severe concussive trauma. Tests become important in choosing those who need specialized therapy. An unsupervised machine learning tool has been used to select two clusters of subjects: one that had chronic vestibular disorders and another that did not. Two tests that were most important in this exercise were the maximum slow-phase velocity on the caloric test and the dynamic visual acuity test.[36]

Posttraumatic Stress Disorder

Dizziness and balance disorder are major causes of disability in posttraumatic stress disorder (PTSD). Resting state fMRI demonstrates differences between PTSD and controls in the following aspects: (1) reduced vestibular connectivity with the left supramarginal gyrus in the PTSD group, (2) negative correlation between symptom severity and functional connectivity with dorsolateral prefrontal cortex and the supramarginal gyrus, and (3) loss of connectivity with the right parietal insular cortex.[37] The interplay between depression, anxiety, and other psychological disorders and symptoms of vertigo and dizziness is described elsewhere in this edition.

Mal de Débarquement

Mal de débarquement is a vestibular disorder that involves a perception of a rocking or swaying motion, relieved by movement and worsened when standing or lying still. This can result in gait imbalance and can be associated with fatigue or changes in mood. The etiology of this disorder and whether it is central or peripheral in nature are uncertain.

INVESTIGATIONS

When a patient presents with symptoms and signs of vestibulopathy, certain investigations can be helpful in distinguishing between central and peripheral etiologies.

Nystagmography

Nystagmus is one of the most frequent and important physical abnormalities associated with vertigo and dizziness. In a recent large study, saccadic smooth pursuit was the most common but least specific type of oculomotor disorder in diseases of the cerebellum. Central fixation nystagmus is seen in a quarter of subjects and gaze-induced nystagmus, rebound nystagmus, or head shaking nystagmus also in 80% of subjects with cerebellar disease.[18]

Nystagmus, noncomitant gaze deficits, convergence deficits, and occasional skew deviation are correlates of vertigo and dizziness, indicating brainstem dysfunction, and may be observed better with Fresnel lenses or by videonystagmography (VNG).

Posturography and Gait Analysis

When the nature of dizziness is unclear, posturography and gait analysis may highlight cerebellar ataxia or an extrapyramidal disorder of reflex correction of posture.

Algorithms

Physical examination in the emergency room is focused on distinguishing between 2 major causes of acute vestibular syndrome: a peripheral vestibular disorder or a central/brainstem or cerebellar disorder. Concise algorithms have been found useful for this purpose. For example, use of the head impulse test (abnormal in peripheral disorder and normal in central disorder), spontaneous nystagmus (either primary position or gaze-induced), and presence of skew deviation (HINTS) score, combined with ABCD2 score of risk for stroke, is successful in predicting a vestibular stroke with highest sensitivity and specificity, particularly if performed using video-oculography.[19]

NEUROPHARMACOLOGY
Implications for Pharmacotherapy in Vestibular Migraine

A distinct difference in neurophysiology and neuropharmacology as well as in chronicity of the underlying disease drives the difference in the choice of preventive pharmacologic treatment of vestibular migraine in comparison to other types of migraine. For example, acute treatment using triptans, which are serotonin receptor (5-HT1B and 5-HT1D) agonists, have their most useful clinical effect by reversing the parasympathetic outflow that causes vasodilatation of meningeal blood vessels—one of the neurophysiologic causes of headache in migraine. They may have no effect or worsen migraine aura, including vertigo of vestibular migraine. Similarly, calcitonin gene–related peptide (CGRP) antagonists have been evaluated by their effect on headache, not aura of migraine. Their effect on the nucleus of the tractus solitaries, however, could be useful for visceral symptoms of nausea and vomiting.[20]

Benzodiazepines and primidone
Because of multiple sites of actions by modulation of GABA function, benzodiazepines and primidone benzodiazepines and primidone potentially are effective in the treatment of dizziness associated with cerebellar disorders.

Propranolol
β-Adrenergic antagonists, particularly propranolol (80–240 mg/d) and metoprolol (50–200 mg/d), not only block the β-receptors in the thalamus but also reduce the discharge of noradrenergic neurons of the locus coeruleus and periaqueductal gray and reduce the sensitization of the trigeminovascular system by action on the rostral ventromedial medulla in a mouse model.[21] Inhibition of nitric oxide synthase and antagonism of 5-HT are other experimentally confirmed mechanisms of action of propranolol.

Antiepileptics
Not all antiepileptics are effective in preventive treatment of migraine. Only topiramate and valproic acid are effective, both of which inhibit sodium ion channels and calcium channels and both modulate GABA/increase GABA concentration.[22,23]

Onabotulinum toxin A
Peripheral action on nociceptive nerve terminal in the meninges and scalp rather than muscle relaxation is the current proposed mechanism of action of botulinum toxin A in treatment of chronic migraine.[24] Onabotulinum toxin A cleaves SNAP-25 to impair vesicular trafficking and release of neurotransmitters between the peripheral nerves. This inhibits those nerve endings that have a heightened state of nociception.

Tricyclic antidepressants

Amitriptyline and nortriptyline have adrenergic depleting actions and anticholinergic activity. These may be expected to act on all levels of the vestibular migraine pathway.

Calcium channel antagonists

Calcium channels are used by excitatory neurotransmitters for neuronal excitation. Calcium channel antagonism is useful in migraine prophylaxis. Verapamil and flunarizine (available in Europe) are 2 that are used. Flunarizine also has dopaminergic antagonism. These may be most useful in modulating thalamocortical activity.

Calcitonin gene–related peptide antagonists

Newer agents against CGRP or its receptor are either small molecular inhibitors or monoclonal antibodies. The monoclonal antibodies presumably are effective on the structures outside the blood-brain barrier in the scalp, meningeal and blood vessels, and cranial/peripheral nerves. Small molecular inhibitors might transfer across the blood-brain barrier to act on the brain parenchyma but have been tested only against pain, not dizziness and vertigo.

Antipsychotics

Dopamine D2 receptor antagonism is the likely primary mechanism of action of quetiapine, olanzapine, and prochlorperazine. But serotonergic and anticholinergic effects also might be important. Wherever the parabrachial, amygdaloid, hippocampal, and hypothalamic network is active with anxiety and sensitivity to stress, this group of medications could be useful.[17]

SUMMARY

Advances in imaging and animal models of migraine have led to an explosion of information relevant to central vestibular migraine. The lack of pharmacologic treatments based on clinical trials hinders choice of medications; standard medications used to treat migraine may be applied to help relieve the symptoms of vestibular migraine.

Most subjects with vestibular disorders seek a specialist after unsuccessful treatments for weeks and months. Chronicity is associated with anxiety, sensitivity to psychological stress, and daily symptoms with loss of employment. The combination of an anticonvulsant and one of the following medication categories: calcium channel antagonist, B-adrenergic antagonist, tricyclic antidepressant, or primidone, shows promise and deserves to be investigated further.

CLINICS CARE POINTS

- Central vestibulopathies include vestibular migraine and certain neurodegenerative disorders and sometimes can feature abnormal brain anatomy.
- Central vestibulopathies can be distinguished from peripheral vestibulopathies by persistence of symptoms and independence from position.
- Central vestibulopathies can be distinguished from peripheral vestibulopathies with certain testing, such as nystagmography or posturography.
- The etiologies of central vestibulopathies are not all understood fully, and some medications indicated for other conditions (eg, migraines) may be used to manage vestibular symptoms.

DISCLOSURE

The authors have no financial conflicts of interest or funding sources to declare.

BIBLIOGRAPHY

1. Zwergal A, Mohwald K, Dieterich M. Vertigo and dizziness in the emergency room. Curr Opin Neurol 2020;33(1):117–25.
2. Lempert T, Olesen J, Furman J, et al. Vestibular migraine: diagnostic criteria. J Vestib Res 2012;22(4):167–72.
3. Balaban CD, Black RD, Silberstein SD. Vestibular neuroscience for the headache specialist. Headache 2019;59(7):1109–27.
4. Helmchen C, Machner B, Rother M, et al. Effects of galvanic vestibular stimulation on resting state brain activity in patients with bilateral vestibulopathy. Hum Brain Mapp 2020;41(9):2527–47.
5. Baier B, Conrad J, Stephan T, et al. Vestibular thalamus: two distinct graviceptive pathways. Neurology 2016;86(2):134–40.
6. Brandt T, Dieterich M. Thalamocortical network: a core structure for integrative multimodal vestibular functions. Curr Opin Neurol 2019;32(1):154–64.
7. Bednarczuk NF, Bonsu A, Ortega MC, et al. Abnormal visuo-vestibular interactions in vestibular migraine: a cross sectional study. Brain 2019;142(3):606–16.
8. Magon S, May A, Stankewitz A, et al. Cortical abnormalities in episodic migraine: a multi-center 3T MRI study. Cephalalgia 2019;39(5):665–73.
9. Amin FM, Hougaard A, Magon S, et al. Altered thalamic connectivity during spontaneous attacks of migraine without aura: a resting-state fMRI study. Cephalalgia 2018;38(7):1237–44.
10. Brennan KC, Pietrobon D. A systems neuroscience approach to migraine. Neuron 2018;97(5):1004–21.
11. Goadsby PJ, Holland PR. An update: pathophysiology of migraine. Neurol Clin 2019;37(4):651–71.
12. Perrenou DA, Mazibrada G, Chauvineau V. Lateropulsion, pushing and verticality perception in hemisphere stroke: a causal relationship? Brain 2008;131(Pt 9):2401–13.
13. Dorobisz K, Dorobisz T, Zatonski T. The assessment of the balance system in cranial artery stenosis. Brain Behav 2020;10(9):e01695.
14. Venhovens J, Meulstee J, Bloem BR, et al. Neurovestibular analysis and falls in Parkinson's disease and atypical parkinsonism. Eur J Neurosci 2016;43(12):1636–46.
15. Marcus HJ, Paine H, Sargeant M, et al. Vestibular dysfunction in acute traumatic brain injury. J Neurol 2019;266(10):2430–3.
16. Balaban CD. Neural substrates linking balance control and anxiety. Physiol Behav 2002;77(4–5):469–75.
17. Eguchi S, Hirose G, Miaki M. Vestibular symptoms in acute hemispheric strokes. J Neurol 2019;266(8):1852–8.
18. Lee SH, Kim JS. Acute diagnosis and management of stroke presenting dizziness or vertigo. Neurol Clin 2015;33(3):687–98, xi.
19. Ahmadi SA, Vivar G, Navab N, et al. Modern machine-learning can support diagnostic differentiation of central and peripheral acute vestibular disorders. J Neurol 2020;267(Suppl 1):143–52.
20. Byun YJ, Levy DA, Nguyen SA, et al. Treatment of vestibular migraine: a systematic review and meta-analysis. Laryngoscope 2020;131(1):186–94.

21. Boyer N, Signoret-Genest J, Artola A, et al. Propranolol treatment prevents chronic central sensitization induced by repeated dural stimulation. Pain 2017; 158(10):2025–34.
22. Naegel S, Obermann M. Topiramate in the prevention and treatment of migraine: efficacy, safety and patient preference. Neuropsychiatr Dis Treat 2010;6:17–28.
23. Cutrer FM, Limmroth V, Moskowitz MA. Possible mechanisms of valproate in migraine prophylaxis. Cephalalgia 1997;17(2):93–100.
24. Burstein R, Zhang XC, Levy D, et al. Selective inhibition of meningeal nociceptors by botulinum neurotoxin type A: therapeutic implications for migraine and other pains. Cephalalgia 2014;34(11):853–69.
25. Argaet EC, Young AS, Bradshaw AP, et al. Cerebellar arteriovenous malformation presenting with recurrent positional vertigo. J Neurol 2019;266(1):247–9.
26. Hong H, Lyu IJ. A case of skew deviation and downbeat Nystagmus induced by Lithium. BMC Ophthalmol 2019;19(1):257.
27. Cortese A, Simone R, Sullivan R, et al. Biallelic expansion of an intronic repeat in RFC1 is a common cause of late-onset ataxia. Nat Genet 2019;51(4): 649–58.
28. Morano A, Carni M, Casciato S, et al. Ictal EEG/fMRI study of vertiginous seizures. Epilepsy Behav 2017;68:51–6.
29. Winawer MR, Connors R, EPGP Investigators. Evidence for a shared genetic susceptibility to migraine and epilepsy. Epilepsia 2013;54(2):288–95.
30. Winawer MR. Phenotype definition in epilepsy. Epilepsy Behav 2006;8(3): 462–76.
31. Romano F, Bockisch CJ, Schuknecht B, et al. Asymmetry in gaze-holding impairment in acute unilateral ischemic cerebellar lesions critically depends on the involvement of the caudal vermis and the dentate nucleus. Cerebellum 2020. https://doi.org/10.1007/s12311-020-01141-7.
32. Chen YS, Chen TS, Huang CW. Non-convulsive seizure clustering misdiagnosed as vertebrobasilar insufficiency. Heliyon 2020;6(11):e05376.
33. Cronin T, Arshad Q, Seemungal BM. Vestibular deficits in neurodegenerative disorders: balance, dizziness, and spatial disorientation. Front Neurol 2017; 8:538.
34. Venhovens J, Meulstee J, Bloem BR, et al. Neurovestibular dysfunction and falls in parkinson's disease and atypical parkinsonism: a prospective 1 year follow-up study. Front Neurol 2020;11:580285.
35. Birdi S, Rajput AH, Fenton M, et al. Progressive supranuclear palsy diagnosis and confounding features: report on 16 autopsied cases. Mov Disord 2002;17(6): 1255–64.
36. Visscher RMS, Feddermann-Demont N, Romano F, et al. Artificial intelligence for understanding concussion: retrospective cluster analysis on the balance and vestibular diagnostic data of concussion patients. PLoS One 2019;14(4): e0214525.
37. Harricharan S, Nicholson AA, Densmore M, et al. Sensory overload and imbalance: resting-state vestibular connectivity in PTSD and its dissociative subtype. Neuropsychologia 2017;106:169–78.

Vestibular Migraine and Its Comorbidities

Ashley Zaleski-King, AuD, PhD*, Ashkan Monfared, MD

KEYWORDS

- Migraine • Headache • Trigeminovascular • Multisensory • Vestibular dysfunction

KEY POINTS

- Vestibular migraine is a common cause of episodic dizziness, described as spinning, a sensation of moving, rocking, or unsteadiness. Often photophobia, phonophobia, motion intolerance, and sensitivity to pressure changes are also associated with VM.
- Patients with VM typically experience episodic attacks; the vertiginous aspect of VM can precede or occur during or after the headache.
- There is a wide range of peripheral and central audiovestibular sequela associated with VM, and VM may coexist with other causes of dizziness. This heterogeneity suggests that subtypes of the condition may exist.
- There are data to show treatment success with basic trigger avoidance, targeted physical therapy, and various pharmacologic approaches for patients with VM.

BACKGROUND

Migraine-associated dizziness, migrainous vertigo, benign recurrent vertigo, migraine-related vestibulopathy, and vestibular migraine (VM) have all been used to describe conditions involving the presence of both migraine and dizziness symptoms.[1–6] Today the term vestibular migraine is most commonly used to describe patients with symptoms associated with vertigo and with migraine. Clinical criteria for patients with both vertigo and migraine were established in 2004 and later validated and revised with the International Headache Society and the Bárány Society committee for the International Classification of Vestibular Disorders (**Table 1**). The International Headache Society described VM as a condition needing further research for full validation.[7]

CLINICAL PRESENTATION

Clinical descriptions of migraine, in particular VM, have evolved significantly over the past decade. Patients with VM commonly describe visual aura, phonophobia

Otolaryngology, GWU Medical Faculty Associates, 2300 M Street Northwest, Washington, DC 20037, USA
* Corresponding author.
E-mail address: asking@mfa.gwu.edu

Otolaryngol Clin N Am 54 (2021) 949–958
https://doi.org/10.1016/j.otc.2021.05.014
oto.theclinics.com
0030-6665/21/© 2021 Elsevier Inc. All rights reserved.

Table 1
International Classification of Headache Disorders, 3rd edition (Beta version) criteria for vestibular migraine

Definite VM	Probable VM
A. At least 5 episodes fulfilling criteria C and D	A. At least 5 episodes with vestibular symptoms of moderate or severe intensity, lasting 5 min to 72 h
B. Current or past history of migraine with or without aura	B. Only B or D of definite vestibular migraine criteria (either migraine history or migraine features during episode)
C. Vestibular symptoms of moderate or severe intensity, lasting 5 min - 72 h	C. Not better accounted for by another ICHD-3 diagnosis or by another vestibular disorder
D. At least 50% of episodes associated with at least one of the following: 1. Headache of unilateral, pulsating, moderate or severe intensity, or aggravated by routine physical activity[a] 2. Photophobia and phonophobia 3. Visual aura	
E. Not better accounted for by another ICHD-3 diagnosis or by another vestibular disorder	

Abbreviation: ICHD, International Classification of Headache Disorders.
[a] Note: To meet D1 criteria to at least 2 of these should apply.

(transient, sound-induced discomfort), and photophobia (visually induced discomfort).[8,9] Up to 40% of patients with VM also describe tinnitus, aural pressure, or fullness in the ears.[1,4,10,11] In addition to these primary features of migraine (with or without aura), patients with VM specifically site vertiginous symptoms. For example, motion sickness and motion sensitivity are common sequelae of VM.[1]

The vertiginous symptoms cited by patients are often nonspecific and analogous to symptoms caused by other forms of dizziness. Common descriptions include spinning, swaying, tilting, floating, fogginess, unsteadiness, rocking, visually induced dizziness, and head-motion-induced dizziness; these symptoms can occur episodically during an attack or during an ictal period, between attacks.[12] Many patients state that the visually induced dizziness and head-motion-induced dizziness aspects of VM are the most problematic and likely causes of impaired participation in work, home, or social activities.[12] Most patients describe more than one symptom during VM attacks with behavioral, sensory, environmental, dietary, and pharmacologic triggers.[12] However, in one recent study, 13% of patients identified with VM had no clear triggers.[12]

The International Classification of Headache Disorders (ICHD) criteria for definite VM necessitate some level of temporal association between vertiginous symptoms and other migrainous symptoms, but as is the case with symptom presentation, the temporal characteristics of VM are variable. Typical migraines last 5 to 60 minutes, whereas vertiginous symptoms can persist for hours.[7,13] Patients with VM may also develop migrainous features in isolation of vertiginous symptoms. Those patients with a history of migraine, but without co-occurrence of migraine and dizziness, may meet the criteria for probable VM.[13,14]

VM can affect individuals throughout the life span. Age of onset is estimated to be between 8 and 50 years, with median age of onset in the third and fourth decades.[5] However, a similar condition may present in children as well. Benign paroxysmal vertigo of childhood has been interpreted as an early expression of migraine, affecting up to 3% of children aged 6 to 12 years.[15,16] Migraine may precede vertigo for many years. The estimated mean lag time between the 2 conditions is about 8 years[17] and may be timed with hormonal changes in women during menopause.[18]

PREVALENCE/INCIDENCE

Migraine and vertigo are 2 prevalent conditions affecting individuals across the life span.[9] It is estimated that approximately 15% of the general population experiences migraines.[19] Up to 15% of visits in general health care settings are due to dizziness concerns.[20] Some argue that migraine is the most common neurologic cause of vertigo,[21,22] with estimated prevalence between 1% and 3% of the adult population.[22] Even still, because symptom presentation overlaps with other causes of dizziness, and in the setting of normal neurologic and neuroimaging data, VM is likely underdiagnosed.[23]

Vertigo is 2 to 3 times more common in patients with migraine when compared with the general population, which is estimated to range from 30% to 50%.[5,6] Of those patients with vertiginous symptoms and migraines, there is likely some proportion that do not meet the diagnostic criteria for other vestibular disorders and are therefore categorized with VM. In sum, the odds of overlap in presentation seem likely just based on the high prevalence of both conditions, the associated symptoms, and lack of diagnostic tools to differentiate the 2 conditions.[14] Even so, it is important to consider the empirical data suggesting a physiologic link beyond symptom coincidence.

PATHOPHYSIOLOGY

Migraine has been classically understood as a headache disorder, triggered by changes in dilation of blood vessels and impaired blood flow. Today, migraine is thought of as a more systemic condition, reflecting more widespread hypersensitivity among central nervous system neurons. It is known that there is overlap between vestibular pathways and brainstem regions that influence sympathetic and parasympathetic regions,[24] which may help explain the anxiety and panic associated with both migraine and dizziness.[24,25] Several theories have been suggested to describe VM pathogenesis, focused on central activation of the vestibular system via the trigeminovascular system, temporoparietal cortical areas related to multisensory processing, and genetic factors.[14]

The trigeminovascular theory of VM emphasizes the activation and sensitization of trigeminal sensory afferent neurons, which stimulate cranial tissues.[26,27] This vasodilation and inflammation is thought to result in pain or "central sensitization" and includes some of the same receptors involved in vestibular system activation (eg, calcitonin gene-related peptide and serotonin).[28–33] Direct central activation of vestibular nuclei by the trigeminovascular system may be a cause of VM.[34] The trigeminal nerve provides afferent input to the contralateral thalamus, which projects to the temporal, parietal, insular, and cingulate cortical regions. It is thought that these reciprocal connections between the trigeminovascular system and the vestibular system generate dizziness symptoms in patients with migraine.[33–35]

Sensory dysregulation is another term used to describe VM pathophysiology. This concept emphasizes the role of multisensory integration in processing and modulating incoming stimuli to derive perception of the environment. Multisensory convergence zones exist within the superior colliculus, basal ganglia, premotor cortex, posterior parietal cortex, inferior prefrontal cortex, and posterior superior temporal sulcus.[35] It is thought that changes within these convergence zones occur in patients with VM, evidenced by comodulation and simultaneous presence and intensity of several different types of symptoms.[36] Imaging studies have provided evidence of increased activity in the thalamus during vestibular stimulation in patients with VM when compared with healthy controls. Gray matter volume abnormalities in pain and multisensory processing cortical areas have also been associated with the presence of VM.[37–39] These data have been interpreted as strong suggestion of a pathophysiological role of these vestibular regions in VM.[40]

Genetic predisposition to VM has been studied based on the high familial reoccurrence of migraine. Genetic mutations linked to hemiplegic migraine or episodic ataxia are not found in VM.[41,42] Polygenic inheritance of VM has not been well studied and is largely unknown.[43,44]

CLINICAL FINDINGS

Vestibular migraine is a diagnosis made primarily based on clinical history. Findings from vestibular and audiological data are divergent across patients and clinics, which is evidence of the variable impact this condition can have on both the peripheral and central nervous systems.[45,46] Even so, vestibular testing can be valuable in characterizing the degree of vestibular involvement, in ruling out other causes of dizziness, and in perhaps directing more customized approaches to physical therapy rehabilitation.

Audiological manifestations of migraine have been studied in smaller patient cohorts. Most recently, when compared with healthy controls without migraine, women with VM were identified with lower loudness discomfort level and delayed frequency following response latencies.[47] These findings led to the conclusion that hyperacusis and delayed temporal processing may be associated with migraine and involve alterations in subcortical auditory pathways, even during the interictal period. Other studies have documented changes to cochlear outer hair cell function[48] and prolonged auditory brainstem response latencies both in between[49] and during[50] migraine attacks. Together these findings suggest that disruption of central auditory sensory processing may contribute to migrainous symptoms and result in a predisposition for increased sensitivity to sensory stimuli.

Vestibular dysfunction is also documented as sequela of migraine. The literature documenting the effects of migraine on clinical vestibular testing shows heterogeneous dysfunction within the central and peripheral vestibular pathways. The neurologic examination is typically normal for patients with VM during the interictal period; nonspecific, nonlocalizing oculomotor deficits have also been associated with VM. Various studies have measured smooth pursuit deficits in 48% of patients with VM, spontaneous nystagmus in about 10%, and central positional or gaze-evoked nystagmus in about 28% of patients with VM.[1–3,51–53] One study measured spontaneous and positional nystagmus in 70% of patients during acute VM, interpreted as evidence of vestibular origin of VM. This same study also described unsteadiness of stance and gait during the symptomatic period.[45]

VM has also been associated with peripheral vestibular end-organ dysfunction, particularly the otolith organs. When assessed by cervical vestibular evoked myogenic potentials, there are data showing impaired saccular function in patients with VM.[54]

Saccular dysfunction may help differentiate VM from other causes of dizziness over time.[55] Other studies demonstrate that saccular function is similar between migrainers with and without vertigo,[56] and when compared with healthy controls.[57] Other studies have identified increased prevalence of bilateral utricular function, assessed through ocular evoked myogenic potentials,[58,59] although this has also been debated.[60] Caloric testing is rarely helpful in differentiating patients with migraine from those with other causes of vertigo.[12] In summary, a variety of symptoms and overlapping clinical vestibular pathologic conditions have been associated with the migraine diagnosis. Peripheral and central patterns of vestibular dysfunction have been associated with VM. The interaction between migraine and other vestibular disorders can be a challenging scenario for diagnosis and treatment.

TREATMENT

There are no existing guidelines to treat VM.[61,62] Even so, promising data are available to show reduction of frequency and severity of VM symptoms with different types of treatments that are often used to treat classic migraine. The first line of treatment of most patients includes trigger management and nutraceuticals. Although not studied specifically for VMs, magnesium, riboflavin, and coenzyme Q10 have demonstrated efficacy for treatment of migraines.[63–66] Considering their low cost and great safety profile they have been widely used for the treatment of VMs as well. However, data on their true efficacy for VMs are still lacking. Many patients show improvement in symptoms after eliminating specific dietary triggers, including artificial sweeteners, processed meats, chocolate, caffeine, monosodium glutamate, alcohol, and aged cheese.[67]

Common pharmacologic treatments could be divided into broad categories of preventative/maintenance and abortive/rescue agents and are included in **Table 2**.[61,68] Typical migraine abortive treatments for classic migraine have been used to treat VM, but clear evidence supporting this approach is lacking, based on a paucity of prospective randomized controlled studies. This is specially the case for the common abortive/rescue medications used for migraines, such as triptans.[10] A recent meta-analysis attempted to clarify available data suggesting therapeutic advantage for patients with VM and focused on the 3 shared, measurable outcome measures, including reduction in the Dizziness Handicap Inventory (DHI), vertigo frequency, and percentage of patients achieving 50% or more symptom resolution.[61] Of the queried studies, all reported pre-post reduction in DHI regardless of the approach, which included serotonin-norepinephrine reuptake inhibitor, calcium channel blocker (CCB), β-blocker (BB), and antiepileptic drugs (AEDs). In the short term, which was defined as 4 to 12 weeks, the largest improvement in DHI was using BB, and the smallest

Table 2 Pharmacologic agents commonly used for VM	
Drug Class	**Name**
β-Blockers	Propranolol, bisoprolol, metoprolol
Calcium channel blockers	Verapamil, amlodipine, flunarizine, cinnarizine
Antiepileptic drugs	Valproic acid, lamotrigine
Tricyclic antidepressants	Amitriptyline, nortriptyline

Data from Byun YJ, Levy DA, Nguyen SA, Brennan E, Rizk HG. Treatment of Vestibular Migraine: A Systematic Review and Meta-analysis. The Laryngoscope. 2021; 131(1):186-94.

improvement was using CCB. In the short term, when measured by vertigo frequency each month, patients receiving BB showed the largest improvement. Patients receiving only physical therapy showed the smallest improvement in the short term, although one study showed interesting changes between short- and long-term vertigo frequency reduction through physical therapy. Of the studies included that focused on symptom improvement of 50% more, approximately 70% noted improvement. The tricyclic acid treatment approach improved symptoms for 68% of patients, diet modification for 75%, and CCB for 76%. One study compared BB with AED treatment and found a significant difference in symptom reduction (73% vs 25%, respectively).

There are data to show that vestibular rehabilitation can improve reported symptoms and vertigo frequency when assessed through questionnaires.[69] There are no clear studies clarifying which subtype of physical therapy, whether it is gaze stabilization, habituation, or alterations to the velocity storage system, explains improvement in symptoms. Similarly more randomized controlled studies are needed to understand appropriate dosing of physical therapy for patients with VM. Owing to heterogeneity of VM, lack of standardized clinical protocols and reporting, and study selection bias, preferred treatment modality has not been determined. The heterogeneity of VM clinical data and the variability of treatment outcomes suggest that subtypes of the condition may exist.

SUMMARY

VM is one of the most common neurologic causes of vertigo. Symptoms and ICHD criteria are used to diagnose VM as no objective tests, imaging or audiologic, have been shown to reliably diagnose this condition. Central auditory, peripheral, and central vestibular pathway involvement has been associated with VM. This heterogeneous clinical presentation and the variability of treatment outcomes suggests that subtypes of the condition may exist. Theories describing VM pathogenesis focus on central activation of the vestibular system via the trigeminovascular system, temporoparietal cortical areas related to multisensory processing, and genetic factors. Although the interaction between migraine and other vestibular disorders can be a challenging scenario for diagnosis and treatment, there are data to show vestibular rehabilitation, and a variety of pharmacologic agents improve reported symptoms and vertigo frequency.

CLINICS CARE POINTS

- VM is common across the life span, especially in females, and can be identified with clinical history and based on published diagnostic criteria.
- VM pathogenesis has been linked to trigeminovascular system, temporoparietal cortical areas related to multisensory processing, and genetic factors.
- Peripheral and central patterns of vestibular dysfunction have been associated with VM. The interaction between migraine and other vestibular disorders can be a challenging scenario for diagnosis and treatment and may suggest that various subtypes of VM exist.
- Although there are no universal standards for treating VM, there are data to support benefit in dietary modification, pharmacologic intervention, and vestibular rehabilitation for patients with VM.

DISCLOSURE

The authors have nothing to disclose.

REFERENCES

1. Cass SP, Ankerstjerne JK, Yetiser S, et al. Migraine-related vestibulopathy. Ann Otol Rhinol Laryngol 1997;106(3):182–9.
2. Cutrer M, Baloh R. Migraine-associated dizziness. Headache 1992;32(6):300–4.
3. Dieterich M, Brandt T. Episodic vertigo related to migraine (90 cases): vestibular migraine? J Neurol 1999;246(10):883–92.
4. Johnson G. Medical management of migraine-related dizziness and vertigo. Laryngoscope 1998;108(S85):1–28.
5. Neuhauser H, Leopold M, Von Brevern M, et al. The interrelations of migraine, vertigo, and migrainous vertigo. Neurology 2001;56(4):436–41.
6. Oh AK, Lee H, Jen JC, et al. Familial benign recurrent vertigo. American Journal of Medical Genetics 2001;100(4):287–91.
7. Headache Classification Committee of the International Headache Society (IHS). The International Classification of Headache Disorders, 3rd edition. Cephalagia 2018;38:1–211.
8. Neuhauser H. The interrelations of migraine, vertigo, and migrainous vertigo. Neurology 2001;56(4):436–41.
9. Zhang Y, Kong Q, Chen J, et al. International Classification of Headache Disorders 3rd edition beta-based field testing of vestibular migraine in China: Demographic, clinical characteristics, audiometric findings and diagnosis statues. Cephalalgia 2016;36(3):240–8.
10. Neuhauser HK, Radtke A, Von Brevern M, et al. Migrainous vertigo: prevalence and impact on quality of life. Neurology 2006;67(6):1028–33.
11. Kayan A, Hood D. Neuro-otological manifestations of migraine. Brain 1984; 107(4):1123–42.
12. Beh SC, Masrour S, Smith SV, et al. The spectrum of vestibular migraine: clinical features, triggers, and examination findings. Headache 2019;59(5):727–40.
13. Lempert T, Olesen J, Furman J, et al. Vestibular migraine: diagnostic criteria. J Vestib Res 2012;22(4):167–72.
14. Huang T-, Wang S-J, Kheradmand A. Vestibular migraine: an update on current understanding and future directions. Cephalalgia 2020;40(1):107–21.
15. Abu-Arafeh I, Russell G. Paroxysmal vertigo as a migraine equivalent in children: a population-based study. Cephalalgia 1995;15(1):22–5.
16. Teggi R, Colombo B, Albera R. Clinical features, familial history, and migraine precursors in patients with definite vestibular migraine: The VM-Phenotypes Projects. Headache 2018;58(4):534–44.
17. Thakar A, Anjaneyulu C, Deka R. Vertigo syndromes and mechanisms in migraine. J Laryngol Otol 2001;115(10):782.
18. Park JH, Viirre E. Vestibular migraine may be an important cause of dizziness/vertigo in perimenopausal period. Med Hypotheses 2010;75(5):409–14.
19. Stovner LJ, Nichols E, Steiner TJ, et al. Global, regional, and national burden of migraine and tension-type headache, 1990–2016: a systematic analysis for the Global Burden of Disease Study 2016. Lancet Neurol 2018;17(11):954–76.
20. Bösner S, Schwarm S, Grevenrath P, et al. Prevalence, aetiologies and prognosis of the symptom dizziness in primary care–a systematic review. BMC Fam Pract 2018;19(1):1–3.
21. Dieterich M, Obermann M, Celebisoy N. Vestibular migraine: The most frequent entity of episodic vertigo. J Neurol 2016;263:S82–9.
22. Formeister EJ, Rizk HG, Kohn MA, et al. The epidemiology of vestibular migraine: A population-based survey study. Otol Neurotol 2018;39:1037–44.

23. Li V, McArdle H, Trip S. Vestibular migraine. BMJ 2019;366:l4213.
24. Balaban C. Vestibular autonomic regulation (including motion sickness and the mechanism of vomiting). Curr Opin Neurol 1999;12(1):29–33.
25. Balaban CD, Thayer JF. Neurological bases for balance–anxiety links. J Anxiety Disord 2001;15(1–2):53–79.
26. Jasmin L, Burkey A, Card J, et al. Transneuronal labeling of a nociceptive pathway, the spino-(trigemino-) parabrachio-amygdaloid, in the rat. J Neurosci 1997;17(10):3751–65.
27. Pietrobon D, Moskowitz M. Pathophysiology of migraine. Annu Rev Physiol 2013; 75:365–91.
28. Durham P. Calcitonin gene-related peptide (CGRP) and migraine. Headache 2006;46:S3–8.
29. Furman J, Marcus D, Balaban C. Migrainous vertigo: development of a pathogenetic model and structured diagnostic interview. Curr Opin Neurol 2003; 16(1):5–13.
30. Schytz H, Olesen J, Ashina M. The PACAP receptor: a novel target for migraine treatment. Neurotherapeutics 2010;7(2):191–6.
31. Ahn SK, Balaban CD. Distribution of 5-HT1B and 5-HT1D receptors in the inner ear. Brain Res 2010;1346:92–101.
32. Ja-Won K, Balaban C. Serotonin-induced plasma extravasation in the murine inner ear: possible mechanism of migraine-associated inner ear dysfunction. Cephalalgia 2006;26(11):1310–9.
33. Balaban CD, Black R, Silberstein SD. Vestibular neuroscience for the headache specialist. Headache 2019;59(7):1109–27.
34. Akerman S, Holland P, Goadsby P. Diencephalic and brainstem mechanisms in migraine. Nat Rev Neurosci 2011;12(10):570–84.
35. Stein B, Stanford T. Multisensory integration: current issues from the perspective of the single neuron. Nat Rev Neurosci 2008;9(4):255–66.
36. Schwedt T. Multisensory integration in migraine. Curr Opin Neurol 2013; 26(3):248.
37. Russo A, Marcelli V, Esposito F, et al. Abnormal thalamic function in patients with vestibular migraine. Neurology 2014;82(23):2120–6.
38. Messina R, Rocca MA, Colombo B, et al. Structural brain abnormalities in patients with vestibular migraine. J Neurol 2017;264(2):295–303.
39. Goadsby PJ, Holland PR, Martins-Oliveira M, et al. Pathophysiology of migraine: a disorder of sensory processing. Physiol Rev 2017;8:553–622.
40. Zhe X, Gao J, Chen L, et al. Altered structure of the vestibular cortex in patients with vestibular migraine. Brain Behav 2020;10(4):e01572.
41. Kim JS, Yue Q, Jen JC, et al. Familial migraine with vertigo: no mutations found in CACNA1A. Am J Med Genet 1998;79(2):148–51.
42. Von Brevern M, Ta N, Shankar A, et al. Migrainous vertigo: mutation analysis of the candidate genes CACNA1A, ATP1A2, SCN1A, and CACNB4. Headache 2006;46(7):1136–41.
43. Lee H, Jen JC, Cha YH, et al. Phenotypic and genetic analysis of a large family with migraine-associated vertigo. Headache 2008;48(10):1460–7.
44. Bahmad F Jr, DePalma SR, Merchant SN, et al. Locus for familial migrainous vertigo disease maps to chromosome 5q35. Ann Otol Rhinol Laryngol 2009;118(9): 670–6.
45. Von Brevern M, Zeise D, Neuhauser H, et al. Acute migrainous vertigo: clinical and oculographic findings. Brain 2005;128(2):365–74.

46. Casani AP, Sellari-Franceschini S, Napolitano A, et al. Otoneurologic dysfunctions in migraine patients with or without vertigo. Otol Neurotol 2009;30(7):961–7.
47. Takeuti AA, Fávero ML, Zaia EH, et al. Auditory brainstem function in women with vestibular migraine: a controlled study. BMC Neurol 2019;19(1):1–7.
48. Hamed SA, Youssef AH, Elattar AM. Assessment of cochlear and auditory pathways in patients with migraine. Am J Otolaryngol 2012;33(4):385–94.
49. Bayazit Y, Yilmaz M, Mumbuc S, et al. Assessment of migraine-related cochleovestibular symptoms. Rev Laryngol Otol Rhinol (Basel) 2001;122(2):85–8.
50. Dash AK, Panda N, Khandelwal G, et al. Migraine and audiovestibular dysfunction: is there a correlation? Am J Otolaryngol 2008;29(5):295–9.
51. Boldingh MI, Ljøstad U, Mygland Å, et al. Comparison of interictal vestibular function in vestibular migraine vs migraine without vertigo. Headache 2013;53(7):1123–33.
52. Celebisoy NE, Gökçay F, Şirin H, et al. Migrainous vertigo: clinical, oculographic and posturographic findings. Cephalalgia 2008;28(1):72–7.
53. von Brevern M. Vestibular migraine: vestibular testing and pathophysiology. Vestibular migraine and related syndromes. Cham (Switzerland): Springer; 2014. p. 83–90.
54. Boldingh MI, Ljøstad U, Mygland Å, et al. Vestibular sensitivity in vestibular migraine: VEMPs and motion sickness susceptibility. Cephalalgia 2011;31(11):1211–9.
55. Dlugaiczyk J, Habs M, Dieterich M. Vestibular evoked myogenic potentials in vestibular migraine and Menière's disease: cVEMPs make the difference. J Neurol 2020;3:1–2.
56. Roceanu A, Allena M, De Pasqua V, et al. Abnormalities of the vestibulo-collic reflex are similar in migraineurs with and without vertigo. Cephalalgia 2008;28(9):988–90.
57. Karatas A, Yüce T, Çebi IT, et al. Evaluation of cervical vestibular-evoked myogenic potential findings in benign paroxysmal positional vertigo. The Journal of International Advanced Otology 2016;12(3):316.
58. Zaleski A, Bogle J, Starling A, et al. Vestibular evoked myogenic potentials in patients with vestibular migraine. Otol Neurotol 2015;36(2):295–302.
59. Makowiec KF, Piker EG, Jacobson GP, et al. Ocular and cervical vestibular evoked myogenic potentials in patients with vestibular migraine. Otol Neurotol 2018;39(7):e561–7.
60. Zuniga MG, Janky KL, Schubert MC, et al. Can vestibular-evoked myogenic potentials help differentiate Ménière disease from vestibular migraine? Otolaryngol Head Neck Surg 2012;146(5):788–96.
61. Byun YJ, Levy DA, Nguyen SA, et al. Treatment of Vestibular Migraine: A Systematic Review and Meta-analysis. Laryngoscope 2021;131(1):186–94.
62. Reploeg MD, Goebel JA. Migraine-associated dizziness: patient characteristics and management options. Otol Neurotol 2002;23(3):364–71.
63. Chiu H-Y, Yeh T-H, Huang Y-C, et al. Effects of intravenous and oral magnesium on reducing migraine: a meta-analysis of randomized controlled trials. Pain Physician 2016;19(1):E97–112.
64. Von Luckner A, Riederer F. Magnesium in migraine prophylaxis—is there an evidence-based rationale? A systematic review. Headache 2018;58(2):199–209.
65. Thompson DF, Saluja HS. Prophylaxis of migraine headaches with riboflavin: a systematic review. J Clin Pharm Ther 2017;42(4):394–403.
66. Slater SK, Nelson TD, Kabbouche MA, et al. A randomized, double-blinded, placebo-controlled, crossover, add-on study of CoEnzyme Q10 in the prevention of pediatric and adolescent migraine. Cephalalgia 2011;31(8):897–905.

67. Mikulec AA, Faraji F, Kinsella LJ. Evaluation of the efficacy of caffeine cessation, nortriptyline, and topiramate therapy in vestibular migraine and complex dizziness of unknown etiology. Am J Otolaryngol 2012;33(1):121–7.

68. Baier B, Winkenwerder E, Dieterich M. Vestibular migraine: effects of prophylactic therapy with various drugs. J Neurol 2009;256(3):436–42.

69. Alghadir A, Shahnawaz A. Effects of vestibular rehabilitation in the management of a vestibular migraine: a review. Front Neurol 2018;9:440.

Progressive and Degenerative Peripheral Vestibular Disorders

Christine Little, BA[a], Jennifer Kelly, DPT[b], Maura K. Cosetti, MD[a,b],*

KEYWORDS

- Meniere's disease • Ototoxicity • Radiation induced vestibulopathy
- Usher syndrome

KEY POINTS

- Peripheral vestibulopathies encompass a heterogenous group of conditions with similar clinical features, making a diagnosis of the underlying etiology difficult.
- Diagnosis often depends on a detailed clinical history with careful attention to the timing and progression of vertigo and associated symptoms.
- Diagnosis may benefit from audiometry, vestibular testing, radiographic imaging, or serologic evaluation.
- Treatment options vary widely between diseases, ranging from observation to medical management or surgical intervention.

 Video content accompanies this article at http://www.pmr.theclinics.com.

MÉNIÈRE'S DISEASE

Introduction

Ménière's disease (MD) is a complex, progressive, chronic peripheral vestibular disorder defined by three cardinal symptoms: episodic vertigo, fluctuating hearing loss, and tinnitus. Although the incidence is rare in the general population, MD is considered the third most common cause of vertigo after benign paroxysmal positional vertigo and vestibular migraine.[1] The incidence of MD has been estimated to be as low as 3.5 per 100,000 individuals and as high as 513 per 100,000 individuals, with a male:female ratio of 1.89:1 suggesting a slight female predominance.[2,3] MD primarily affects

[a] Department of Otolaryngology–Head and Neck Surgery, Icahn School of Medicine at Mount Sinai, 1 Gustave Levy Place, New York, NY 10029, USA; [b] Ear Institute, New York Eye and Ear Infirmary of Mount Sinai, 380 Second Avenue, 9th Floor, New York, NY 10010, USA
* Corresponding author. Department of Otolaryngology-Head and Neck Surgery, Ear Institute of NYEE of Mount Sinai, 380 Second Avenue, 9th Floor, New York, NY 10010.
E-mail address: Maura.Cosetti@mountsinai.org

Otolaryngol Clin N Am 54 (2021) 959–971
https://doi.org/10.1016/j.otc.2021.05.015   oto.theclinics.com
0030-6665/21/© 2021 Elsevier Inc. All rights reserved.

middle-aged adults, with mean onset of age occurring between 40 and 50 years of age.[4]

MD is a multifaceted condition with a variety of proposed etiologies, including morphologic variations in the temporal bone, autoimmune conditions, genetics, and environmental factors. The primary histologic feature underlying MD is endolymphatic hydrops (EH), defined as an increased accumulation of endolymph in the cochlea and vestibular system of the inner ear.[1] EH is thought to occur because of impaired intra-labyrinthine fluid homeostasis, secondary to a wide variety of factors including excessive production or decreased absorption of endolymph, ionic imbalances, and genetic abnormalities.[5]

Clinical Presentation

In addition to episodic vertigo, fluctuating hearing loss, and tinnitus, many patients describe aural fullness, gait or postural instability, and nausea.[6] The hallmark of the disease is the fluctuating nature of symptoms, with remission of symptoms between attacks. Numerous environmental and hormonal factors have been implicated in precipitating MD attacks including stress, sleep deprivation, menstruation, and barometric pressure changes.[1] It is estimated that only 40% of MD patients have the classic symptom triad at initial presentation.[7] Rather, most patients present with vertigo as the initial symptom, with or without aural fullness or tinnitus.[8]

Recurrent, episodic, nonpositional vertigo is the most prevalent and disabling symptom of MD, present in 96.2% of patients.[9] Vertigo attacks typically last between 5 minutes and 4 hours, but can be longer.[10] Data on the natural history of MD show that the intensity and length of vertigo attacks often increase over time.[10] Sensorineural hearing loss (SNHL) and tinnitus accompany vertigo attacks in 77% and 83% of patients, respectively.[11] Hearing loss classically affects the low frequencies, may be mild in the initial stages of the disease, and often improves between attacks.[12] However, over time, repeated attacks of MD result in progressive SNHL that does not return to baseline.[12]

MD is typically unilateral at presentation, with only 11% of patients showing symptoms of bilateral MD at initial diagnosis.[13] The risk of bilateral MD involvement increases with duration of the disease and is estimated as 24%, with an average interval to bilateral conversion of 7.6 years.[13]

Diagnosis

MD is a clinical diagnosis, requiring a detailed history and physical examination. The current diagnostic criteria were developed through a joint partnership between the Bárány Society and several international organizations as part of the International Classification of Vestibular Disorders. The classification has two categories: definite and probable MD.[14] Definite MD requires two or more episodes of vertigo lasting between 20 minutes and 12 hours, low- to medium-frequency SNHL and fluctuating aural symptoms (hearing loss, tinnitus, or fullness). In contrast, probable MD is a broader diagnosis, defined by episodes of vertigo lasting between 20 minutes and 24 hours in conjunction with fluctuating aural symptoms in the affected ear.

Pure tone audiometry

As described previously, SNHL in MD typically affects the lower frequencies (250 and 500 Hz) to a much greater degree (**Fig. 1**). However, over time, SNHL may progress to moderate or severe and affect all frequencies.[15] In contrast, bilateral MD can present with a flat pattern even in the initial stages of disease.[15] Although hearing loss may have a variable configuration, it is a crucial component of MD diagnosis, and

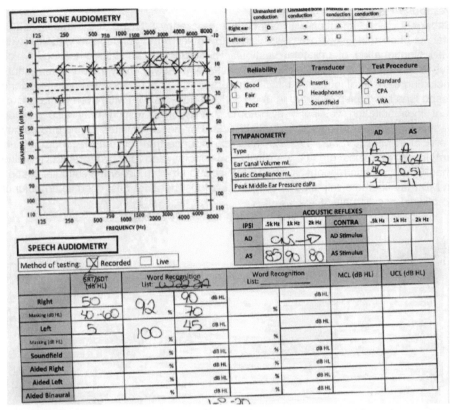

Fig. 1. Comprehensive audiometry including pure-tones, immittance, and word recognition testing in a patient with Ménière's disease of the right ear. The audiogram depicts severe upsloping right sensorineural hearing loss predominately affecting the lower frequencies. VT, vibrotactile.

audiometry should be performed in all patients.[16] In addition to diagnosis, audiometry plays a crucial role in treatment decision-making and understanding disease progression over time.

Electrocochleography

Abnormalities in electrocochleography (ECoG) testing have been reported in MD patients, including an increase in the summating potential (SP), an enlarged SP to action potential (AP) ratio, and a prolonged AP waveform.[1] However, recent studies have shown that ECoG has a low sensitivity and negative predictive value in patients with MD when compared with imaging modalities such as MRI.[17]

MRI

Advances in gadolinium-enhanced MRI over the past decade have provided exciting breakthroughs in MD diagnosis.[18] Primarily used to rule out other pathology that could be mimicking MD, imaging findings of EH have been demonstrated in MD patients on MRI.[19] While not yet widely available, MRI may have important implications for MD diagnosis in the future.

Vestibular testing

Bithermal caloric irrigation with videonystagmography (VNG) is the primary vestibular function test used to assess vestibulo-ocular reflex function in patients with MD. Confirmation of unilateral vestibular hypofunction on caloric testing, which has been reported in up to 75% of patients with MD, may guide intervention, including the use of intratympanic (IT) therapy or surgery.[20] However, normal caloric responses have been reported in up to 50% of patients with MD, even with concurrent incapacitating vestibular symptoms.[21] Vestibular testing may also include vestibular-evoked myogenic potentials (VEMPs), ideally including multifrequency cervical VEMPs (cVEMP) (**Fig. 2**). There is evidence that the cVEMP 1000/500 Hz amplitude ratio has greater sensitivity, specificity, and positive predictive value than ECoG, caloric responses, and VEMP at 500 Hz.[22] In general, vestibular testing in MD may fluctuate with time or symptoms and is therefore best used as an adjunct to clinical assessment.[22]

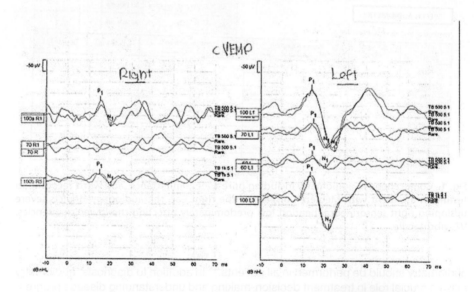

cVEMP	RIGHT	LEFT	ASYMMETRY
Latency of P1 @ 500 Hz	15.33 ms	14 ms	
Latency of N1 @ 500Hz	20.33 ms	25 ms	
500Hz amplitude @ 100 dB	117.8 uV	280.4 uV	*0.41- significant*
Threshold @ 500 Hz	CNT	*60 dB*	
Latency of P1 @ 1k Hz	15 ms	13.33 ms	
Latency of N1 @ 1k Hz	20.33 ms	22.33 ms	
1000 Hz amplitude @ 100 dB	57 uV	236.4 uV	*0.61- significant*
1000/500 Hz Ratio	0.48	0.8	

Fig. 2. Cervical vestibular-evoked myogenic potential testing (cVEMPs) in Ménière's disease (MD). Tracings from multifrequency cVEMPs performed in the right and left ear on a patient with clinical suspicion for MD of the right ear. Data have shown that the cVEMP 1000/500 Hz amplitude ratio has greater sensitivity, specificity, and positive predictive value than electrocochleography (ECoG) or bithermal caloric responses during videonystagmography (VNG). (*Data from* Angeli SI, Goncalves S. Cervical VEMP tuning changes by Meniere's disease stages. Laryngoscope Investig Otolaryngol. 2019;4(5):543-549.)

Treatment

Acute attacks of MD can be treated with vestibular suppressants such as benzodiazepines or dimenhydrinate, as well as antidopaminergic agents for management of nausea and vomiting.[23] A short course of oral corticosteroids may be used during periods of frequent MD episodes to lessen occurrence of attacks.[23] The mainstay of MD treatment aims to reduce attacks of MD and improve quality of life through diet and lifestyle modifications, pharmacotherapy, and surgical intervention.

Dietary and lifestyle modifications

Dietary restrictions are commonly given as first line of treatment for patients with MD and include reduction in salt, caffeine, and alcohol intake. However, there is no high level evidence on which to base these recommendations.[24]

Medications

Oral diuretics, such as hydrochlorothiazide and acetazolamide, are the primary choice for pharmacologic treatment.[1,23] Betahistine (commonly available in countries outside the United States and compounded in the US) has shown possible efficacy, as have other oral medications such as acyclovir and calcium channel blockers.[4] IT steroids (ie, dexamethasone) and gentamicin (low and high dose) may be used as an adjunct or alternative to oral therapy. Steroids are categorized as "hearing sparing" interventions and are titrated to symptom control.[25]

Surgical intervention

Surgical treatment is typically considered after pharmacologic management, and lifestyle modifications have failed to control symptoms. Surgical options for hearing preservation include endolymphatic sac surgery and vestibular neurectomy. Ablative procedures induce destruction of the labyrinth (eg, labyrinthectomy, with expected hearing loss), vestibular nerve, or hair cells to prevent the ear from generating or transmitting the sensation of vertigo.

AUTOIMMUNE VESTIBULOPATHY

Autoimmune-mediated vestibular disorders can be classified into two groups: isolated immune-mediated vestibular disorders and vestibular disorders associated with systemic autoimmune disease.

Immune Mediated Vestibular Disorders

The primary isolated immune-mediated vestibular disorders associated with the development of vertigo include autoimmune inner ear disease (AIED) and MD.

Autoimmune-mediated inner ear disease

Introduction. AIED is a condition of rapidly progressive, bilateral, asymmetric SNHL evolving usually over a period of weeks to months. Generalized imbalance, positional vertigo, and episodic vertigo are estimated to occur in up to 50% of patients with AIED.[26] AIED is a rare disease, estimated to affect between 5 and 30 per 100,000 individuals with an estimated prevalence of 45,000 cases in the United States.[27] The pathogenesis of AIED likely involves both T-cell responses and autoantibody development against specific antigens of the inner ear, leading to inflammation of the cochlear and vestibular system, EHs, neuronal degeneration, and impaired signaling.[28]

Clinical presentation. The clinical presentation of AIED is characterized by fluctuating, bilateral SNHL often associated with tinnitus and/or vertigo, which typically benefits from immunosuppressive therapy. The onset of hearing loss is rapid and typically occurs over a period of 3 to 90 days.[29] Vertigo is present in nearly half of all patients, whereas tinnitus and aural fullness are described in 25% to 50% of patients.[29] Audiometry usually reveals a flat audiogram with multifrequency involvement, although low frequencies may be affected more.[30]

Diagnosis. Currently, there remains no standardized criteria or definitive tests for the diagnosis of AIED. Therefore, diagnosis relies on clinical symptoms, diagnostic workup, and positive response to corticosteroids. Workup should include detailed serologic evaluation to rule out other underlying systemic immune disorders and MRI to rule out retrocochlear pathologies.[30] Clinicians should pay careful attention to the timing and progression of symptoms, specifically the presence of bilateral, asymmetric hearing loss greater than 30 dB developing rapidly over a short interval of 3 to 90 days.

Treatment. The mainstay of treatment for AIED is corticosteroids, although data suggest only 15% to 30% of patients respond to steroid therapy.[31] Immunosuppressive and immunomodulatory drugs can be used as second-line agents, although the benefit of these medications remains controversial.

Vestibular Disorders Associated with Systemic Autoimmune Disease

Numerous systemic autoimmune disorders are associated with the development of vertigo. The onset of vertigo in these conditions is heterogenous and may be a presenting symptom or occur at any time during the course of the disease (**Table 1**).

Table 1		
Systemic autoimmune diseases associated with the development of vestibular dysfunction		
Autoimmune Disorder	**Estimated Prevalence of Vestibular Symptoms (%)**	**Citation**
Behçet's disease	15–47	31
Sarcoidosis	20	32
Vogt-Koyanagi-Harada Syndrome	4	31
Relapsing polychondritis	6–13	31
Ankylosing spondylitis	34–40	33,34
Systemic lupus erythematosus	9–30	35,36
Granulomatosis with polyangiitis	8–9	37,38
Multiple sclerosis	7–30	28
Cogan's syndrome	Not assessed	
Polyarteritis nodosa	Not assessed	
Sjogren's syndrome	Not assessed	
Lyme disease	Not assessed	
Autoimmune thyroid disease	Not assessed	
Antiphospholipid syndrome	Not assessed	

Diagnosis and treatment

A multidisciplinary approach is essential to detecting and managing vestibular dysfunction associated with systemic autoimmune disease. Audiovestibular testing in patients with autoimmune disease and vertigo may impact treatment, as early targeted therapy with corticosteroid has been shown to improve vestibular function if promptly initiated.[26,31] Management of AIED ideally involves partnership with rheumatologic specialists to assist with identification and management of the underlying systemic autoimmune condition.[28]

GENETIC AND CONGENITAL PERIPHERAL VESTIBULOPATHY
Ushers Syndrome

Introduction

Usher syndrome (USH) encompasses a group of recessively inherited disorders characterized by sensory impairment of the audiovestibular and visual systems. USH is the leading cause of combined sight and hearing loss, with an estimated prevalence of 4 to 17 per 100,000 individuals worldwide.[39] The Usher genes encode a variety of proteins critical for the development and maintenance of hair cells of the vestibulocochlear system and maintenance of retinal photoreceptors.[39]

Clinical presentation

USH is classified into three distinct clinical subtypes according to the severity of hearing loss and the presence or absence of vestibular dysfunction. Visual loss due to retinitis pigmentosa is a common feature of all three subtypes.

Usher syndrome type 1 (USH1) is the most severe subtype of USH, characterized by profound congenital SNHL with vestibular areflexia. Vestibular dysfunction typically manifests in early childhood as delay in motor development, especially in walking and activities requiring coordination or balance. Usher syndrome type 3 (USH3) is extremely rare, accounting for only 2% to 4% of all cases of USH.[39] Vestibular dysfunction is estimated to occur in approximately 50% of patients, although is typically milder and occurs later in development than USH1.[39] Usher syndrome type 2 (USH2) is defined by the absence of vestibular symptoms and therefore will not be discussed further.

Diagnosis

Diagnosis of USH1 is typically detected through the newborn screen or is suspected in infants with profound SNHL and delays in motor development. Owing to the later onset of SNHL and milder vestibular symptoms, diagnosis of USH3 is often delayed until the onset of visual symptoms, usually occurring after puberty.[39] Clinical classification into USH1, USH2, or USH3 is based on the clinical history in combination with audiovestibular and ophthalmologic testing. Advances in genetic sequencing have yielded promise into achieving a molecular diagnosis of USH, although genetic testing is not yet a diagnostic criterion for USH.[40]

POSTRADIATION VESTIBULOPATHY
Introduction

The auditory-vestibular system of the inner ear is particularly susceptible to radiation toxicity. It is estimated that nearly half of all patients who undergo radiation therapy (RT) for head and neck cancers (including external beam and fractionated stereotactic radiotherapy) will develop signs of auditory or vestibular dysfunction.[41] Data suggest that post-RT vestibulopathy is the result of either peripheral labyrinthine disorder or central vestibular lesions, with the former being more common.[42] Although the mechanism is not fully understood, it has been proposed to result from either direct radiation injury to the inner ear or labyrinthitis secondary to radiation-induced otitis media.[42]

Clinical presentation

Vertigo may present acutely after RT, or months to years after therapy has been completed. Approximately 30% of patients receiving RT to the temporal bone for head and neck cancer report vertigo.[41] Of patients experiencing subjective vertigo, VNGs were abnormal in 83%.[43]

Stereotactic radiosurgery (SRS) is a common modality for treatment of vestibular schwannomas. Posttreatment vestibulopathy in this group is well-described and may result from injury to the peripheral or retrocochlear vestibular apparatus.[44] Evidence from the literature suggests that vertigo most commonly occurs within the first 6 months after SRS and typically resolves with or without treatment within 2 years, although progressively worsening vertigo that does not resolve has been described in a small subset of patients.[45]

Diagnosis and treatment

The diagnosis of RT vestibulopathy relies on clinical findings and a history of prior RT therapy. The treatment of these patients includes vestibular suppressants for short-term relief of acute symptoms and vestibular rehabilitation for treatment of residual dizziness and imbalance. Vestibular symptoms are often worst in the first 6 months after RT because of posttreatment inflammation and may self-resolve as the inflammation subsides.[46] Early prevention and control of radiation otitis media may prevent labyrinthitis and subsequent development of post-RT vertigo.[42]

OTOTOXIC VESTIBULOPATHY
Introduction

Ototoxicity refers to drugs that cause functional impairment or cellular damage to the tissues of the inner ear, including both the cochlear and vestibular system. Vestibulotoxicity refers specifically to injury of the vestibular system and has been associated with various pharmaceutical agents[47] (**Box 1**). The mechanism by which these medications cause injury to the vestibular system is multifaceted and not fully understood, although destruction of vestibular hair cells and degeneration of vestibular ganglion neurons are thought to play a major role.[48,49]

Box 1
Pharmacologic agents with known vestibulotoxicity[49,50]

Medication

Aminoglycosides
  Gentamicin
  Tobramycin
  Dibekacin
  Streptomycin

Cancer
  Cisplatin
  Carboplatin

Antimalarials
  Chloroquine
  Hydroxychloroquine

The risk of vestibulotoxic effects vary widely between studies, likely due to differences in dosage and duration of medication use, but have been reported to be as high as 60% in patients treated with aminoglycosides[51] and 50% in patients receiving platinum-based cancer therapeutics.[52]

Clinical Presentation

Vestibulotoxicity typically manifests as dizziness, vertigo, oscillopsia, or imbalance.[53] Symptoms are more often bilateral because of the systemic administration of these medications. Vestibular dysfunction may be accompanied by signs of cochleotoxicity, such as SNHL or tinnitus. Platinum-based cancer drugs and aminoglycosides, especially cisplatin and gentamicin, are associated with irreversible damage to the inner ear, and vestibulotoxic effects are usually permanent.[47,50] In contrast, the vestibulotoxic effects of chloroquine and hydroxychloroquine are usually reversable with discontinuation of the offending agent.[47,50]

Diagnosis

Early recognition and diagnosis are imperative to prevent further damage to the vestibular system and preserve function. Evidence confirms frequent delays between symptom onset of and recognition by physicians, likely due to the insidious and progressive nature of vestibulotoxicity.[54] This may be counteracted by frequent monitoring of audiovestibular function in patients receiving known offending agents, including audiometry, VNG, VEMP, and rotatory chair testing.[50,55]

Treatment

When identified, vestibulotoxic effects may be reversed or mitigated by stopping the offending agent. In addition, administration of steroids, such as dexamethasone and methylprednisolone, has been shown to help improve the symptoms of cisplatin-, chloroquine-, and hydroxychloroquine-induced ototoxicity.[56,57]

PERILYMPHATIC FISTULA

A perilymphatic fistula (PLF) is characterized by egress of perilymphatic fluid from the inner ear, specifically the oval and/or round windows.[58] It may follow head trauma, barotrauma, or have an idiopathic onset and is characterized by some combination of fluctuating or nonfluctuating symptoms of vertigo, SNHL, aural fullness, and tinnitus. Classically, patients may complain of sound- or pressure-induced vertigo (Tullio or Hennebert signs, respectively) as well as intermittent nausea triggered by movement of the head or changes in air pressure.[59,60] Chronic symptoms may be treated surgically, although the condition may heal spontaneously in rare cases.[60] Controversy regarding the incidence, etiology, and diagnosis is longstanding and reflects the lack of sensitivity and specificity of available testing. For most patients, PLF diagnosis is confirmed with intraoperative visualization of perilymphatic leakage from the inner ear and subsequent symptomatic improvement after surgical repair[58] (Video 1). However, recent diagnostic criteria use newly available perilymph biomarker testing in combination with a supportive traumatic history as "definite" PLFs; lack of antecedent events may support a "probable" PLF diagnosis.

SUMMARY

Progressive and degenerative peripheral vestibular disorders may be caused by a wide variety of underlying conditions, including MD, autoimmune conditions, congenital pathologies, ototoxic medications, RT, and trauma. Many of these vestibulopathies present with similar clinical symptoms, making a diagnosis of the underlying etiology difficult. Diagnosis often depends on a detailed clinical history, including the timing and progression of vertigo and associated symptoms, in combination with specific questioning about antecedent trauma, medication or radiation exposure, systemic autoimmune disease, and family history of hearing and balance disorders. In addition to audiometry, differentiation among entities may require vestibular testing, radiographic imaging, or serologic evaluation. Treatment options are disparate and disease-specific, ranging from observation to medical management or surgical intervention, underscoring the need for astute investigation and diagnosis.

CLINICS CARE POINTS

- Ménière's disease (MD) remains a clinical diagnosis; however, data for improved sensitivity and specificity of MRI and multifrequency cervical vestibular-evoked myogenic potential for MD may supplant the use of videonystagmography and electrocochleography in evaluation of this disease.

- Autoimmune inner ear disease remains a diagnostic challenge but is supported by bilateral symptomatology and concurrent systemic autoimmune disease.

- A high level of clinical suspicion for vestibular injury is appropriate for vertigo after radiation or ototoxic medication exposure; early intervention may have important implications for outcome and symptom resolution.

- Concern for a congenital, progressive peripheral vestibulopathy should prompt investigation for Usher syndrome.

- Perilymphatic fistula may present with or without antecedent trauma and may be idiopathic; diagnosis was historically confirmed with surgical intervention, although more recently available biomarker testing may now play a role.

DISCLOSURE

The authors declare that there are no conflicts of interest.

SUPPLEMENTARY DATA

Supplementary data to this article can be found online at https://doi.org/10.1016/j.otc.2021.05.015.

REFERENCES

1. Espinosa-Sanchez JM, Lopez-Escamez JA. Meniere's disease. Handb Clin Neurol 2016;137:257–77.
2. Alexander TH, Harris JP. Current epidemiology of Meniere's syndrome. Otolaryngol Clin North Am 2010;43(5):965–70.
3. Harris JP, Alexander TH. Current-day prevalence of Meniere's syndrome. Audiol Neurootol 2010;15(5):318–22.
4. Nakashima T, Pyykko I, Arroll MA, et al. Meniere's disease. Nat Rev Dis Primers 2016;2:16028.
5. Merchant SN, Adams JC, Nadol JB Jr. Pathophysiology of Meniere's syndrome: are symptoms caused by endolymphatic hydrops? Otol Neurotol 2005;26(1):74–81.
6. Gurkov R, Pyyko I, Zou J, et al. What is Meniere's disease? A contemporary re-evaluation of endolymphatic hydrops. J Neurol 2016;263(Suppl 1):S71–81.

7. Belinchon A, Perez-Garrigues H, Tenias JM. Evolution of symptoms in Meniere's disease. Audiol Neurootol 2012;17(2):126–32.

8. Pyykko I, Nakashima T, Yoshida T, et al. Meniere's disease: a reappraisal supported by a variable latency of symptoms and the MRI visualisation of endolymphatic hydrops. BMJ Open 2013;3(2).

9. Paparella MM, Mancini F. Vestibular Meniere's disease. Otolaryngol Head Neck Surg 1985;93(2):148–51.

10. Havia M, Kentala E. Progression of symptoms of dizziness in Meniere's disease. Arch Otolaryngol Head Neck Surg 2004;130(4):431–5.

11. Lopez-Escamez JA, Dlugaiczyk J, Jacobs J, et al. Accompanying Symptoms Overlap during Attacks in Meniere's Disease and Vestibular Migraine. Front Neurol 2014;5:265.

12. Vassiliou A, Vlastarakos PV, Maragoudakis P, et al. Meniere's disease: Still a mystery disease with difficult differential diagnosis. Ann Indian Acad Neurol 2011; 14(1):12–8.

13. House JW, Doherty JK, Fisher LM, et al. Meniere's disease: prevalence of contralateral ear involvement. Otol Neurotol 2006;27(3):355–61.

14. Lopez-Escamez JA, Carey J, Chung WH, et al. Diagnostic criteria for Meniere's disease. J Vestib Res 2015;25(1):1–7.

15. Belinchon A, Perez-Garrigues H, Tenias JM, et al. Hearing assessment in Meniere's disease. Laryngoscope 2011;121(3):622–6.

16. Basura GJ, Adams ME, Monfared A, et al. Clinical Practice Guideline: Ménière's Disease. Otolaryngol Head Neck Surg 2020;162(2_suppl):S1–55.

17. Ziylan F, Smeeing DP, Stegeman I, et al. Click Stimulus Electrocochleography Versus MRI With Intratympanic Contrast in Meniere's Disease: A Systematic Review. Otol Neurotol 2016;37(5):421–7.

18. Naganawa S, Nakashima T. Visualization of endolymphatic hydrops with MR imaging in patients with Meniere's disease and related pathologies: current status of its methods and clinical significance. Jpn J Radiol 2014;32(4):191–204.

19. Lingam RK, Connor SEJ, Casselman JW, et al. MRI in otology: applications in cholesteatoma and Meniere's disease. Clin Radiol 2018;73(1):35–44.

20. Wang HM, Tsai SM, Chien CY, et al. Analysis of auditory and vestibular function in patients with unilateral Meniere's disease. Acta Otolaryngol 2012;132(12): 1246–51.

21. de Sousa LC, Piza MR, da Costa SS. Diagnosis of Meniere's disease: routine and extended tests. Otolaryngol Clin North Am 2002;35(3):547–64.

22. Angeli SI, Goncalves S. Cervical VEMP tuning changes by Meniere's disease stages. Laryngoscope Investig Otolaryngol 2019;4(5):543–9.

23. Espinosa-Sanchez JM, Lopez-Escamez JA. The pharmacological management of vertigo in Meniere disease. Expert Opin Pharmacother 2020;21(14):1753–63.

24. Hussain K, Murdin L, Schilder AG. Restriction of salt, caffeine and alcohol intake for the treatment of Meniere's disease or syndrome. Cochrane Database Syst Rev 2018;12:CD012173.

25. Sajjadi H, Paparella MM. Meniere's disease. Lancet 2008;372(9636):406–14. https://doi.org/10.1016/S0140-6736(08)61161-7.

26. Bovo R, Aimoni C, Martini A. Immune-mediated inner ear disease. Acta Otolaryngol 2006;126(10):1012–21.

27. Vambutas A, Pathak S. AAO: Autoimmune and Autoinflammatory (Disease) in Otology: What is New in Immune-Mediated Hearing Loss. Laryngoscope Investig Otolaryngol 2016;1(5):110–5.

28. Russo FY, Ralli M, De Seta D, et al. Autoimmune vertigo: an update on vestibular disorders associated with autoimmune mechanisms. Immunol Res 2018;66(6): 675–85.
29. Ciorba A, Corazzi V, Bianchini C, et al. Autoimmune inner ear disease (AIED): A diagnostic challenge. Int J Immunopathol Pharmacol 2018;32. 2058738418808680.
30. Das S, Bakshi SS, Seepana R. Demystifying autoimmune inner ear disease. Eur Arch Otorhinolaryngol 2019;276(12):3267–74.
31. Girasoli L, Cazzador D, Padoan R, et al. Update on Vertigo in Autoimmune Disorders, from Diagnosis to Treatment. J Immunol Res 2018;2018:5072582.
32. Colvin IB. Audiovestibular manifestations of sarcoidosis: a review of the literature. Laryngoscope 2006;116(1):75–82.
33. Erbek SS, Erbek HS, Yilmaz S, et al. Cochleovestibular dysfunction in ankylosing spondylitis. Audiol Neurootol 2006;11(5):294–300.
34. Kapusuz Gencer Z, Ozkiris M, Gunaydin I, et al. The impact of ankylosing spondylitis on audiovestibular functions. Eur Arch Otorhinolaryngol 2014;271(9): 2415–20.
35. Di Stadio A, Ralli M. Systemic Lupus Erythematosus and hearing disorders: Literature review and meta-analysis of clinical and temporal bone findings. J Int Med Res 2017;45(5):1470–80.
36. Batuecas-Caletrio A, del Pino-Montes J, Cordero-Civantos C, et al. Hearing and vestibular disorders in patients with systemic lupus erythematosus. Lupus 2013; 22(5):437–42.
37. Seccia V, Fortunato S, Cristofani-Mencacci L, et al. Focus on audiologic impairment in eosinophilic granulomatosis with polyangiitis. Laryngoscope 2016; 126(12):2792–7.
38. Wojciechowska J, KreCicki T. Clinical characteristics of patients with granulomatosis with polyangiitis and microscopic polyangiitis in ENT practice: a comparative analysis. Acta Otorhinolaryngol Ital 2018;38(6):517–27.
39. Toms M, Pagarkar W, Moosajee M. Usher syndrome: clinical features, molecular genetics and advancing therapeutics. Ther Adv Ophthalmol 2020;12. 2515841420952194.
40. Aparisi MJ, Aller E, Fuster-Garcia C, et al. Targeted next generation sequencing for molecular diagnosis of Usher syndrome. Orphanet J Rare Dis 2014;9:168.
41. Bhandare N, Mendenhall WM, Antonelli PJ. Radiation effects on the auditory and vestibular systems. Otolaryngol Clin North Am 2009;42(4):623–34.
42. Young YH, Ko JY, Sheen TS. Postirradiation vertigo in nasopharyngeal carcinoma survivors. Otol Neurotol 2004;25(3):366–70.
43. Bhandare N, Mendenhall W, Morris CG, et al. Vestibular Apparatus Dysfunction after External Beam Radiation Therapy for Head and Neck Cancers. Otolaryngol Head Neck Surg 2013;149(2_suppl):P239.
44. Werner-Wasik M, Rudoler S, Preston PE, et al. Immediate side effects of stereotactic radiotherapy and radiosurgery. Int J Radiat Oncol Biol Phys 1999;43(2): 299–304.
45. Wackym PA, Hannley MT, Runge-Samuelson CL, et al. Gamma Knife surgery of vestibular schwannomas: longitudinal changes in vestibular function and measurement of the Dizziness Handicap Inventory. J Neurosurg 2008;109(Suppl): 137–43.
46. Young YH, Cheng PW, Ko JY. A 10-year longitudinal study of tubal function in patients with nasopharyngeal carcinoma after irradiation. Arch Otolaryngol Head Neck Surg 1997;123(9):945–8.

47. Lanvers-Kaminsky C, Zehnhoff-Dinnesen AA, Parfitt R, et al. Drug-induced ototoxicity: Mechanisms, Pharmacogenetics, and protective strategies. Clin Pharmacol Ther 2017;101(4):491–500.

48. Sedo-Cabezon L, Boadas-Vaello P, Soler-Martin C, et al. Vestibular damage in chronic ototoxicity: a mini-review. Neurotoxicology 2014;43:21–7.

49. Gans RE, Rauterkus G, Research A. Vestibular Toxicity: Causes, Evaluation Protocols, Intervention, and Management. Semin Hear 2019;40(2):144–53.

50. DiSogra RM. Common Aminoglycosides and Platinum-Based Ototoxic Drugs: Cochlear/Vestibular Side Effects and Incidence. Semin Hear 2019;40(2):104–7.

51. Van Hecke R, Van Rompaey V, Wuyts FL, et al. Systemic Aminoglycosides-Induced Vestibulotoxicity in Humans. Ear Hear 2017;38(6):653–62.

52. Prayuenyong P, Taylor JA, Pearson SE, et al. Vestibulotoxicity Associated With Platinum-Based Chemotherapy in Survivors of Cancer: A Scoping Review. Front Oncol 2018;8:363.

53. Handelsman JA. Vestibulotoxicity: strategies for clinical diagnosis and rehabilitation. Int J Audiol 2018;57(sup4):S99–107.

54. Ahmed RM, Hannigan IP, MacDougall HG, et al. Gentamicin ototoxicity: a 23-year selected case series of 103 patients. Med J Aust 2012;196(11):701–4.

55. Association AS-L-H. Audiologic management of individuals receiving cochleotoxic drug therapy. Available at: https://www.asha.org/policy/gl1994-00003/. Accessed November 29, 2020.

56. Hammill TL, Campbell KC. Protection for medication-induced hearing loss: the state of the science. Int J Audiol 2018;57(sup4):S67–75.

57. Prayuenyong P, Kasbekar AV, Baguley DM. Clinical Implications of Chloroquine and Hydroxychloroquine Ototoxicity for COVID-19 Treatment: A Mini-Review. Front Public Health 2020;8:252.

58. Sarna B, Abouzari M, Merna C, et al. Perilymphatic Fistula: A Review of Classification, Etiology, Diagnosis, and Treatment. Front Neurol 2020;11:1046.

59. Fife TD, Giza C. Posttraumatic vertigo and dizziness. Semin Neurol 2013;33(3):238–43.

60. Kolev OI, Sergeeva M. Vestibular disorders following different types of head and neck trauma. Funct Neurol 2016;31(2):75–80.

The Dizzy Child

Elizabeth A. Kelly, MD[a],*, Kristen L. Janky, AuD, PhD[b],
Jessie N. Patterson, AuD, PhD[b]

KEYWORDS

- Pediatric • Children • Dizziness • Vestibular disorders • Vestibular testing

KEY POINTS

- Vestibular disorders occur in pediatric patients and may impact gross motor function and visual acuity.
- Vestibular function testing can be completed in children with minor modifications
- Children with greater severity of hearing loss are more likely to have vestibular loss
- Vestibular migraine is the most common etiology of pediatric dizziness

INTRODUCTION

The prevalence of imbalance or dizziness in childhood is reported to range from 0.45% to 15.0%.[1–3] Vestibular disorders may impact gross motor skill development, visual acuity, and contribute to psychological distress.[4–6] Vestibular disorders in childhood is a growing area of research and clinical medicine. In a retrospective review evaluating the prevalence of vestibular and balance disorders, the largest subgroup consisted of the diagnosis of unspecified dizziness, suggesting the need for increased awareness and improvement of appropriate diagnosis and management of these conditions in children.[1]

Understanding the development and maturation of the vestibular system may provide further insight into the vestibular testing results and etiology of dizziness at different age groups. Compared with the cochlea, the vestibular organs develop earlier and faster.[7] Although the vestibular aqueduct is still growing up until the 39th week of gestation,[8] the remaining vestibular organs are fully developed around 25 weeks gestational age.[9] Vestibular receptors such as otoconia and types I and II hair cells are fully developed by the end of the second trimester.[7,10] The end organs seem to be adult-like at full term or shortly after, but efferent connections are not fully mature until several months or years later. The vestibulo-ocular reflex, which allows for stable gaze with head movements demonstrates stable slow component velocity of nystagmus by 12 months of age[11]; however, vestibulo-ocular reflex gain is high in

[a] Department of Otolaryngology, Boys Town National Research Hospital, 555 N 30th St., Omaha, NE 68131, USA; [b] Department of Audiology, Boys Town National Research Hospital, 555 N 30th St., Omaha, NE 68131, USA
* Corresponding author.
E-mail address: elizabethkelly22@gmail.com

Otolaryngol Clin N Am 54 (2021) 973–987
https://doi.org/10.1016/j.otc.2021.06.002
0030-6665/21/© 2021 Elsevier Inc. All rights reserved.

young children, which continues to normalize until 11 years of age.[12] The vestibulospinal reflex, which is vital for postural control, continues to mature until at least 15 years of age.[7] Furthermore, the vestibulocollic reflex, which allows for stabilizing the head, continues to mature through adolescence.[13,14]

CLINICAL EVALUATION

The medical history is often the most important aspect of evaluating a patient with dizziness. However, obtaining a history in pediatric patients can be challenging because children may not have the language to appropriately describe the sensations that are experienced. Often the history depends on a caregiver's observations. If possible, having the patient describe the sensation that they experience can help differentiate peripheral dizziness from nonperipheral dizziness related to other health conditions. Characterizing the frequency and timing of dizziness can be helpful in determining potential etiologies. Delays in gross motor milestones (**Table 1**) can be seen in patients with vestibular dysfunction and may warrant additional investigation with vestibular testing.[15] Patients with vestibular loss may have a decrease in motor function performance.[16] Associations with hearing loss, otitis media (OM), cranial nerve abnormalities, and headaches should be investigated.

A Pediatric Dizziness Handicap Inventory for patient caregivers was introduced in 2015 as a tool that identifies the impact dizziness symptoms have on the pediatric patient.[17] The Pediatric Vestibular Symptom Questionnaire can be administered to determine presence and degree of severity of subjective vestibular symptoms in children (ages 6–17 years).[18] Those that have symptoms owing to vestibular disorders or dizziness post-concussion are predicted to have higher scores (more severe symptoms) compared with healthy children.[18] With further development, these questionnaires may also have a role in assessing effectiveness and progress in treatment.

A head and neck examination should be completed specifically focusing on the eye examination (eg, to evaluate for nystagmus), otologic examination (eg, to rule out middle ear disease), and neurologic examination. A bedside head impulse test should be completed by moving the child's head to each side while maintaining focus on a stable object and observing for a deviation from the target followed by a rapid refixation onto the target. The presence of a refixation saccade suggests an abnormality of the ipsilateral horizontal semicircular canal. Gross motor skills are assessed during the visit

Table 1	
Normal developmental gross motor milestones[67,68]	
Developmental Motor Milestone	**Expected Age to Reach Milestone**
Head control	4 mo
Sit without support	6–9 mo
Crawling	6–9 mo
Walking	12–18 mo
Standing on 1 foot	30 months—briefly 36 months—2 s 4 years old—5 s 5 years old—10 s

Data from Gerber RJ, Wilks T, Erdie-Lalena C. Developmental milestones: motor development. Pediatr Rev 2010; 31:267-276; quiz 277., Syed MI, Rutka JA, Sharma A, Cushing SL. The 'dizzy child': a 12-minute consultation. Clin Otolaryngol 2014; 39:228-234.

(see **Table 1**). The Bruininks–Oseretsky Test of Motor Proficiency 2, a test of postural stability assessing the static and dynamic balance function with 9 separate tasks (4 with eyes open and then with eyes closed), can be undertaken in those patients with limited access to vestibular testing. Results have been correlated with vestibular testing results, specifically the rotary chair.[18]

VESTIBULAR FUNCTION TESTING

Vestibular function testing can be completed in children; however, appropriateness of testing varies by patient age and may require minor modification. We provide a brief description of common vestibular function tests and an overview of modifications to be considered when testing children, including the age at which each test is recommended. For a more in-depth discussion, see Janky and Rodriguez.[19]

VESTIBULAR EVOKED MYOGENIC POTENTIAL

Vestibular evoked myogenic potentials (VEMPs) are electromyographic (EMG) responses to loud acoustic stimulation. The most common VEMP responses are the cervical VEMP, measured on the contracted sternocleidomastoid (SCM) muscle and the ocular VEMP measured on the inferior oblique extraocular muscle.

The cervical VEMP is an inhibitory, ipsilateral response; thus, it measures release of the SCM from contraction. The cervical VEMP reflects the pathway extending from the saccule, inferior vestibular nerve, vestibular nuclei to motoneurons of the SCM.[20] **Fig. 1**A shows the electrode configuration with active electrodes on the SCM belly (in line with the chin), EMG electrodes below the active electrodes, a reference electrode on the manubrium of the sternum and a ground electrode on the nose. Cervical

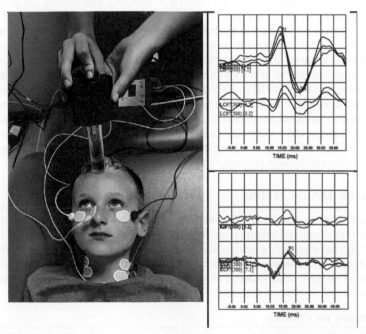

Fig. 1. (*A*) Electrode montage for cervical and ocular VEMP, (*B*) characteristic cervical VEMP waveform (upper tracing), and (*C*) characteristic ocular VEMP waveform (lower tracing).

VEMP outcome parameters are the P13 and N23 latency and the P13/N23 peak-to-peak amplitude (see **Fig. 1**B). The cervical VEMP peak-to-peak amplitude is affected by degree of SCM contraction, larger SCM contractions result in larger amplitudes; therefore, a normalized amplitude is often calculated where EMG is divided by the peak-to-peak amplitude.[21,22]

The ocular VEMP is an excitatory, contralateral response; thus, measures contraction of the inferior oblique extraocular muscle. The ocular VEMP reflects the pathway extending from the utricle, superior vestibular nerve, vestibular nuclei, and motoneurons of the inferior oblique muscle.[23,24] **Fig. 1**A shows the electrode configuration with active electrodes over the muscle belly of the inferior oblique muscle, a reference electrode on the nose and a ground electrode on the manubrium of the sternum. Ocular VEMP outcome parameters are the N10 and P16 latency and the N10/P16 peak-to-peak amplitude (see **Fig. 1**C). The ocular VEMP peak-to-peak amplitude is affected by degree of inferior oblique contraction; larger contractions result in larger amplitudes. The degree of inferior oblique contraction is controlled by standardizing the degree of up-gaze during testing. This maneuver is typically completed by giving patients a set target at approximately 30° up gaze to view during testing.[25]

Modifications for Children

Cervical and ocular VEMP are optimal tests of vestibular function in children because they are fast, do not induce dizziness, and provide information about both otolith organs and both branches of the vestibular nerve. Cervical VEMP have been recorded in newborns and infants,[26] although ocular VEMP are not reliably recorded until age 3 to 4 years.[27] For cervical VEMP, children often have difficulty maintaining SCM contraction, which can be alleviated by laying supine, propped up on their elbows with the head turned. EMG monitoring is recommended in children who need frequent breaks during testing. For ocular VEMP, children have difficulty maintaining up gaze, which can be alleviated by using a smart phone, tablet, or sticker placed at 30° up gaze.

VEMPs can be completed in response to either air- or bone-conducted stimuli. A 125 dB SPL, 500 Hz toneburst is a common stimulus used for VEMP testing. Children have smaller ear canal volumes compared with adults; therefore, stimulus intensities are on average 3 dB higher in children's ears.[28,29] Tympanometry is recommended before VEMP testing and a 120 dB SPL, 500 Hz toneburst is recommended for children with ear canal volumes of less than 0.9 mL to ensure safe sound exposure.[28] Bone conduction stimuli can also be considered, which is safer in terms of sound exposure, requires less time and bypasses the middle ear in cases of conductive hearing loss. Compared with adults, VEMP amplitudes are not significantly different; however, latencies are shorter, and thresholds are lower in children.[30] VEMPs are reliable in children.[31,32]

VIDEO HEAD IMPULSE TESTING

Video head impulse testing (vHIT) assesses each semicircular canal and each branch of the vestibular nerve. Patients wear a pair of tight-fitting goggles while the examiner delivers high acceleration head impulses in the plane of each semicircular canal. There are 2 outcome parameters: gain (the ratio of eye to head movement) and corrective saccades. The vHIT is considered abnormal when gain is less than 0.8 coupled with the presence of corrective saccades.[33]

Modifications for Children

The vHIT is advantageous in children because it is fast (10–15 minutes) and does not induce dizziness. Goggles for vHIT need to be worn tightly. For children with smaller head size, a piece of foam can be inserted in the back of the head for a more secure fit. Children as young as 3 years can complete standard vHIT. For children who cannot wear vHIT goggles, remote video systems can be used.[34] A smart phone, tablet, or sticker can be used as a fixation point to keep children engaged. The vHIT is reliable in children[35]; however, does take longer to administer.[36]

Fig. 2 shows a typical vHIT set up and an example of normal vHIT gain output and tracings. Many studies document similar gain values between children and young adults[16,33]; however, age-related changes have been found with gain increasing up to age 6.[34] Nonetheless, vHIT is not considered to be abnormal unless gain values are less than 0.8 and coupled with repeatable corrective saccades.

ROTARY CHAIR

The rotary chair is a motorized chair in which patients rotate without fixation. Fixation is removed by either a darkened enclosure or light occluding goggles. Nystagmus in response to rotation is measured by either electrodes or infrared goggles. The rotary chair assesses the horizontal canal and superior branch of the vestibular nerve and takes approximately 10 to 15 minutes to complete. Two paradigms are used: sinusoidal harmonic acceleration, where the chair moves gently back and forth at various frequencies or step testing, where the chair rotates for approximately 45 seconds and then comes to an abrupt stop. With either paradigm, there are 3 outcome parameters: gain, phase (time constant), and symmetry. Gain is the ratio of eye velocity to chair velocity, phase (time constant) is the relationship in timing between eye and chair movement, and asymmetry is the comparison between the velocity of right and left beating nystagmus.

Modifications for Children

Infants and small children may sit on a parent's lap while rotating in the dark (**Fig. 3**). The rotary chair can be completed in children as young as 2 months of age. Because

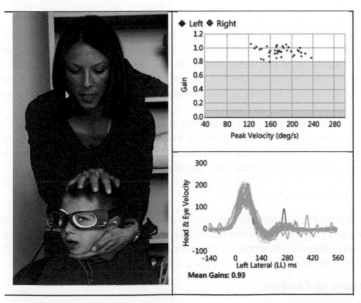

Fig. 2. (*A*) A typical vHIT set up. (*B* and *C*) Example of normal vHIT gain output and tracings, respectively.

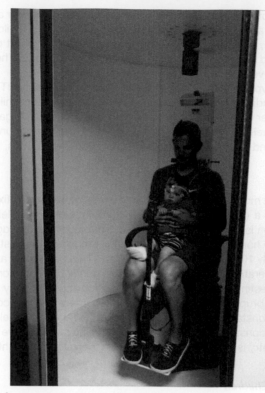

Fig. 3. Depiction of rotary chair set up with an infant seated on the parent's lap. The door is closed, while the child and parent rotate in the dark. The child is monitored via the chair mounted camera.

drowsiness can affect gain, children need to remain awake and alert during testing, which is easier in older children. Alertness is generally maintained by singing songs. Owing to maturation of the vestibulo-ocular reflex, some infants less than 9 months of age with normal vestibular function do not generate nystagmus in response to rotation; therefore, repeat testing is recommended when responses are absent in infants.[37] The most common paradigm used in children is sinusoidal harmonic acceleration. We recommend completing a low (0.01 Hz), mid (0.04 Hz), and high (0.16 Hz) frequency first. If normal, these frequencies are enough. If abnormal, 0.08, 0.02, and 0.32 Hz would then be completed. Tympanometry is recommended before rotary chair because rotary chair can be affected by active OM.[38]

VIDEONYSTAGMOGRAPHY

Videonystagmography primarily consists of an ocular motor battery, positional testing, and calorics. Eye movements are monitored by either electrodes or infrared goggles. Description of these tests exceeds the scope of this article. For an in-depth description of each test, see Janky and Shepard (2019).[39]

Modifications for Children

For ocular motor testing, fun, colorful targets can be helpful when assessing children. Children should be able to achieve normal smooth pursuit by age 5,[40] normal saccades by age 12,[41] and normal optokinetic nystagmus by age 7.[42] Caloric testing provides a low frequency assessment of the horizontal semicircular canal; however, it can be scary because vision is occluded, the ear is filled with water, and dizziness is a side effect. In our clinic, caloric testing is not attempted until age 6 or 7. Children may require additional reassurance by either positive feedback or hand holding by a parent during testing. Caloric irrigations can be decreased in duration or limited to monothermal irrigations.

IMAGING

A detailed history and physical examination are important aspects of the assessment of the dizzy patient and provide information needed to determine if additional testing or imaging is indicated. The majority of patients evaluated for dizziness have normal findings on imaging.[43,44] In patients with auditory and vestibular symptoms, anatomic anomalies such as a cochleovestibular dysplasia or enlarged vestibular aqueduct can be identified on either MRI or computed tomography scan. Focal neurologic symptoms, cranial nerve deficits, or worsening/persistent dizziness are often important indicators for imaging and these central findings can be assessed with MRI. A computed tomography scan of the temporal bone can often be helpful in the setting where there are concerns for chronic ear disease or cholesteatoma, defects in bony labyrinth, or temporal bone fracture or trauma. However, further research is needed to characterize the role of imaging in these patients.

ETIOLOGIES OF PEDIATRIC DIZZINESS

The etiology and prevalence of vestibular disorders in children differs from that seen in the adult population. A summary of etiologies from recent clinical studies is presented in **Table 2**. We have highlighted a few of the more common diagnoses.

Migraine disorders are often the most common reported cause of dizziness in the pediatric population (30%–35%).[43,45] There are 3 migraine variant disorders described: benign paroxysmal torticollis of infancy, benign paroxysmal vertigo of childhood (BPVC), and vestibular migraine.[46] Patients with benign paroxysmal torticollis of infancy have associations with OM, balance concerns, and motor delay; 43% progress to BPVC.[47] BPVC is predominant in preschool aged children and progresses to vestibular migraine in 15% of cases.[47,48] Recently, a new diagnostic criteria consensus document and classification was reported to aid in diagnosis, research, and management strategies for children with migraine and vertigo.[49] The 3 classifications, including vestibular migraine of childhood, probable vestibular migraine of childhood and recurrent vertigo of childhood, are suggested to replace use of BPVC.[49]

Pediatric patients with vestibular migraine often describe true rotary vertigo with variations in episode duration. These symptoms can be accompanied by photophobia, phonophobia, and nausea and vomiting.[44] vHIT may show higher levels of gain in patients with vestibular migraine but often vestibular testing is normal.[44,50] Behavioral modifications, avoidance of triggers, and diet management are often suggested in treatment for adults with vestibular migraine. There are reports in pediatric literature that good sleep hygiene, routine exercise, and a balanced diet may provide benefit in children.[51] Symptom improvement was noted in 70% in those who received triptans for acute management of symptoms.[44] Ibuprofen is shown to provide some benefit in small studies in treatment of acute migraine pain in pediatric patients.[52] Typically, patients are responsive to prophylactic medications.[44] Medications shown to be most beneficial include tricyclics, cyproheptadine, and topiramate.[44]

Table 2
Etiology of pediatric dizziness

	Brodsky[2] 2020- Dizziness,[a] %	Brodsky[2] 2020- Imbalance,[b] %	Wang[43] 2020	Ciolek[69] 2018	Sommerfleck[70] 2016	O'Reilly[45] 2011	O'Reilly[1] 2010
Total n	9247[c]	9247[c]	1021	169	206	132	2546
Age range	3–17 y	3–17 y	9 mo – 21 y	2–17 y	1–18 y	1–17 y	Newborn – 18 y
Migraine/headache	0	0	357 (35%)	45 (27%)	87 (42%)	23 (17%)	
BPVC	1.3%	0.7%	58 (6%)	8 (5%)	16 (8%)	6 (5%)	
BPTI						3 (2%)	
Motion sickness					2 (1%)		25 (1%)
CNS structural lesion				5 (3%)	4 (2%)	12 (9%)	
Dysautonomia			160 (16%)	17 (10%)			
Other central causes	5%	2%		11 (7%)	19 (9%)	3 (2%)	73 (3%)
BPPV	5%	2%	221 (22%)	3 (2%)	8 (4%)	3 (2%)	42 (2%)
Labyrinthitis				5 (3%)	6 (3%)	1 (1%)	15 (0.6%)
Vestibular neuritis			50 (5%)		4 (2%)	2 (2%)	7 (0.3%)
Meniere's disease	0	0		9 (5%)		3 (2%)	11 (0.4%)
Otitis media	0	1.5%	42 (4%)	5 (3%)	4 (2%)	3 (2%)	
Other otologic disorder	0	2%		3 (2%)	4 (2%)	23 (17%)	
Other vestibulopathy				14 (8%)	17 (9%)	4 (3%)	77 (3%)
Concussion/TBI	8%	6%	264 (26%)	7 (4%)	13 (6%)	13 (10%)	
Behavioral health conditions	12%	6%	138 (14%)	9 (5%)	9 (4%)	8 (6%)	
Other health condition	70%	60%	41 (4%)	9 (5%)	9 (4%)	6 (5%)	6 (0.2%)
Unspecified dizziness	1%	9%		32 (18%)	4 (2%)	4 (3%)	2283 (90%)
PPPD	8%	4%	114 (11%)				
Movement disorder/Motor delay	8%	4%		3 (2%)	3 (2%)	18 (14%)	

Abbreviations: BPPV, benign paroxysmal positional vertigo; BPTI, benign paroxysmal torticollis of infancy; BPVC, benign paroxysmal vertigo of childhood; CNS, central nervous system; PPPD-persistent postural-perceptual dizziness; TBI, traumatic brain injury.

[a] Diagnosis in patients reporting dizziness.
[b] Diagnosis in patients reporting imbalance.
[c] Raw sample, weighted projections used to estimate prevalence rates on national scale.

Behind headaches, dizziness and imbalance are the most common symptoms seen after concussion and have been found to predict a protracted recovery.[53–55] Dizziness ranges from imbalance to true vertigo. Often, the vestibular system is physiologically intact, but rather functional deficits are observed presumably owing to a central disruption of appropriate integration of afferent sensory information for clear vision and postural control.[56–58] However, there is evidence that peripheral vestibular dysfunction does occur in 25% of children with concussion and the most common peripheral finding is BPPV.[47] Furthermore, abnormalities with smooth pursuit, saccades and near-point convergence are also observed and have also been found to predict protracted recovery, which can help to direct rehabilitation needs, including physical therapy and/or vision therapy, in addition to adjustments at school.[55]

Dizziness has been found to be associated with OM[59] and OM is proposed to be among the most common causes of dizziness in young children.[17,60] However, OM is more frequent in young children whose ability to describe their symptoms is often limited; therefore, dizziness is not accurately documented[17] and vestibular function is not routinely assessed. Thus, it is difficult to determine if OM causes dizziness. Given the concomitant conductive hearing loss, vHIT is useful for assessing children with OM to identify potential vestibular deficits secondary to the OM.[61,62]

Vestibular disorders seen in adults can also be observed in children. BPPV is more common in older children and in children with other conditions such as concussion or vestibular migraine.[43,47] There is typically a triggering event. Like adults, the posterior semicircular canal is the most common canal involved and children often respond to 1 to 2 repositioning maneuvers; however, horizontal, superior, and multicanal involvement is more common in children than adults. Children with vestibular migraine have higher rates of recurrence.[47] Few pediatric patients develop vestibular neuritis and Meniere disease; thus, there is little evidence to support differences in treatment strategies for children compared with adults.

The etiology of dizziness in children varies based on age and location of evaluation (**Table 3**). In children presenting with dizziness in the emergency department, there was an increased incidence of central nervous system and infectious disease etiology in the youngest age group (preschool) compared with older children.[63] More than 1 vestibular disorder can occur in a single patient; therefore, it is important to be vigilant to assess for all potential contributions to the patient's symptoms to direct the appropriate management. In a retrospective review, one-half of pediatric patients receive 2 or more diagnoses, more often in children who are greater than 12 years of age. Vestibular migraine, BPPV, persistent postural–perceptual dizziness was the most common combination of diagnoses in children without trauma or concussion.[43] Age should be considered when determining etiology.

Brodsky and colleagues[2] completed an interview survey through the National Center for Health Statistics to identify the prevalence of pediatric dizziness. Parental report indicated that a large percentage of dizziness or imbalance was due to other health conditions (see **Table 2**). For the purposes of this review, we also included diagnoses of diabetes and low blood pressure under this heading. These diagnoses were provided by the parent report and may represent the difficulty in providing a definitive diagnosis and lack of expertise in the identification and management of pediatric vestibular disorders.[2]

AUDITORY AND VESTIBULAR DYSFUNCTION

There is a significant association between vestibular loss and sensorineural hearing loss. Children with greater severity of hearing loss are more likely to have vestibular

Table 3
Etiology of dizziness based on age

Preschool aged	Grasso[63] 2020 n (%)[a]	Sommerfleck[70] 2016 n (%)[b]	Lee[48] 2017 n (%)[c]
Total n	113	54	31
Age	≤6 year old	1–5 year olds	≤6 year old
PVC		16 (29.6%)	22 (70.9%)
Acute migraine or BPPV	16 (14.2%)	2 (3.7%)	VM- 6 (19.4%) BPPV- 1 (3.2%)
Vasovagal vertigo	8 (7.2%)		
Infectious disease	27 (23.8%)	4 (7.4%)	
Psychogenic	7 (6.2%)		1 (3.2%)
CNS	26 (23%)	16 (29.6%)	
Peripheral nervous system	4 (3.6%)	4 (7.4%)	
Post-traumatic	25 (3.3%)	6 (11.1%)	
Not classifiable vertigo	21 (18.5%)		
Other		6 (11.1%)	1 (3.2%)

Elementary school aged	Grasso[63] 2020 n (%)[a]	Sommerfleck[70] 2016 n (%)[b]	Lee[48] 2017 n (%)[c]	Wang[43] 2020 n (%)[d]
Total n	251	82	133	383
Age	7–12 y	6–11 y	7–12 y	<12 y
BPVC			40 (30.1%)	54 (14.1%)
Vestibular migraine or BPPV	49 (18.5%)	VM-28 (34.1%) BPPV- 1 (1.2%)	VM- 39 (29.3%) BPPV- 6 (4.5%)	VM- 83 (21.7%) BPPV- 52 (13.6%)
Psychogenic (includes anxiety, PPPD)	32 (12.7%)	4 (4.9%)	8 (6%)	39 (10.2%)
CNS	8 (3.1%)	5 (6.1%)		
Peripheral nervous system (vestibular neuritis, labyrinthitis)	6 (2.4%)	4 (4.9%)	6 (4.5%)	13 (3.4%)
Cardiogenic (orthostatic dizziness, vasovagal syncope)	53 (19.7%)	1 (1.2%)	5 (3.8%)	25 (6.5%)
Post-traumatic/concussion	6 (2.4%)	5 (6.1%)		36 (9.4%)
Infectious disease	42 (16.2%)			
Pharmacologic causes	2 (0.8%)			
Not classifiable vertigo	53 (21.1%)	10 (12.1%)		
Multiple			8 (6%)	
Others		24 (29.2%)	21 (15.8%)	

Adolescent aged	Grasso[63] 2020[a]	Sommerfleck[70] 2016[b]	Lee[48] 2017[c]	Wang[43] 2020[d]
Total n	393	70	247	638
Age	>12 y	12–18 y	13–18 y	≥12 y

(continued on next page)

Table 3
(continued)

	Grasso[63] 2020[a]	Sommerfleck[70] 2016[b]	Lee[48] 2017[c]	Wang[43] 2020[d]
BPVC			32 (12.9%)	4 (0.6%)
Vestibular migraine or BPPV	87 (22.2%)	VM- 20 (28.6%) BPPV- 7 (10%)	VM- 75 (30.5%) BPPV- 14 (5.7%)	VM-274 (42.9%) BPPV-169 (26.5%)
Psychogenic (includes anxiety, PPPD)	63 (16%)	6 (8.6%)	16 (6.5%)	213 (33.4%)
CNS	4 (1%)	9 (12.9%)		
Peripheral nervous system (vestibular neuritis, Meniere's disease)	22 (5.6%)	3 (4.3%)	52 (21%)	37 (5.8%)
Cardiogenic (orthostatic dizziness, vasovagal syncope)	79 (20.2%)	1 (1.4%)	33 (13.4%)	135 (21.2%)
Post-traumatic/concussion	16 (4.1%)	2 (2.9%)		228 (35.7%)
Infectious disease	57 (14.5%)			
Pharmacologic causes	4 (1%)			
Not classifiable vertigo	61 (15.5%)	4 (5.7%)		
Multiple			9 (3.6%)	
Others		18 (25.7%)	16 (6.5%)	

Abbreviations: BPPV, benign paroxysmal positional vertigo; BPVC, benign paroxysmal vertigo of childhood; CNS, central nervous system; PPPD, persistent postural-perceptual dizziness; VM, vestibular migraine.
[a] Children admitted to the emergency department.
[b] Children seen in otolaryngology department.
[c] Children seen at dizziness clinic.
[d] Children seen at pediatric balance and vestibular program.

loss.[15] In a retrospective review of audiometric and rotary chair findings, children with mild hearing loss did not have vestibular loss, whereas children with bilateral pure tone averages of more than 40 dB were found to have unilateral vestibular loss and those with bilateral puretone average of more than 66 dB were found to have bilateral vestibular loss.[15]

Specific conditions associated with sensorineural hearing loss such as congenital cytomegalovirus or auditory neuropathy spectrum disorder have reported concurrent vestibular dysfunction. A retrospective analysis demonstrated that 90% of patients with congenital cytomegalovirus have canal dysfunction and 86% have otolithic dysfunction; one-half of the patients had progressive vestibular deterioration over time.[64] Patients diagnosed with auditory neuropathy spectrum disorder had probable or definite vestibulopathy based on vestibular function testing in 43% of cases.[65] Anatomic anomalies, specifically enlarged vestibular aqueduct, are also associated with vestibular dysfunction. Although hearing loss is primarily the predominant symptom, more than one-half of patients may have vestibular symptoms.[66]

SUMMARY

Vestibular disorders occur in pediatric patients with potential impact on motor development, visual acuity and mental health. Vestibular testing is feasible and effective in pediatric patients with minor modifications. The differential diagnosis for pediatric dizziness is extensive. Increased awareness and further investigation in this area will help improve our diagnosis and management of children with dizziness.

CLINICS CARE POINTS

- The prevalence of imbalance or dizziness in childhood ranges from 0.45% to 15.0%.
- Children with dizziness can have delays in gross motor skills, visual acuity concerns, and psychological distress
- Vestibular testing is feasible and effective in pediatric patients
- The list of potential etiologies of dizziness in children is large and varies from common causes of dizziness in adults.

DISCLOSURE

The authors have no disclosures to report.

REFERENCES

1. O'Reilly RC, Morlet T, Nicholas BD, et al. Prevalence of vestibular and balance disorders in children. Otol Neurotol 2010;31:1441–4.
2. Brodsky JR, Lipson S, Bhattacharyya N. Prevalence of pediatric dizziness and imbalance in the United States. Otolaryngol Head Neck Surg 2020;162:241–7.
3. Russell G, Abu-Arafeh I. Paroxysmal vertigo in children–an epidemiological study. Int J Pediatr Otorhinolaryngol 1999;49(Suppl 1):S105–7.
4. Braswell J, Rine RM. Evidence that vestibular hypofunction affects reading acuity in children. Int J Pediatr Otorhinolaryngol 2006;70:1957–65.
5. Inoue A, Iwasaki S, Ushio M, et al. Effect of vestibular dysfunction on the development of gross motor function in children with profound hearing loss. Audiol Neurootol 2013;18:143–51.
6. Lee CH, Lee SB, Kim YJ, et al. Utility of psychological screening for the diagnosis of pediatric episodic vertigo. Otol Neurotol 2014;35:e324–30.
7. O'Reilly R, Grindle C, Zwicky EF, et al. Development of the vestibular system and balance function: differential diagnosis in the pediatric population. Otolaryngol Clin North Am 2011;44:251–71, vii.
8. Richard C, Laroche N, Malaval L, et al. New insight into the bony labyrinth: a microcomputed tomography study. Auris Nasus Larynx 2010;37:155–61.
9. Jeffery N, Spoor F. Prenatal growth and development of the modern human labyrinth. J Anat 2004;204:71–92.
10. Wright CG, Hubbard DG. SEM observations on development of human otoconia during the first trimester of gestation. Acta Otolaryngol 1982;94:7–18.
11. Eviatar L, Eviatar A. The normal nystagmic response of infants to caloric and per-rotatory stimulation. Laryngoscope 1979;89:1036–45.
12. Ornitz EM, Kaplan AR, Westlake JR. Development of the vestibulo-ocular reflex from infancy to adulthood. Acta Otolaryngol 1985;100:180–93.
13. Valente M. Maturational effects of the vestibular system: a study of rotary chair, computerized dynamic posturography, and vestibular evoked myogenic potentials with children. J Am Acad Audiol 2007;18:461–81.
14. Kelsch TA, Schaefer LA, Esquivel CR. Vestibular evoked myogenic potentials in young children: test parameters and normative data. Laryngoscope 2006;116:895–900.

15. Janky KL, Thomas MLA, High RR, et al. Predictive factors for vestibular loss in children with hearing loss. Am J Audiol 2018;27:137–46.

16. Janky KL, Givens D. Vestibular, visual acuity, and balance outcomes in children with cochlear implants: a preliminary report. Ear Hear 2015;36:e364–72.

17. McCaslin DL, Jacobson GP, Lambert W, et al. The development of the Vanderbilt pediatric dizziness handicap inventory for patient caregivers (DHI-PC). Int J Pediatr Otorhinolaryngol 2015;79:1662–6.

18. Pavlou M, Whitney S, Alkathiry AA, et al. The pediatric vestibular symptom questionnaire: a validation study. J Pediatr 2016;168:171–7.e1.

19. Janky KL, Rodriguez AI. Quantitative vestibular function testing in the pediatric population. Semin Hear 2018;39:257–74.

20. Colebatch JG, Halmagyi GM, Skuse NF. Myogenic potentials generated by a click-evoked vestibulocollic reflex. J Neurol Neurosurg Psychiatry 1994;57:190–7.

21. Bogle JM, Zapala DA, Criter R, et al. The effect of muscle contraction level on the cervical vestibular evoked myogenic potential (cVEMP): usefulness of amplitude normalization. J Am Acad Audiol 2013;24:77–88.

22. McCaslin DL, Fowler A, Jacobson GP. Amplitude normalization reduces cervical vestibular evoked myogenic potential (cVEMP) amplitude asymmetries in normal subjects: proof of concept. J Am Acad Audiol 2014;25:268–77.

23. Rosengren SM, McAngus Todd NP, Colebatch JG. Vestibular-evoked extraocular potentials produced by stimulation with bone-conducted sound. Clin Neurophysiol 2005;116:1938–48.

24. Todd NP, Rosengren SM, Aw ST, et al. Ocular vestibular evoked myogenic potentials (OVEMPs) produced by air- and bone-conducted sound. Clin Neurophysiol 2007;118:381–90.

25. Govender S, Rosengren SM, Colebatch JG. The effect of gaze direction on the ocular vestibular evoked myogenic potential produced by air-conducted sound. Clin Neurophysiol 2009;120:1386–91.

26. Sheykholeslami K, Megerian CA, Arnold JE, et al. Vestibular-evoked myogenic potentials in infancy and early childhood. Laryngoscope 2005;115:1440–4.

27. Wang SJ, Hsieh WS, Young YH. Development of ocular vestibular-evoked myogenic potentials in small children. Laryngoscope 2013;123:512–7.

28. Rodriguez AI, Thomas MLA, Fitzpatrick D, et al. Effects of high sound exposure during air-conducted vestibular evoked myogenic potential testing in children and young adults. Ear Hear 2018;39:269–77.

29. Thomas MLA, Fitzpatrick D, McCreery R, et al. Big stimulus, little ears: safety in administering vestibular-evoked myogenic potentials in children. J Am Acad Audiol 2017;28:395–403.

30. Rodriguez AI, Thomas MLA, Janky KL. Air-conducted vestibular evoked myogenic potential testing in children, adolescents, and young adults: thresholds, frequency tuning, and effects of sound exposure. Ear Hear 2019;40: 192–203.

31. Fuemmeler E, Rodriguez AI, Thomas M, et al. Vestibular evoked myogenic potential (VEMP) test-retest reliability in children. Otol Neurotol 2020;41:e1052–9.

32. Greenwalt NL, Patterson JN, Rodriguez AI, et al. Bone conduction vibration vestibular evoked myogenic potential (VEMP) testing: reliability in children, adolescents, and young adults. Ear Hear 2020;42:355–63.

33. Janky KL, Patterson J, Shepard N, et al. Video head impulse test (VHIT): the role of corrective saccades in identifying patients with vestibular loss. Otol Neurotol 2018;39:467–73.

34. Wiener-Vacher SR, Wiener SI. Video head impulse tests with a remote camera system: normative values of semicircular canal vestibulo-ocular reflex gain in infants and children. Front Neurol 2017;8:434.
35. Ross LM, Helminski JO. Test-retest and interrater reliability of the video head impulse test in the pediatric population. Otol Neurotol 2016;37:558–63.
36. Hulse R, Hormann K, Servais JJ, et al. Clinical experience with video head impulse test in children. Int J Pediatr Otorhinolaryngol 2015;79:1288–93.
37. Staller SJ, Goin DW, Hildebrandt M. Pediatric vestibular evaluation with harmonic acceleration. Otolaryngol Head Neck Surg 1986;95:471–6.
38. Casselbrant ML, Furman JM, Mandel EM, et al. Past history of otitis media and balance in four-year-old children. Laryngoscope 2000;110:773–8.
39. Janky KL, Shepard NT. Pediatric vestibular testing. In: Jacobson S, Barin B, Janky MC, editors. Balance function assessment and management. 3rd ed. San Diego, CA: Plural Publishing; 2019. p. 457–77.
40. Levens SL. Electronystagmography in normal children. Br J Audiol 1988;22:51–6.
41. Bucci MP, Seassau M. Saccadic eye movements in children: a developmental study. Exp Brain Res 2012;222:21–30.
42. D'Agostino R, Melagrana A, Pasquale G, et al. The study of optokinetic 'look' nystagmus in children: our experience. Int J Pediatr Otorhinolaryngol 1997;40:141–6.
43. Wang A, Zhou G, Lipson S, et al. Multifactorial characteristics of pediatric dizziness and imbalance. Laryngoscope 2021;131:E1308–14.
44. Brodsky JR, Cusick BA, Zhou G. Evaluation and management of vestibular migraine in children: experience from a pediatric vestibular clinic. Eur J Paediatr Neurol 2016;20:85–92.
45. O'Reilly RC, Greywoode J, Morlet T, et al. Comprehensive vestibular and balance testing in the dizzy pediatric population. Otolaryngol Head Neck Surg 2011;144:142–8.
46. Headache Classification Committee of the International Headache Society. The International Classification of Headache Disorders, 3rd edition (beta version). Cephalalgia 2013;33:629–808.
47. Brodsky J, Kaur K, Shoshany T, et al. Benign paroxysmal migraine variants of infancy and childhood: transitions and clinical features. Eur J Paediatr Neurol 2018;22:667–73.
48. Lee JD, Kim CH, Hong SM, et al. Prevalence of vestibular and balance disorders in children and adolescents according to age: a multi-center study. Int J Pediatr Otorhinolaryngol 2017;94:36–9.
49. van de Berg R, Widdershoven J, Bisdorff A, et al. Vestibular migraine of childhood and recurrent vertigo of childhood: diagnostic criteria consensus document of the Committee for the Classification of Vestibular Disorders of the Barany Society and the International Headache Society. J Vestib Res 2021;31:1–9.
50. Rodriguez-Villalba R, Caballero-Borrego M, Villarraga V, et al. Vestibulo-ocular reflex assessed with video head impulse test in children with vestibular migraine: our experience. Int J Pediatr Otorhinolaryngol 2020;137:110161.
51. Langhagen T, Landgraf MN, Huppert D, et al. Vestibular migraine in children and adolescents. Curr Pain Headache Rep 2016;20:67.
52. Richer L, Billinghurst L, Linsdell MA, et al. Drugs for the acute treatment of migraine in children and adolescents. Cochrane Database Syst Rev 2016;4:CD005220.
53. Eisenberg MA, Meehan WP 3rd, Mannix R. Duration and course of post-concussive symptoms. Pediatrics 2014;133:999–1006.

54. Guerriero RM, Proctor MR, Mannix R, et al. Epidemiology, trends, assessment and management of sport-related concussion in United States high schools. Curr Opin Pediatr 2012;24:696–701.

55. Master CL, Master SR, Wiebe DJ, et al. Vision and vestibular system dysfunction predicts prolonged concussion recovery in children. Clin J Sport Med 2018;28: 139–45.

56. Guskiewicz KM. Balance assessment in the management of sport-related concussion. Clin Sports Med 2011;30:89–102, ix.

57. Reed-Jones RJ, Murray NG, Powell DW. Clinical assessment of balance in adults with concussion. Semin Speech Lang 2014;35:186–95.

58. Zhou G, Brodsky JR. Objective vestibular testing of children with dizziness and balance complaints following sports-related concussions. Otolaryngol Head Neck Surg 2015;152:1133–9.

59. Schaaf RC. The frequency of vestibular disorders in developmentally delayed preschoolers with otitis media. Am J Occup Ther 1985;39:247–52.

60. Koyuncu M, Saka MM, Tanyeri Y, et al. Effects of otitis media with effusion on the vestibular system in children. Otolaryngol Head Neck Surg 1999;120:117–21.

61. Fujiwara K, Morita S, Fukuda A, et al. Usefulness of the video head impulse test for the evaluation of vestibular function in patients with otitis media with antineutrophil cytoplasmic antibody-associated vasculitis. Otol Neurotol 2021;42: e483–8.

62. Comert E, Sencan Z, Kocak FM, et al. Clinical evaluation of the vestibular impairment using video head impulse test in children with acute otitis media. Int J Pediatr Otorhinolaryngol 2021;141:110568.

63. Grasso A, Poropat F, Kamagni Vodie T, et al. How age matters in the assessment of vertigo in the pediatric emergency department: a 10-year age-stratified etiology survey. Pediatr Emerg Care 2020.

64. Bernard S, Wiener-Vacher S, Van Den Abbeele T, et al. Vestibular disorders in children with congenital cytomegalovirus infection. Pediatrics 2015;136:e887–95.

65. Nash R, Veness J, Wyatt M, et al. Vestibular function in children with auditory neuropathy spectrum disorder. Int J Pediatr Otorhinolaryngol 2014;78:1269–73.

66. Song JJ, Hong SK, Lee SY, et al. Vestibular manifestations in subjects with enlarged vestibular aqueduct. Otol Neurotol 2018;39:e461–7.

67. Gerber RJ, Wilks T, Erdie-Lalena C. Developmental milestones: motor development. Pediatr Rev 2010;31:267–76, quiz 277.

68. Syed MI, Rutka JA, Sharma A, et al. The 'dizzy child': a 12-minute consultation. Clin Otolaryngol 2014;39:228–34.

69. Ciolek PJ, Kang E, Honaker JA, et al. Pediatric vestibular testing: tolerability of test components in children. Int J Pediatr Otorhinolaryngol 2018;113:29–33.

70. Sommerfleck PA, Gonzalez Macchi ME, Weinschelbaum R, et al. Balance disorders in childhood: Main etiologies according to age. Usefulness of the video head impulse test. Int J Pediatr Otorhinolaryngol 2016;87:148–53.

The Neuropsychology of Dizziness and Related Disorders

Shin C. Beh, MD

KEYWORDS

• Vertigo • Dizziness • Cognition • Anxiety • Depression • Mood

KEY POINTS

- The vestibular system plays an important role in cognition, particularly visuospatial abilities such as self-motion perception, spatial learning, spatial memory, and body image awareness.
- There is a reciprocal relationship between vestibular and psychiatric disorders. The incidence of psychiatric disorders is higher among people with vertigo/dizziness, and vice versa.
- The psychiatric and cognitive impact of vestibular disorders results in significant impact on sufferers' quality of life and job productivity.

INTRODUCTION

The relationship between vertigo/dizziness, psychiatric disorders, and cognitive dysfunction has been recognized for millennia. Classical Greek words for vertigo also carried additional connotations of mental agitation and gloom; furthermore, ancient medical texts also associated vertigo and dizziness with melancholia, mania, anxiety, and a tendency to "madness."[1]

Compared with the general population, the incidence of depression, anxiety, and panic is much higher among people with vestibular disorders (ranging from 20% to over two-thirds).[2–15] There is a two-way ("chicken-and-egg") relationship between vestibular and psychiatric disorders. People suffering from vertigo and dizziness are at higher risk of depression, anxiety, and panic.[2,4,6–11] By the same token, people with psychiatric disorders such as anxiety, panic, depression, and obsessive-compulsive disorder are at higher risk of experiencing vertigo/dizziness.[12–14] A functioning peripheral vestibular system may be important in the development of anxiety. People with bilateral vestibular failure (BVF) have a much lower incidence of anxiety even though they suffer from significant balance difficulties, vertigo,

Department of Neurology, Vestibular & Neuro-Visual Disorders Clinic, University of Texas Southwestern Medical Center at Dallas, 5323 Harry Hines Boulevard, Dallas, TX 75390, USA
E-mail address: scjbeh@gmail.com

Otolaryngol Clin N Am 54 (2021) 989–997
https://doi.org/10.1016/j.otc.2021.05.016
oto.theclinics.com

dizziness, and oscillopsia.[16] However, there remains a high incidence of depression and reduced quality of life in BVF.[17] Furthermore, vestibular stimulation can alter the mood[18]; the influence of vestibular stimulation on mood is not necessarily negative but may be beneficial.[19] On the other hand, anxiety and depression can influence vestibular responses, by altering the duration of caloric responses, the severity of directional preponderance, and slow-phase velocity of the vestibulo-ocular reflex.[20–22]

PATHOPHYSIOLOGICAL CORRELATES

A neurobiological explanation underlies the close relationship between vestibular and psychiatric disorders, specifically the interconnections between limbic, autonomic, and vestibular centers.[14] The parabrachial nucleus (PBN) plays a key role in conditioned fear and anxiety responses and interoception.[23–25] The PBN connects vestibular and emotion processing centers, sharing reciprocal connections between the vestibular nuclei, central amygdaloid nucleus, thalamus (midline and intralaminar nuclei), hypothalamus, and infralimbic cortex.[14] Other brainstem loci that are interconnected with the vestibular nuclei and play key roles in psychiatric conditions include the locus coeruleus, nucleus subcoeruleus, and raphe nuclei. The vestibular nuclei receive noradrenergic projections from the locus coeruleus and nucleus subcoeruleus.[26,27] The densest projections supply the superior and lateral vestibular nuclei, and the rostral nucleus prepositus hypoglossi.[14] Serotonergic input to the vestibular nuclei arises from the dorsal raphe nuclei and nuclei raphe pallidus and obscurus.[28] One-quarter of dorsal raphe nuclei projections to the vestibular nuclei ascend to the amygdala, indicating coordinated serotonergic modulation of vestibular and central amygdaloid nuclei in dizziness-related anxiety.[14] These serotonergic and noradrenergic pathways not only support the link between vertigo/dizziness and psychiatric disorders but also explain why antidepressant therapies are effective for a variety of vestibular disorders.

IMPACT ON QUALITY OF LIFE

The prevalence of psychiatric disorders among people with vestibular disorders can also be attributed to the impact of vertigo/dizziness on various aspects of patients' lives. The impact of vertigo/dizziness on quality of life correlates with greater anxiety levels.[29] Among people with vestibular disorders, 50% report reduced work productivity, 27% changed jobs, and 21% quit their jobs because of the impact of vertigo/dizziness.[30] Furthermore, vertigo/dizziness disrupted social activities in 57% and impacted family life in 35%.[30] Illness uncertainty may also account for the prevalence of psychiatric disorders in people with vertigo/dizziness. Illness uncertainty is defined as the perception of the ambiguities surrounding an illness and is associated with a heavy emotional toll in chronic illnesses.[31] Illness intrusiveness is also another factor responsible for the higher psychiatric comorbid burden among people with vertigo/dizziness. Illness intrusiveness refers to how illness and its treatment(s) interferes with one's valued activities and interests and correlates with anxiety and depression.[31] Unsurprisingly, illness intrusiveness is greater in unpredictable diseases, such as vestibular migraine and Meniere's disease.[31] A recent study found vertigo more intrusive than 33 out of 37 chronic illnesses, including multiple sclerosis, laryngeal cancer, rheumatoid arthritis, and end-stage renal disease.[31] Vertigo was only surpassed by HIV, fibromyalgia, anxiety disorders, and chronic fatigue syndrome/myalgic encephalomyelitis.[31]

PERSISTENT POSTURAL PERCEPTUAL DIZZINESS

Persistent postural-perceptual dizziness (PPPD)[32] is a disorder that underscores the intimate relationship between anxiety and dizziness. PPPD is characterized by pervasive dizziness, unsteadiness, and/or nonspinning vertigo, that may wax and wane, and is aggravated by upright posture, motion, and visual stimuli.[33] This disorder is usually triggered by conditions that manifest with vertigo/dizziness, medical illness, or emotional stressors. The symptoms can last for months or even years and be highly disabling. Neuroimaging in PPPD reveals reduced connectivity from the left hippocampus (which controls egocentric spatial navigation) to multiple regions, increased connections between the frontal and occipital cortices (indicating greater reliance on visual cues for balance), diminished dominant vestibular hemispheric activity (with decreased connectivity with frontal regulatory areas, visual cortices, and the hippocampus), and failure to activate the central insular sulcus (responsible for resolving motion trajectories in gravity) when presented with visual motion.[33,34] Default-mode network abnormalities are also present in PPPD, involving regions that also regulate emotional processing, self-referential mental activity, and recollection of previous experiences.[35]

Freud observed that some patients' focus on specific somatic symptoms during anxiety attacks formed the basis of the psychodynamic formulation of psychogenic dizziness as either a symptom associated with anxiety, or an anxiety equivalent (ie, the manifestation of anxiety such as dizziness, without the conscious perception of anxiety).[36] However, it is important to point out that PPPD is not just a somatoform condition (ie, an anxiety equivalent) but a complex and underdiagnosed otoneuropsychiatric disorder that underscores the complicated interconnected relationship between anxiety and dizziness. Individuals with neurotic temperaments, or pre-existing anxiety disorders, are at higher risk for developing PPPD,[33] supporting observations that those with anxiety and obsessive-compulsive disorder are more vulnerable to dizziness.[14] Even though PPPD symptoms improve with antidepressants and cognitive behavioral therapy, these improvements may occur independent of mood changes and at antidepressant doses lower than that used for anxiety or depression.[33] In addition, anxiety alters vestibular responses,[20,21] and anxious people have more difficulty with multisensory integration, resulting in overreliance on visual cues, and the fear of falling (or space and motion discomfort).[37–39] Visual, vestibular, and proprioceptive cues are often processed subconsciously and, as such, may trigger fear or anxiety without a person being aware of the provoking cues.[14] In PPPD and anxiety, patients demonstrate heightened vigilance and a fear or anxiety of bodily sensations and thoughts related to anxiety.[40,41] Therefore, because vestibular sensations such as palpitations, nausea, and vague visceral sensations also occur in anxiety and panic disorders,[14] the hypervigilance to, and misinterpretation of, interoceptive vestibular sensations often leads to anxiety, or a fear of being anxious.

MAL DE DEBARQUEMENT SYNDROME

Mal de debarquement syndrome (MDDS)[42] is an underdiagnosed condition characterized by a pervasive rocking, swaying, or bobbing motion that begins after prolonged exposure to passive motion (eg, being on a ship) but persists even after returning to an earth-stable environment.[43] One unique characteristic of MDDS is that the persistent illusory motion subsides temporarily when the patient is re-exposed to passive motion (eg, being in a car, boat, or plane)[43]; this distinct feature separates it from PPPD, which tends to be aggravated by passive motion.[33] MDDS could arguably be considered a disorder of higher vestibular function that affects motion perception. An intriguing explanation for MDDS is dysfunctional central velocity storage mechanisms generating a persistent memory of an internal representation of motion.[44] Indeed, gray matter changes are observed in the visual-vestibular processing region, default mode network, somatosensory network, and central executive areas.[45] The incidence of anxiety and depression is high in people with MDDS, particularly those with coexisting vestibular migraine.[43,46] It is associated with high levels of illness intrusiveness and diminished quality of life.[47,48] MDDS also responds favorably to antidepressant therapy.[43]

COGNITIVE EFFECTS AND VISUOSPATIAL ORIENTATION

Many cognitive impairments occur in vestibular disorders, including dysfunctions of learning, memory, executive function, and visuospatial ability.[7,9,42,49–52] People with vertigo have a 3.9-fold increased risk of suffering limitation of activities due to memory difficulties.[7] Those with vertigo are 8.3-times more likely to endorse "serious difficulty concentrating, remembering, or making decisions."[7] While depression, anxiety, and panic account for 32% of the effect of vertigo on cognition,[7] the relationship between cognition and the vestibular system extends beyond the impact of vertigo/dizziness on mood.

The vestibular system plays an important role in cognition, particularly self-motion perception, interoception, body image awareness, social cognition, processing speed, spatial navigation, spatial learning, spatial memory, motivation, numerical cognition, and object recognition.[53,54] Of particular interest, the vestibular system plays a central role in visuospatial cognition. Vestibular cortical regions important in spatial cognition include the parietoinsular vestibular cortex, anterior parietal cortex, posterior parietal cortex, medial superior temporal cortex, cingulate gyrus, retrosplenial cortex, and hippocampal and parahippocampal cortices.[53,54] The pathways involved in vestibular cognition include (1) vestibulo-thalamo-cortical pathway, which conveys spatial information to the hippocampus, and are associated with spatial representations and distinguishing self-versus-object motion; (2) the dorsal tegmental nucleus-lateral mammillary nucleus-thalamic anterodorsal nucleus-entorhinal cortex pathway which conveys head-direction information; (3) the nucleus reticularis pontis oralis-supramammillary nucleus-hippocampal medial septum pathway which carries information for hippocampal theta rhythm and memory; (4) the cerebellum-thalamic ventral lateral nucleus-parietal cortex pathway, which mediates spatial learning; and (5) the vestibulo-basal ganglial-hippocampal pathway.[53]

Constant, real-time vestibular and visual information is needed for spatial navigation to provide an accurate representation of a person's location and movement within a 3D environment. Accordingly, visuospatial ability is impaired in vestibular dysfunction, particularly in BVF.[9,54–58] Attesting to the importance of the vestibular system in spatial memory and navigation, BVF patients demonstrate structural and functional changes in the hippocampus, mirroring their navigational and visuospatial deficits.[54] Such changes do not occur with unilateral vestibular loss.[59] The impact of BVF on cognition indicates that peripheral vestibular disorders, and not just central vestibular disorders, can lead to neuropsychological deficits.

Vestibular input influences the processing of information that is typically represented in a specific spatial order. For example, as numbers of lesser value are represented on the left and larger values on the right, alterations in vestibular information can affect the generation of numbers. Turning the head to the left facilitates the random generation of smaller numbers.[19] Rotating the body to the left and downward improved small number generation; rotating the body to the right and upward improves large number generation.[60,61] Climbing stairs or going up an elevator improved the ability to perform additions; descending stairs or an elevator improved the ability to perform subtractions.[62] Similarly, vestibular input can influence the perception of one's mental time line, where past events are associated with the left or moving backwards, and future events with the right or moving forwards.[19] Contemplating the past is accompanied by backward sway, and forward sway with thinking about the future.[63] Processing speed of future-oriented words increases with forward, versus backward, passive whole-body movement.[19] These fascinating effects are most likely due to the shift in spatial attention in the direction of motion; leftward rotation facilitates perception of visual and tactile information on the left, and vice versa.[19] Altering vestibular input or rotating body position can impact how a person mentally manipulates objects or their body parts.[19] Cognitive processes can also alter the perception of vestibular information. Imagining whole-body rotations can produce corresponding nystagmus.[64] Visualizing motion also alters the perception of horizontal or vertical.[65,66]

DISORDERS OF HIGHER VESTIBULAR FUNCTION

Disorders of higher vestibular function include pusher syndrome, hemispatial neglect, topographagnosia, and room-tilt illusion.[59] Hemispatial neglect arises from impaired awareness of visual stimuli in the egocentric hemifield contralateral to an acute right temporoparietal insult, usually affecting the right superior temporal cortex and insula.[54] Patients with hemispatial neglect have intact visual fields but direct their spatial attention and corresponding head-eye movements to the ipsilesional visual field, ignoring all stimuli in the contralateral hemifield.[59] Interestingly, right vestibular stimulation in those with right hemispheric lesions improves hemispatial neglect,[67,68] particularly when combined with left neck muscle vibration.[69] Similarly, vestibular stimulation effectively attenuates disorders of body representation, including hemianesthesia, somatoparaphrenia, phantom limb sensations, and macrosomatognosia.[19]

Pusher syndrome is characterized by a tendency of an acute stroke patient to actively push the body to the hemiparetic (ie, contralesional) side with the intact arm and leg; infarcts involving the posterior insula and thalamus are usually to blame.[54,59] Pusher syndrome and hemispatial neglect usually arise from right-sided lesions in right-handers, attesting to the effect of vestibular hemispheric dominance.[54] Room-tilt illusion causes paroxysmal 180-degree or 90-degree tilts of the visual environment. It results from cortical dysfunction of vestibular-vestibular interaction, resulting in a mismatch between the visual and vestibular perception of verticality; it is usually due to subcortical vestibular lesions, at the level of the brainstem or periphery, but manifests with visual symptoms.[54,59]

The ability to orient oneself requires not only real-time visuospatial information but also recollection of previously acquired environmental information.[70] This previously acquired information can be represented as landmarks ("beacons" in the environment), route (memory of paths that connect the landmarks, organized according to an egocentric frame of reference), and survey (a map-like representation of the environment encoding directions and distances between landmarks regardless of one's location).[70] Topographagnosia (or topographic disorientation) refers to the inability to orient to one's surroundings. It can be categorized as (1) egocentric disorientation (inability to represent locations of objects in relationship to oneself); (2) heading disorientation (inability to derive directional information from landmarks); (3) landmark agnosia (difficulty recognizing and using landmarks for navigation); and (4) anterograde disorientation (navigational deficits limited to novel environments).[71] Most cases are associated with left-sided visual field deficits. Lesions that cause topographic disorientation are usually localized to the right temporal or occipital lobes.[71] Right hippocampal or parahippocampal lesions may also cause topographagnosia,[71] most likely by disrupting access to previously acquired environmental information.

SUMMARY

In summary, the neuropsychiatric and cognitive effects of vertigo and dizziness are a critical component of the debility experienced by people with vestibular disorders. There is a reciprocal relationship between vertigo/dizziness and psychiatric disorders; people with vertigo/dizziness are at higher risk of mood disorders, and vice versa. Vestibular input also influences cognitive abilities, particularly visuo-spatial skills. Centrally, supratentorial lesions result in disorders of higher vestibular function, such as pusher syndrome and hemispatial neglect. Peripherally, BVF impairs visuospatial ability and hippocampal atrophy. Of note, the peripheral and central dichotomy is somewhat simplistic; peripheral vestibular disorders such as Meniere's disease, benign paroxysmal positional vertigo, and vestibular neuritis can cause central conditions such as PPPD. It is essential for clinicians to be aware of the psychiatric and cognitive impact of vertigo/dizziness when treating people with vestibular disorders.

CLINICS CARE POINTS

- Recognizing the existence of psychiatric comorbidities among people with vertigo/dizziness is vital to proper care.
- Cognitive impairment in people with vertigo/dizziness can be due to the impact of psychiatric disorders, but vestibular input plays an important role in cognitive skills as well.

DISCLOSURE

The author has nothing to disclose.

REFERENCES

1. Balaban CD, Jacob RG. Background and history of the interface between anxiety and vertigo. J Anxiety Disord 2001;15:27–51.
2. Eagger S, Luxon LM, Davies RA, et al. Psychiatric morbidity in patients with peripheral vestibular disorder: a clinical and neuro-otological study. J Neurol Neurosurg Psychiatry 1992;55:383–7.
3. Grunfeld EA, Gresty MA, Bronstein AM. Screening for depression among neuro-otology patients with and without identifiable vestibular lesions. Int J Audiol 2003; 42:161–5.
4. Godemann F, Linden M, Neu P, et al. A prospective study on the course of anxiety after vestibular neuronitis. J Psychosom Res 2004;56:351–4.
5. Ketola S, Havia M, Appelberg B, et al. Depressive symptoms underestimated in vertiginous patients. Otolaryngol Head Neck Surg 2007;137:312–5.
6. Eckhardt-Henn A, Best C, Bense S, et al. Psychiatric comorbidity in different organic vertigo syndromes. J Neurol 2008;255:420–8.
7. Bigelow RT, Semenov YR, du Lac S, et al. Vestibular vertigo and comorbid cognitive and psychiatric impairment: the 2008 National Health Interview Survey. J Neurol Neurosurg Psychiatry 2016;87:367–72.

8. Garcia FV, Coelho MH, Figueira ML. Psychological manifestations of vertigo: a pilot prospective observational study in a Portuguese population. Int Tinnitus J 2003;9:42–7.
9. Guidetti G, Monzani D, Trebbi M, et al. Impaired navigation skills in patients with psychological distress and chronic peripheral vestibular hypofunction without vertigo. Acta Otorhinolaryngol Ital 2008;28:21–5.
10. Gazzola JM, Aratani MC, Doná F, et al. Factors relating to depressive symptoms among elderly people with chronic vestibular dysfunction. Arq Neuropsiquiatr 2009;67:416–22.
11. Lahmann C, Henningsen P, Brandt T, et al. Psychiatric comorbidity and psychosocial impairment among patients with vertigo and dizziness. J Neurol Neurosurg Psychiatry 2014;86:302–8.
12. Teggi R, Caldirol D, Colombo B, et al. Dizziness, migrainous vertigo and psychiatric disorders. J Laryngol Otol 2010;24:285–90.
13. Staab JP, Ruckenstein MJ. Which comes first? Psychogenic dizziness versus otogenic anxiety. Laryngoscope 2003;113:1714–8.
14. Coelho CM, Balaban CD. Visuo-vestibular contributions to anxiety and fear. Neurosci Biobehav Rev 2015;48:148–59.
15. Beh SC, Masrour S, Smith SV, et al. The spectrum of vestibular migraine: clinical features, triggers, and examination findings. Headache 2019;59:727–40.
16. Decker J, Limburg K, Henningsen P, et al. Intact vestibular function is relevant for anxiety related to vertigo. J Neurol 2019;266:89–92.
17. Lucieer F, Duijn s, Van Rompaey V, et al. Full spectrum of reported symptoms of bilateral vestibulopathy needs further investigation – a systematic review. Front Neurol 2018;9:352.
18. Preuss N, Hasler G, Mast FW. Caloric vestibular stimulation modulates affective control and mood. Brain Stimul 2014;7:133–40.
19. Mast FW, Preuss N, Hartmann M, et al. Spatial cognition, body representation and affective processes: the role of vestibular information beyond ocular reflexes and control of posture. Front Integr Neurosci 2014;8:44.
20. Hallpike C, Harrison M, Slater E. Abnormalities of the caloric test results in certain varieties of mental disorder. Acta Oto-Laryngol 1951;39:151–9.
21. Yardley L, Masson E, Verschuur C, et al. Symptoms, anxiety and handicap in dizzy patients: development of the vertigo symptom scale. J Psychosom Res 1992;36:731–41.
22. Ried AMS, Aviles M. Asymmetries of vestibular dysfunction in major depression. Neuroscience 2007;144:128–34.
23. Charney DS, Deutch A. A functional neuroanatomy of anxiety and fear: implications for the pathophysiology and treatment of anxiety disorders. Crit Rev Neurobiol 1996;10:3–4.
24. Goddard AW, Charney DS. Toward an integrated neurobiology of panic disorder. J Clin Psychiatry 1997;58:4–11.
25. Gauriau C, Bernard JF. Pain pathways and parabrachial circuits in the rat. Exp Physiol 2002;87:251–8.
26. Schuerger RJ, Balaban CD. Immunohistochemical demonstration of regionally selective projections from locus coeruleus to the vestibular nuclei in rats. Exp Brain Res 1993;92:351–9.
27. Schuerger RJ, Balaban CD. Organization of the coeruleo-vestibular pathway in rats, rabbits, and monkeys. Brain Res Rev 1999;30:189–217.
28. Halberstadt A, Balaban C. Organization of projections from the raphe nuclei to the vestibular nuclei in rats. Neuroscience 2003;120:573–94.

29. Erlandsson SL, Eriksson-Mangold M, Weinberg A. Meniere's Disease: trauma, distress and adaptation studied through interview analyses. Scand Audiol 1996;25:45–56.

30. Bronstein AM, Golding JF, Gresty MA. The social impact of dizziness in London and Siena. J Neurol 2010;257:183–90.

31. Arroll M, Dancey CP, Attree EA, et al. People with symptoms of Meniere's disease: the relationship between illness intrusiveness, illness uncertainty, dizziness handicap, and depression. Otol Neurotol 2012;33:816–23.

32. Staab JP, Eckhardt-Henn A, Horii A, et al. Diagnostic criteria for persistent postural-perceptual dizziness (PPPD): Consensus document of the committee for the Classification of Vestibular Disorders of the Bárány Society. J Vestib Res 2017;27(4):191–208.

33. Staab J. Persistent postural-perceptual dizziness. Semin Neurol 2020;40:130–7.

34. Popp P, zu Eulenberg P, Stephan T, et al. Cortical alterations in phobic postural vertigo – a multimodal imaging approach. Ann Clin Transl Neurol 2018;5:717–29.

35. Huber J, Flanagin AL, Popp P, et al. Network changes in patients with phobic postural vertigo. Brain Behav 2020;10:e01622.

36. Magnusson PA, Nilsson A, Hendriksson NG. Psychogenic vertigo with an anxiety frame of reference: an experimental study. Br J Med Psychol 1977;50:187–201.

37. Yardley L, Luxon L, Lear S, et al. Vestibular and posturographic test results in people with symptoms of panic and agoraphobia. J Audiol Med 1994;3:48–65.

38. Jacob RG, Furman JM, Durrant JD, et al. Surface dependence: a balance control strategy in panic disorder with agoraphobia. Psychosom Med 1997;59:323–30.

39. Viaud-Delmon I, Berthoz A, Jouvent R. Multisensory integration for spatial orientation in trait anxiety subjects: absence of visual dependence. Eur Psychiatry 2002;17:194–9.

40. Heinrichs N, Edler C, Eskens S, et al. Predicting continued dizziness after an acute peripheral vestibular disorder. Psychosom Med 2007;69:700–7.

41. Trinidade A, Harman P, Stone J, et al. Assessment of potential risk factors for the development of persistent postural-perceptual dizziness: a case-control pilot study. Front Neurol 2021;11:601883.

42. Cha YH, Baloh RW, Cho C, et al. Mal de débarquement syndrome diagnostic criteria: Consensus document of the Classification Committee of the Bárány Society. J Vestib Res 2020;30(5):285–93.

43. Claessen MHG, van der Ham IJM. Classification of navigation impairment: a systematic review of neuropsychological case studies. Neurosci Biobehav Rev 2017;73:81–97.

44. Van Ombergen A, Van Rompaey V, Maes LK, et al. Mal de debarquement syndrome: a systematic review. J Neurol 2016;263:843–54.

45. Moeller L, Lempert T. Mal de debarquement: pseudo-hallucinations from vestibular memory? J Neurol 2007;254:813–5.

46. Cha YH, Chakrapani S. Voxel based morphometry alterations in Mal de debarquement syndrome. PLoS One 2015;10:e0135021.

47. Beh SC, Chiang HS, Sanderson C. The interconnections of mal de debarquement syndrome and vestibular migraine. Laryngoscope 2021;131(5):E1653–61.

48. Arroll MA, Attree EA, Cha YH, et al. The relationship between symptom severity, stigma, illness intrusiveness and depression in Mal de Debarquement syndrome. J Health Psychol 2016;21:1339–50.

49. Ayres AJ. Learning Disabilities and the Vestibular System. J Learn Disabil 1978;11:18–29.

50. Byl NN, Byl FM, Rosenthal JH. Interaction of spatial perception, vestibular function, and exercise in young school age boys with learning disabilities. Percept Mot Skills 1989;68:727–38.
51. Grimm RJ, Hemenway WG, Lebray PR, et al. The perilymph fistula syndrome defined in mild head trauma. Acta Otolaryngol Suppl 1989;464:1–40.
52. Risey J, Briner W. Dyscalculia in patients with vertigo. J Vestib Res 1990;1:31–7.
53. Black FO, Pesznecker S, Stallings V. Permanent gentamicin vestibulotoxicity. Otol Neurotol 2001;25:559–69.
54. Hitier M, Besnard S, Smith PF. Vestibular pathways involved in cognition. Front Integr Neurosci 2014;8:59.
55. Dieterich M, Brandt T. The parietal lobe and the vestibular system. Handb Clin Neurol 2018;151:119–40.
56. Candidi M, Micarelli A, Viziano A, et al. Impaired mental rotation in benign paroxysmal positional vertigo and acute vestibular neuritis. Front Hum Neurosci 2013; 7:783.
57. Zheng Y, Darlington CL, Smith PF. Bilateral labyrinthectomy causes long-term deficit in object recognition in rat. Neuroreport 2004;15:1913–6.
58. Zheng Y, Goddard M, Darlington CL, et al. Bilateral vestibular deafferentation impairs performance in a spatial forced alternation task in rats. Hippocampus 2007; 17:253–6.
59. Brandt T. Vestibular loss causes hippocampal atrophy and impaired spatial memory in humans. Brain 2005;128:2732–41.
60. Brandt T, Strupp M, Dieterich M. Towards a concept of disorders of "higher vestibular function". Front Integr Neurosci 2014;8:47.
61. Hartmann M, Farkas R, Mast FW. Self-motion perception influences number processing: evidence from a parity task. Cogn Process 2012;13:189–92.
62. Hartmann M, Grabherr L, Mast FW. Moving along the mental number line: interactions between whole-body motion and numerical cognition. J Exp Psychol Hum Percept Perform 2012;38:1416–27.
63. Lugli L, Baroni G, Anelli F, et al. Counting is easier while experiencing a congruent motion. PLoS One 2013;8:e64500.
64. Miles LK, Nind LK, Macrae CN. Moving through time. Psychol Sci 2010;21:222–3.
65. Rodionov V, Zislin J, Elidan J. Imaginatino of body rotation can induce eye movements. Acta Otolaryngol 2004;124:684–9.
66. Mast FW, Berthoz A, Kosslyn SM. Mental imagery of visual motion modifies the perception of roll-vection stimulation. Perception 2001;30:945–57.
67. Mertz S, Lepecq JC. Imagined body orientation and perception of the visual vertical. Psychol Res 2001;65:64–70.
68. Cappa S, Storzi R, Vallar G. Remission of hemineglect and anosognosia during vestibular stimulation. Neuropsychologia 1987;25:775–82.
69. Vallar G, Bottini G, Rusconi ML. Exploring somatosensory hemineglect by vestibular stimulation. Brain 1993;116:71–86.
70. Karnath HO. Subjective body orientation in neglect and the interactive contribution of neck muscle proprioception and vestibular stimulation. Brain 1994;117: 1001–12.
71. Wolbers T, Wiener JM. Challenges for identifying the neural mechanisms that support spatial navigation: the impact of spatial scale. Front Hum Neurosci 2014;8:571.

Nonvestibular Dizziness

Nicole T. Jiam, MD[a], Olwen C. Murphy, MBBCh, MRCPI[b],
Daniel R. Gold, DO[b], Erin Isanhart, PT, DPT, NCS[c], Dong-In Sinn, MD[d,1],
Kristen K. Steenerson, MD[d,e,2], Jeffrey D. Sharon, MD[f,*]

KEYWORDS

- Non-vestibular dizziness • Autonomic disorders • Visual disturbances
- Cervicogenic disorders • Medications • Vertigo

KEY POINTS

- Dizziness is a common patient complaint that may be due to vestibular or nonvestibular etiologies.
- There are many causes of nonvestibular dizziness including visual disturbances, autonomic dizziness, cervicogenic dizziness, medication-induced dizziness, metabolic dysregulation, thyroid diseases, and cardiovascular conditions.
- A detailed understanding of these medical conditions will help aid diagnosis and appropriate management.

 Video content accompanies this article at http://www.oto.theclinics.com.

INTRODUCTION

Dizziness is a common symptom, accounting for an estimated 5% of all primary care visits.[1] In fact, approximately 35% of Americans report a lifetime prevalence of dizziness.[2,3] Determining the root cause of a patient's dizziness, however, is a diagnostic challenge for many providers. During history taking, patients use the terms "dizziness" and "vertigo" interchangeably to describe a broad range of sensations.[4] Although

[a] Department of Otolaryngology–Head & Neck Surgery, University of California San Francisco School of Medicine, 2233 Post Street, UCSF Box 3213, San Francisco, CA 94115, USA; [b] Department of Neurology, Johns Hopkins University School of Medicine, 600 N Wolfe Street, Pathology 2-210, Baltimore, MD 21287, USA; [c] Angular Momentum Physical Therapy, 4459 Scottsfield Drive, San Jose, CA 95136-1630, USA; [d] Department of Neurology & Neurological Sciences, Stanford University School of Medicine, Palo Alto, CA 94304, USA; [e] Department of Otolaryngology–Head & Neck Surgery, Stanford University School of Medicine, Palo Alto, CA 94303, USA; [f] Department of Otolaryngology–Head & Neck Surgery, University of California San Francisco School of Medicine, 2233 Post Street, Room 315, San Francisco, CA 94115, USA
[1] Present address: 213 Quarry Road, Palo Alto, CA 94304.
[2] Present address: 2452 Watson Court, Suite 1700, Palo Alto, CA 94303.
* Corresponding author.
E-mail address: jeffrey.sharon@ucsf.edu

Otolaryngol Clin N Am 54 (2021) 999–1013
https://doi.org/10.1016/j.otc.2021.05.017
0030-6665/21/© 2021 Elsevier Inc. All rights reserved.

typical American usage defines dizziness as an umbrella term with vertigo as a subset category, the Barany Society delineates these two terms to be nonhierarchical.[5] Dizziness refers to a distorted sense of spatial orientation without a false sense of motion, whereas vertigo describes the sensation of self-motion when there is no movement or the perception of distorted self-motion with normal head movement. Owing to the confusion patients may face with distinguishing between dizziness versus vertigo, some providers find it helpful to ask patients to describe what they are feeling to determine whether they are experiencing true vertigo, presyncope/syncope, unsteadiness, anxiety, lightheadedness, and so forth. Broadly speaking, the differential diagnosis for dizziness may be broken down into two categories: (1) vestibular (central or peripheral) versus (2) nonvestibular sources of dizziness. This article focuses on common causes of nonvestibular dizziness such as visual disturbances, autonomic dizziness, cervicogenic dizziness (CGD), medication-induced dizziness, and other miscellaneous medical conditions. Within each subsection, we will provide an overview of these disorders with the goal of increasing awareness, diagnosis, and management of nonvestibular dizziness.

DIZZINESS AND OSCILLOPSIA IN VISION DISORDERS
Superior Oblique Myokymia

Superior oblique myokymia (SOM) is a monocular disorder characterized by episodic involuntary contraction of the superior oblique muscle. As the primary action of the superior oblique muscle is intorsion, SOM results in torsional high-frequency low-amplitude eye movements (Video 1).[6] This may be experienced by the patient as episodes of oscillopsia (shifting, shimmering, jumping, or fluttering of vision), vertical or oblique diplopia (since the secondary action of the superior oblique muscle is depression), or occasionally vague symptoms of dizziness. The frequency and duration of symptoms can vary greatly between individual patients. Typically, a patient may report multiple daily occurrences over a period of weeks or months, with each episode lasting seconds.[7,8] Symptoms may occur more frequently with stress or fatigue and may spontaneously remit and then recur months or years later.[8]

Diagnosis of SOM can be challenging. Patients with SOM may end up in an otology clinic because the associated oscillopsia can be misinterpreted as a vestibular symptom. The monocular nature of the disorder is an important clinical clue, and SOM should be considered in any patient reporting dizziness or oscillopsia which resolves when the affected eye is covered. In most patients, there are no abnormal signs between episodes.[7,8] Episodes can sometimes be induced by downgaze or by a head tilt toward the affected side. In some patients, the high-frequency low-amplitude eye movements may be difficult to appreciate on bedside examination and may be better seen with binocular video-oculography or with the fundoscopic examination (to observe oscillation of the retinal structures).[7] Notably, monocular video-oculography may not capture SOM episodes if the camera is viewing the unaffected eye.

MR imaging is often normal in patients with SOM,[7,8] although vascular contact with the 4th cranial nerve (which innervates the superior oblique muscle) has been identified and proposed as a pathophysiologic mechanism in some patients,[9] and other structural pathologies have been rarely described.[6] Where treatment of SOM is required, carbamazepine or carbamazepine derivatives are most commonly used.[10] Other medications that have also been used empirically include gabapentin, pregabalin, baclofen, memantine, phenytoin, clonazepam, and beta-blockers (topically or orally).[6,7] In some patients with refractory symptoms, extraocular surgery has been undertaken.[11] In addition, microvascular decompression has been reported as a successful treatment in some individuals with neurovascular contact.[12]

Visual Vertigo

Dizziness in some patients may be triggered by visual motion or complex visual environments, for example, traffic on a street, a grocery store aisle, or watching fast-moving sports on television. These patients do not describe visual symptoms, but rather a sense of disequilibrium, dizziness, or vertigo in response to these triggers.[13] Patients with visual vertigo often have a preceding vestibular injury (such as vestibular neuritis), vestibular migraine, or an underlying disorder of balance, for example, cerebellar disease.[14,15] Increased visual dependence in response to the underlying disorder is a unifying feature in these patient groups and is thought to be an important pathophysiological trigger for the development of visual vertigo.[15] Similar to other patient groups with chronic dizziness, patients with visual vertigo often have comorbid anxiety or depression, and episodes of visual vertigo can sometimes be erroneously attributed to panic attacks.[13] The presence of an underlying balance disorder along with sensitivity to multiple types of visual motion can help differentiate visual vertigo from panic attacks or specific phobias. In addition, an ophthalmology assessment may be useful to rule out an ocular disorder.

Visual vertigo can be treated with a multifaceted approach. Vestibular physical therapy is an essential component of treatment and should focus on underlying balance or dizziness alongside visual desensitization approaches. Visual desensitization typically includes exposure to optokinetic stimuli while the patient is stationary, eventually progressing to exposure while in active motion.[13] Some of these exercises can now be completed by patients remotely, using appropriate online video material. Pharmacologic therapies may be helpful for the treatment of the underlying disorder (eg, vestibular migraine or Meniere's disease) or managing comorbid anxiety or depression that can exacerbate symptoms.

Medial Longitudinal Fasciculus Brainstem Syndromes

The medial longitudinal fasciculus (MLF) is a paired white matter tract close to the midline in the dorsal brainstem linking several brainstem nuclei, and injury to this tract can result in several clinical manifestations relevant to otologists, including an internuclear ophthalmoplegia (INO), skew deviation, spontaneous nystagmus, and abnormalities of the vertical vestibulo-ocular reflex (VOR).

The MLF links the horizontal gaze centers in the pons (sixth cranial nerve nucleus and the paramedian pontine reticular formation) and the third cranial nerve nucleus in the midbrain (including the medial rectus subnucleus).[16] In the normal state, horizontal gaze in one direction is triggered by the ipsilateral pons, and signals are transmitted through decussating fibers to the contralateral MLF, and in turn, the contralateral 3rd cranial nerve nucleus in the midbrain, allowing for the contraction of the ipsilateral lateral rectus muscle and contralateral medial rectus muscle, thus facilitating conjugate horizontal gaze.[17] A lesion of the MLF can cause disruption of this pathway, resulting in an INO—defined as an abnormality of adduction (slowed adduction, limited range of adduction, or complete failure of adduction) during horizontal gaze (Video 2). An INO is described as right or left according to the abnormal adducting eye (which is ipsilateral to the MLF lesion) and may be associated with nystagmus of the abducting eye. On bedside examination, a subtle INO may be most apparent as an adduction lag during large horizontal saccades (slowness of the adducting saccade relative to the abducting saccade).[16]

An INO can cause a variety of symptoms or may indeed be asymptomatic. Patients may describe double vision, blurred vision, oscillopsia, visual lag, and difficulty tracking moving objects.[18] In the clinical history, patients may find these symptoms hard to differentiate and simply describe dizziness when looking in a particular direction. Dizziness triggered by horizontal gaze can thus often be confused with head-motion-induced dizziness, for example, a patient with an INO may describe dizziness triggered when vehicles approach from the right while driving, making it important for the physician to try and differentiate head movement from eye movement triggers in the history. In some cases, an INO can actually be associated with typical vestibular dizziness/vertigo and spontaneous nystagmus (with head-movement-independent oscillopsia) acutely, and an abnormal vertical VOR (with head-movement dependent oscillopsia) which can persist over time, because the vertical semicircular canal pathways (linking the vertical semicircular canals to the vertical gaze centers in the midbrain) also travel within the MLF and can be affected by lesions in this tract.[19] A skew deviation can commonly occur in association with an INO because the utricle pathways (contributing to vertical alignment of the eyes through the physiologic ocular tilt reaction responding to head tilt) also travel within the MLF.[16]

The most common causes of an INO are stroke (most frequently unilateral INO) and multiple sclerosis (most frequently bilateral INO).[20] A myriad of other causes have also been described including trauma, neoplasms, infection, neuroimmune disorders, iatrogenic injury, vasculitis, and vascular malformations.[20] There is no specific treatment for INO, so management should focus on identification and treatment of the etiologic cause. Some patients report that diplopia improves when wearing spectacles with thick frames, which can block the image from the abducting eye in horizontal gaze. This can also mitigate any oscillopsia associated with the abducting nystagmus.

AUTONOMIC DIZZINESS

Standing positions can be challenging for patients with cardiovascular autonomic dysregulation and may cause various symptoms including dizziness. Within a few minutes after standing up, gravity shifts about 500 mL of intravascular fluid (blood) down below the heart, mainly in the splanchnic and large muscular vasculatures. After approximately 20 to 30 minutes of standing, plasma volume decreases due to fluid shift into the interstitial spaces by about 450 mL, which intensifies orthostatic stress.[21] Orthostatic stress can cause various hemodynamic abnormalities with inadequate blood flow to the brain and other organs. The decreased perfusion results in dizziness, vision changes, tinnitus, near-fainting, and syncope.[22] Patients can also experience nausea, sweating, flushing, and palpitations due to compensatory sympathetic hyperactivation.

Orthostatic hypotension (OH) is defined as a drop in systolic blood pressure (BP) by at least 20 mm Hg (diastolic by 10 mm Hg) within 3 minutes of standing (**Fig. 1**A).[23] OH is not always symptomatic, and management of this condition should be based on symptoms, not BP measurements only[24]; there is no association between the severity of BP changes or absolute standing BP and clinical symptoms.[25] Nonetheless, a study involving patients with Parkinson's disease reported a standing mean arterial pressure of 75 mm Hg as an objective threshold for pharmacologic interventions.[26]

Postural orthostatic tachycardia syndrome (POTS) is a heterogeneous autonomic syndrome with exaggerated postural tachycardia and relevant orthostatic symptoms. An exaggerated postural tachycardia is defined as a sustained increase in heart rate of 30 or greater beats per minute (bpm) without OH within 10 minutes of standing (>40 bpm for 12- to 19-year-old populations) (**Fig. 1**B).[23] An exaggerated postural

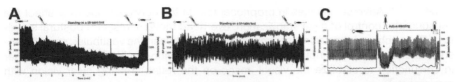

Fig. 1. Various hemodynamic changes to orthostatic stress measured by continuous beat-to-beat blood pressure and heart rate monitoring. A tilt-table test on a patient with a neuro-degenerative disease revealed supine hypertension and orthostatic hypotension that persisted during the test (*A*). A patient with postural orthostatic tachycardia syndrome showed a sustained increase in heart rate without a significant drop in blood pressure during a 10-minute-long tilt-table test (*B*). A person with initial orthostatic hypotension may show a transient drop in systolic blood pressure by 40 mm Hg or more within 15 seconds of *active* standing (*C*) (marked with *). An active standing test is not sensitive, but specific, for initial orthostatic hypotension. Please note a different time scale on the x axis (*C*). Black lines show continuous beat-to-beat blood pressure measurements with upper and lower margins indicating systolic and diastolic blood pressure, respectively. Red lines indicate heart rate.

tachycardia alone is not diagnostic of POTS. Chronic orthostatic intolerance for at least 3 months (ideally 6 months) that improves significantly upon sitting/lying down should be present for the diagnosis.[27] Possible immunologic triggers such as infection often precede POTS. Patients may have autonomic symptoms of sudomotor (sweating), bladder, and/or gastrointestinal involvement. Other associated conditions include hypermobile joints syndrome, chronic fatigue syndrome, gastrointestinal dysmotility, and migraine. Their causal relationship with POTS remains unclear.

Patients with initial OH, defined as a transient drop in systolic BP by >40 mm HG and/or in diastolic BP by >20 mm Hg within 15 seconds after standing report short-lived symptoms right after standing (**Fig. 1**C).[28] Because the BP changes are transient, symptoms often present right after standing up. Initial OH is considered benign in adolescents and young adults. Patients with autonomic neuropathy or on BP-lowering agents may report similar symptoms.[29] Patients with mild or intermittent autonomic disorders may become symptomatic only in situations that amplify orthostatic stress or cause shifts and stasis of plasma volume. Common scenarios include prolonged standing, alcohol, BP-lowering medications, exposure to warm weather, postprandial period, and exercise.

CERVICOGENIC DIZZINESS

CGD, formerly referred to as cervical vertigo, is described as a nonspecific sensation of altered orientation in space and disequilibrium originating from abnormal afferent activity from the neck, but not necessarily the illusion of motion.[30] It is characterized by the presence of disequilibrium, lightheadedness, imbalance, unsteadiness, disorientation, visual disturbances, and neck pain and may be accompanied by a headache.[31–35] Dizziness is described as lasting minutes to hours, lower in intensity, episodic, and rarely involves true vertigo compared with dizziness from the vestibular system.[35] Symptoms can result in anxiety, depression, and inability to perform activities of daily living and occupation duties, which contributes to decreased quality of life.[36]

The pathophysiology of CGD remains to be fully understood. In many cases of CGD, there is a diagnosis of whiplash-associated disorder, spondylosis, degenerative disc disease, inflammation, degeneration, or mechanical dysfunction of the cervical spine.[31,33,37] Adverse changes in proprioceptors in the cervical spine may affect the sensorimotor control of gaze stabilization, eye-head movements, and postural stability.[37] These changes result in a sensory mismatch between the vestibular, somatosensory, and visual afferent inputs.[35,37] The VOR and cervico-ocular reflex work together in conjunction to stabilize the visual image on the retina creating clear vision with movement.[38]

CGD is often a diagnosis of exclusion secondary to a lack of appropriate diagnostic tests and the potential overlap into other etiologies.[31] A clinician must perform a proper examination and demonstrate sound clinical decision-making to lead to a diagnosis of CGD. The examination must assess for other causes of dizziness including the peripheral or central vestibular system and visual system.[35] A clinical cervical assessment includes ligament stability, vertebrobasilar blood flow, manual spinal examination of facet joint dysfunction, palpation for segmental tenderness, traction, strength, clinical tests, proprioception, and postural alignment (**Fig. 2**; **Table 1**).[33,39,40]

Treatment for CGD includes both orthopedic and vestibular physical therapy. Manual orthopedic techniques, including Maitland's passive mobilizations and Mulligan's sustained natural apophyseal glides, address hypomobility of the cervical spine and produce a significant improvement in the frequency of dizziness.[35,36,41,42] The performance of strengthening and neuromuscular recruitment of the deep cervical flexors combined with cervical proprioception enable fine motor movement patterns of the upper cervical spine which leads to an improvement in range of motion and activity with a decrease in dizziness and pain.[39]

Despite the paucity of studies performing vestibular physical therapy and orthopedic physical therapy, Wrisley and colleagues[43] and Lystad and colleagues[42] support the combination of both therapies to fully address all the patient's symptoms. Future research investigating the benefits of orthopedic and vestibular physical therapy is imperative for efficient diagnosis and treatment of CGD.

MEDICATION-INDUCED DIZZINESS

Dizziness is a common side effect of many medications, and misuse of these medications is associated with an increased risk of falls in older adults.[44] In an effort to

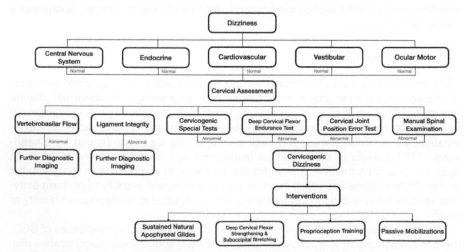

Fig. 2. Clinical assessment and management of cervicogenic dizziness.

Table 1
Clinical tests for cervicogenic dizziness

Test	Purpose	Performance	Abnormal	Specificity	Sensitivity
Alar Ligament Stress Test[69]	Alar ligament integrity at the atlas and axis.	Assess in the supine position. The clinician stabilizes the spinous process of C2 and passively performs side bending bilaterally.	The C2 spinous process has a lack of movement.	96%–100%	69%–72%
Sharp-Purser Test[39]	Transverse ligament integrity to maintain the position of the odontoid process on the atlas.	Assess is in the seated position. The clinician places their thumb on the C2 spinous process. Their other hand on the patient's forehead. The patient flexes their cervical spine while the clinician pushes on the forehead posteriorly.	A clunk or click with symptoms of dizziness.	96%	69%
Vertebrobasilar blood flow[39,70]	Assess blood flow in the vertebral artery	Assess in the seated position for signs of vertebrobasilar insufficiency during symptom provocation. Patient performs sustained end range rotation or end range rotation with extension. Can be performed passively in the supine position.	Patient complains of dizziness, diplopia, dysarthria, or drop attacks.	76%–100%	0%–57%
Smooth Pursuit Neck Torsion Test[71]	Cervicogenic dizziness	Patient is seated on a swivel chair with their neck in a neutral position. The clinician holds their head stable. The patient performs smooth pursuits in the neutral position, body rotation 45° right with neutral head, and body rotation 45° left with neutral head.	Abnormal pursuits or symptoms of dizziness.	91%	90%

(continued on next page)

Table 1
(continued)

Test	Purpose	Performance	Abnormal	Specificity	Sensitivity
Head-Neck Differentiation Test[72]	Cervicogenic dizziness	Patient is seated on a swivel chair with neck in a neutral position with their eyes closed. Clinician holds their head stable while the patient moves their body side to side 45° from center at 60 beats per minute.	Patient has symptoms of dizziness.	90%	N/A
Cervical Torsion Test[72]	Cervicogenic dizziness	Patient is seated on a swivel chair with neck in a neutral position with their eyes closed. Clinician holds their head stable while the patient moves their body side to right 90° for 30 s. Repeat with the body rotating to the left 90° for 30 s.	Patient has symptoms of dizziness.	98%	N/A
Cervical Joint Position Error Test[39]	Cervical proprioception	Patient is seated with a head laser 90 cm from a bullseye target. Patient will either rotate, extend, or flex their neck with their eyes closed and then return to the bullseye.	Patient has a difference of >4.5° from the bullseye.	N/A	N/A
Deep Cervical Flexor Endurance Test[73]	Strength of deep cervical flexor muscles (longus capitis and longus colli) during craniocervical flexion.	Patient is in the supine position. The clinician passively moves the patient into craniocervical flexion with the head lifted 2 cm from the surface. Patient is required to maintain this position independently as long as they are able.	<39.9 s for men <29.4 s for women	N/A	N/A

improve medication selection and to minimize adverse drug events among the elderly, the American Geriatrics Society (AGS) began publishing the Beers Criteria of Potentially Inappropriate Medication (PIM) use.[45] This is an evidence-based list of PIMs that should be avoided in most older adults, and incorporation of the AGS Beers Criteria into clinical prescribing patterns would likely help mitigate medication-induced dizziness and falls.

As discussed, there is an extensive list of medications that could cause dizzy symptoms. In general, medications that are more prone to this side-effect are antidepressants, antiseizure drugs, antihypertensive medications, antibiotics, anti-inflammatory medications, and diuretics.[46,47] Antidepressants are a common offender. The abrupt discontinuation of selective serotonin reuptake inhibitors (SSRIs) frequently causes dizziness. Paradoxically, SSRIs have also been shown to relieve dizziness in patients with major or minor anxiety disorders, major depressions, and undifferentiated somatoform dizziness.[48] For a detailed table of common medications that may induce dizziness or vertigo as an adverse drug reaction, please refer to Chimirri and colleagues.[46] In order to minimize incidences of medication-induced dizziness, medication reconciliation should be performed regularly during provider outpatient visits, and drugs that do not offer benefit to the patient should be discontinued in a timely fashion.

OTHER FORMS OF NONVESTIBULAR DIZZINESS

Symptoms of metabolic dysregulation may include dizziness. Hyperventilation is defined as rapid, deep breathing exceeding metabolic needs.[49] The process of over-breathing increases serum pH and lowers the concentration of ionized calcium. Subsequent arterial vasoconstriction reduces both cerebral and inner ear circulation, thereby decreasing the tissue oxygenation and inducing lightheadedness. Another metabolic-related condition is hypoglycemia. Glycemic variability is common in people who use insulin or take certain tablets to reduce high blood sugar, and this patient population is more vulnerable to hypoglycemia.[50] Because the brain relies on blood sugar as its primary source of energy, hypoglycemia can cause neuronal death.[51] Signs of hypoglycemia include headache, fatigue, anxiety, confusion, cold sweats, pale face, and dizziness. Carbon monoxide has also been reported to cause dizziness. Lumio first described hearing loss and vertigo from chronic carbon monoxide poisoning in 1948, which may have arisen from neurotoxicity, lactate acidosis, and cochlear and vestibular nerve damage.[52] Although the exact pathophysiology remains unclear, carbon monoxide has also been shown to affect cochlear electrophysiology and blood flow.[53,54]

In addition to metabolic conditions, dizziness may also manifest from autoimmune thyroid diseases. Hypothyroidism may result in low BP and bradycardia leading to dizziness. Conversely, hyperthyroidism may cause heart palpitations, arrhythmia, and lightheadedness. These symptoms typically resolve with medical management of the underlying thyroid disease. Interestingly, thyroid diseases such as goiter, hypothyroidism, and hyperthyroidism are associated with Meniere's disease[55]—a medical condition clinically diagnosed by recurrent vertigo attacks and cochlear symptoms of fluctuating hearing loss, tinnitus, and/or aural fullness.[56] As such, patients with a thyroid disorder and dizziness complaints should also be evaluated for peripheral vestibular dysfunction.

During a clinic visit, an alcohol drinking history should be solicited. Alcohol consumption can cause dizziness through central, peripheral, and autonomic mechanisms. Ethanol induces cerebellar dysfunction and ataxia by disrupting molecular neurotransmission, inducing dendritic regression, provoking neuronal inflammation/

toxicity, and modifying brain input functionality.[57,58] Alcohol can also induce peripheral neuropathy, resulting in sensory ataxia and alcohol-related dizziness/imbalance.[59] Positional alcohol nystagmus can also occur when alcohol diffuses into the cupula and transforms the semicircular canal into gravity-sensitive receptors because of the difference of specific gravities of alcohol and the vestibular endolymph.[60] Last but not least, alcohol ingestion may induce dehydration and orthostatic dizziness by inhibiting the release of antidiuretic hormones.[61] This effect is even more pronounced and prolonged in chronic alcoholics.

Although dizziness resulting from a primary cardiovascular disorder (eg, arrhythmia, carotid sinus reflex, defective heart valve, embolism, myocardial infarction, vascular anomaly, anemia) could also be classified as a form of nonvestibular dizziness, it is more frequently framed as presyncope (impending faint) or syncope among clinicians.[62] Seminal syncope studies have explicitly excluded patients with dizziness or vertigo.[63–65] We did not delve into cardiovascular-associated dizziness in the present article; however, this should be kept on the differential diagnosis whenever a patient presents with dizziness.

Disuse disequilibrium, otherwise known as deconditioning, is a common cause of nonvestibular dizziness.[66,67] Elderly adults are more prone to disuse disequilibrium because of a greater incidence of immobilizing surgeries, chronic illnesses, near-falls or falls, and fatigue.[68] Unfortunately, fear of falling and disuse disequilibrium can perpetuate a vicious cycle of a sedentary lifestyle and reduce a patient's willingness to participate in physical rehabilitation. Although there are no large controlled studies of the management of disuse disequilibrium, this condition is generally responsive to gait and balance physical therapy.[66]

SUMMARY

Dizziness is a common symptom that arises from various disorders. Determining whether a patient is experiencing central, peripheral, or nonvestibular dizziness is an important aspect of history taking and physical examination. Here, we described many forms of nonvestibular dizziness including visual disturbances, autonomic dysfunction, CGD, medication-induced side effects, metabolic dysregulation, autoimmune diseases, and alcohol consumption. An understanding of each of these medical conditions will improve the likelihood of diagnosis and appropriate management of these patients.

CLINICS CARE POINTS

- Patients who demonstrate monocular oscillopsia, vertical or oblique diplopia, and vague symptoms of dizziness should be evaluated for superior oblique myokymia via downgaze examination during a fundoscopic examination or binocular video-oculography (to observe oscillations of the retinal structure). Treatment options include medications (eg, carbamazepine) or extraocular surgery for those who are refractory to medical management.

- Visual vertigo often presents as dizziness triggered by visual motion or complex visual environments. Patients with visual vertigo often have had preceding vestibular injury, vestibular migraine, or an underlying balance disorder. Treatment should be multifaceted and include vestibular physical therapy, visual desensitization, and pharmacologic therapies (if appropriate) for the underlying or comorbid disorders.

- Medial longitudinal fasciculus (MLF) brainstem syndromes occur when there is injury to a paired white matter tract linking the horizontal gaze centers in the pons and the third cranial nerve nucleus in the midbrain. Disruption of the MLF pathway can result in internuclear ophthalmoplegia, which may be described as diplopia, blurred vision, oscillopsia, visual lag, difficult tracking moving objects, or dizziness when looking in a particular direction. Differentiation between dizziness induced by head movements versus eye movements is important for diagnosis and treatment of the underlying cause.

- Orthostatic hypotension is defined as a drop in systolic blood pressure by at least 20 mm Hg (diastolic by 10 mm Hg) within 3 minutes of standing and should be treated if a patient is symptomatic. Medications such as fludrocortisone, midodrine, and pyridostigmine are considered in patients who do not respond to maximized lifestyle modifications.

- Postural orthostatic tachycardia syndrome (POTS) is a heterogeneous autonomic syndrome with exaggerated postural tachycardia and chronic orthostatic intolerance. Patients with POTS are generally treated with graded exercise program, hydration, modified high-sodium diet, medications, and compression garments.

- Initial orthostatic hypotension is defined by a transient drop in systolic blood pressure by >40 mm HG and/or in diastolic BP by >20 mm Hg within 15 seconds after standing. Patients are typically treated with lifestyle modifications.

- To patients with autonomic dizziness, it is recommended to avoid their own triggers such as abrupt/prolonged standing, alcohol, antihypertensive medications, warm weather, large meals, and strenuous exercise.

- Cervicogenic dizziness is often a diagnosis of exclusion due to the lack of appropriate diagnostic tests and is a nonspecific sensation of altered orientation in space and disequilibrium originating from abnormal afferent activity from the neck but not necessarily the illusion of motion. Treatment involves orthopedic and vestibular physical therapy.

- Antidepressants, antiseizure drugs, anti-hypertensive medications, antibiotics, anti-inflammatory medications, and diuretics are medications that commonly induce dizziness as a side effect. Medication reconciliation should be regularly performed for potentially inappropriate use (Beers Criteria), particularly in the elderly population.

- Hyperventilation, hypoglycemia, carbon monoxide poisoning, and thyroid disorders may induce metabolic or homeostatic dysregulation that can result in dizziness. Treatment of these underlying metabolic conditions generally resolves symptoms. Hypothyroidism and hyperthyroidism are also associated with an increased incidence of Meniere's disease (a form of peripheral vestibular dizziness); therefore, clinicians should also assess for peripheral vestibulopathies.

- Disuse disequilibrium is associated with a fear of falling, resulting in deconditioning. This medical condition is common among the elderly population and generally responds well to physical therapy exercises.

DISCLOSURE

The authors have nothing to disclose.

SUPPLEMENTARY DATA

Supplementary data to this article can be found online at https://doi.org/10.1016/j.otc. 2021.05.017.

REFERENCES

1. Post RE, Dickerson LM. Dizziness: a diagnostic approach. Am Fam Physician 2010;82(4):361–8, 369.
2. Bigelow RT, Semenov YR, du Lac S, et al. Vestibular vertigo and comorbid cognitive and psychiatric impairment: the 2008 National Health Interview Survey. J Neurol Neurosurg Psychiatry 2016;87(4):367–72.
3. Neuhauser HK. Epidemiology of vertigo. Curr Opin Neurol 2007;20(1):40–6.

4. Newman-Toker DE, Cannon LM, Stofferahn ME, et al. Imprecision in patient reports of dizziness symptom quality: a cross-sectional study conducted in an acute care setting. Mayo Clin Proc 2007;82(11):1329–40.

5. Bisdorff A, Von Brevern M, Lempert T, et al. Classification of vestibular symptoms: towards an international classification of vestibular disorders. J Vestib Res 2009; 19(1–2):1–13.

6. Tandon A, Oliveira C. Superior oblique myokymia, a review. Curr Opin Ophthalmol 2019;30(6):472–5.

7. Thinda S, Chen Y-R, Liao YJ. Cardinal features of superior oblique myokymia: an infrared oculography study. Am J Ophthalmol Case Rep 2017;7:115–9.

8. Brazis PW, Miller NR, Henderer JD, et al. The natural history and results of treatment of superior oblique myokymia. Arch Ophthalmol 1994;112(8):1063–7.

9. Yousry I, Dieterich M, Naidich TP, et al. Superior oblique myokymia: magnetic resonance imaging support for the neurovascular compression hypothesis. Ann Neurol 2002;51(3):361–8.

10. Williams PE, Purvin VA, Kawasaki A. Superior oblique myokymia: efficacy of medical treatment. J AAPOS 2007;11(3):254–7.

11. Agarwal S, Kushner BJ. Results of extraocular muscle surgery for superior oblique myokymia. J AAPOS 2009;13(5):472–6.

12. Fam MD, Scott C, Forster A, et al. Microvascular decompression for superior oblique myokymia: case report. Br J Neurosurg 2014;28(4):552–5.

13. Bronstein AM, Golding JF, Gresty MA. Vertigo and dizziness from environmental motion: visual vertigo, motion sickness, and drivers' disorientation. Semin Neurol 2013;33(3):219–30.

14. Lempert T. Vestibular migraine. Semin Neurol 2013;33(3):212–8.

15. Bronstein AM. Visual vertigo syndrome: clinical and posturography findings. J Neurol Neurosurg Psychiatry 1995;59(5):472–6.

16. Virgo JD, Plant GT. Internuclear ophthalmoplegia. Pract Neurol 2017;17(2): 149–53.

17. Pierrot-Deseilligny C. Nuclear, internuclear, and supranuclear ocular motor disorders. Handb Clin Neurol 2011;102:319–31.

18. Nij Bijvank JA, van Rijn LJ, Balk LJ, et al. Diagnosing and quantifying a common deficit in multiple sclerosis: internuclear ophthalmoplegia. Neurology 2019; 92(20):e2299–308.

19. Lee S-H, Kim S-H, Kim S-S, et al. Preferential impairment of the contralesional posterior semicircular canal in internuclear ophthalmoplegia. Front Neurol 2017; 8:502.

20. Keane JR. Internuclear ophthalmoplegia: unusual causes in 114 of 410 patients. Arch Neurol 2005;62(5):714–7.

21. Robertson D. The pathophysiology and diagnosis of orthostatic hypotension. Clin Auton Res 2008;18(Suppl 1):2–7.

22. Freeman R. Clinical practice. Neurogenic orthostatic hypotension. N Engl J Med 2008;358(6):615–24.

23. Freeman R, Wieling W, Axelrod FB, et al. Consensus statement on the definition of orthostatic hypotension, neurally mediated syncope and the postural tachycardia syndrome. Auton Neurosci 2011;161(1–2):46–8.

24. Freeman R, Abuzinadah AR, Gibbons C, et al. Orthostatic hypotension: JACC state-of-the-art review. J Am Coll Cardiol 2018;72(11):1294–309.

25. Freeman R, Illigens BMW, Lapusca R, et al. Symptom recognition is impaired in patients with orthostatic hypotension. Hypertension 2020;75(5):1325–32.

26. Palma J-A, Gomez-Esteban JC, Norcliffe-Kaufmann L, et al. Orthostatic hypotension in Parkinson disease: how much you fall or how low you go? Mov Disord 2015;30(5):639–45.

27. Olshansky B, Cannom D, Fedorowski A, et al. Postural Orthostatic Tachycardia Syndrome (POTS): a critical assessment. Prog Cardiovasc Dis 2020;63(3): 263–70.

28. Wieling W, Krediet CTP, van Dijk N, et al. Initial orthostatic hypotension: review of a forgotten condition. Clin Sci 2007;112(3):157–65.

29. Lindqvist A, Torffvit O, Rittner R, et al. Artery blood pressure oscillation after active standing up: an indicator of sympathetic function in diabetic patients. Clin Physiol 1997;17(2):159–69.

30. Ryan GM, Cope S. Cervical vertigo. Lancet 1955;269(6905):1355–8.

31. Thompson-Harvey A, Hain TC. Symptoms in cervical vertigo. Laryngoscope Investig Otolaryngol 2019;4(1):109–15.

32. Cook C, Hegedus E. Orthopedic physical examination tests: pearson new international edition: an evidence-based approach. London (UK): Pearson; 2013.

33. Reiley AS, Vickory FM, Funderburg SE, et al. How to diagnose cervicogenic dizziness. Arch Physiother 2017;7:12.

34. Ahadi M, Naser Z, Abolghasemi J. Vestibular-balance rehabilitation in patients with whiplash-associated disorders. Int Tinnitus J 2019;23(1):42–6.

35. Alsaif AA, Johnson EG. Cervicogenic dizziness: implications for physical therapy. Indian J Physiother Occup Ther 2011;5(4):6–11.

36. Hoppes CW, Romanello AJ, Gaudette KE, et al. Physical therapy interventions for cervicogenic dizziness in a military-aged population: protocol for a systematic review. Syst Rev 2020;9(1):62.

37. Jung FC, Mathew S, Littmann AE, et al. Clinical decision making in the management of patients with cervicogenic dizziness: a case series. J Orthop Sports Phys Ther 2017;47(11):874–84.

38. Ischebeck BK, de Vries J, van Wingerden JP, et al. The influence of cervical movement on eye stabilization reflexes: a randomized trial. Exp Brain Res 2018;236(1):297–304.

39. Sung Y-H. Upper cervical spine dysfunction and dizziness. J Exerc Rehabil 2020; 16(5):385–91.

40. Olson LE, Millar AL, Dunker J, et al. Reliability of a clinical test for deep cervical flexor endurance. J Manipulative Physiol Ther 2006;29(2):134–8.

41. Reid SA, Rivett DA, Katekar MG, et al. Efficacy of manual therapy treatments for people with cervicogenic dizziness and pain: protocol of a randomised controlled trial. BMC Musculoskelet Disord 2012;13:201.

42. Lystad RP, Bell G, Bonnevie-Svendsen M, et al. Manual therapy with and without vestibular rehabilitation for cervicogenic dizziness: a systematic review. Chiropr Man Therap 2011;19(1):21.

43. Wrisley DM, Sparto PJ, Whitney SL, et al. Cervicogenic dizziness: a review of diagnosis and treatment. J Orthop Sports Phys Ther 2000;30(12):755–66.

44. Berdot S, Bertrand M, Dartigues J-F, et al. Inappropriate medication use and risk of falls–a prospective study in a large community-dwelling elderly cohort. BMC Geriatr 2009;9:30.

45. By the 2019 American Geriatrics Society Beers Criteria® Update Expert Panel. American geriatrics society 2019 updated AGS beers criteria® for potentially inappropriate medication use in older adults. J Am Geriatr Soc 2019;67(4): 674–94.

46. Chimirri S, Aiello R, Mazzitello C, et al. Vertigo/dizziness as a Drugs' adverse reaction. J Pharmacol Pharmacother 2013;4(Suppl 1):S104–9.

47. Altissimi G, Colizza A, Cianfrone G, et al. Drugs inducing hearing loss, tinnitus, dizziness and vertigo: an updated guide. Eur Rev Med Pharmacol Sci 2020; 24(15):7946–52.

48. Staab JP, Ruckenstein MJ, Solomon D, et al. Serotonin reuptake inhibitors for dizziness with psychiatric symptoms. Arch Otolaryngol Head Neck Surg 2002; 128(5):554–60.

49. Sakellari V, Bronstein AM, Corna S, et al. The effects of hyperventilation on postural control mechanisms. Brain 1997;120(Pt 9):1659–73.

50. Weinstock RS, Aleppo G, Bailey TS, et al. The role of blood glucose monitoring in diabetes management. American Diabetes Association; 2021.

51. Suh SW, Hamby AM, Swanson RA. Hypoglycemia, brain energetics, and hypoglycemic neuronal death. Glia 2007;55(12):1280–6.

52. Lumio JO. Otoneurological studies of chronic carbon monoxide poisoning in Finland. Acta Otolaryngol Suppl 1948;67:65–75.

53. Fechter LD, Thorne PR, Nuttall AL. Effects of carbon monoxide on cochlear electrophysiology and blood flow. Hear Res 1987;27(1):37–45.

54. Seale B, Ahanger S, Hari C. Subacute carbon monoxide poisoning presenting as vertigo and fluctuating low frequency hearing loss. J Surg Case Rep 2018; 2018(8):rjy205.

55. Kim SY, Song YS, Wee JH, et al. Association between Ménière's disease and thyroid diseases: a nested case-control study. Sci Rep 2020;10(1):18224.

56. Goebel JA. 2015 Equilibrium Committee Amendment to the 1995 AAO-HNS guidelines for the definition of ménière's disease. Otolaryngol Head Neck Surg 2016;154(3):403–4.

57. Luo J. Effects of ethanol on the cerebellum: advances and prospects. Cerebellum 2015;14(4):383–5.

58. Gruol DL, Melkonian C, Ly K, et al. Alcohol and IL-6 alter expression of synaptic proteins in cerebellum of transgenic mice with increased astrocyte expression of IL-6. Neuroscience 2020;442:124–37.

59. Julian T, Glascow N, Syeed R, et al. Alcohol-related peripheral neuropathy: a systematic review and meta-analysis. J Neurol 2019;266(12):2907–19.

60. Money KE, Myles WS. Heavy water nystagmus and effects of alcohol. Nature 1974;247(5440):404–5.

61. Roberts KE. Mechanism of dehydration following alcohol ingestion. Arch Intern Med 1963;112:154–7.

62. Newman-Toker DE, Dy FJ, Stanton VA, et al. How often is dizziness from primary cardiovascular disease true vertigo? A systematic review. J Gen Intern Med 2008; 23(12):2087–94.

63. Ammirati F, Colivicchi F, Santini M. Diagnosing syncope in clinical practice. Implementation of a simplified diagnostic algorithm in a multicentre prospective trial - the OESIL 2 study (Osservatorio Epidemiologico della Sincope nel Lazio). Eur Heart J 2000;21(11):935–40.

64. Oh JH, Hanusa BH, Kapoor WN. Do symptoms predict cardiac arrhythmias and mortality in patients with syncope? Arch Intern Med 1999;159(4):375–80.

65. Sarasin FP, Louis-Simonet M, Carballo D, et al. Prospective evaluation of patients with syncope: a population-based study. Am J Med 2001;111(3):177–84.

66. Cameron ID, Dyer SM, Panagoda CE, et al. Interventions for preventing falls in older people in care facilities and hospitals. Cochrane Database Syst Rev 2018;9:CD005465.

67. Herdman SJ, Clendaniel R. Vestibular rehabilitation. F.A. Davis; 2014.
68. Bortz WM 2nd. Disuse and aging. JAMA 1982;248(10):1203–8.
69. Hutting N, Scholten-Peeters GGM, Vijverman V, et al. Diagnostic accuracy of upper cervical spine instability tests: a systematic review. Phys Ther 2013;93(12):1686–95.
70. Hutting N, Verhagen AP, Vijverman V, et al. Diagnostic accuracy of premanipulative vertebrobasilar insufficiency tests: a systematic review. Man Ther 2013;18(3):177–82.
71. L'Heureux-Lebeau B, Godbout A, Berbiche D, et al. Evaluation of paraclinical tests in the diagnosis of cervicogenic dizziness. Otol Neurotol 2014;35(10):1858–65.
72. Treleaven J, Joloud V, Nevo Y, et al. Normative responses to clinical tests for cervicogenic dizziness: clinical cervical torsion test and head-neck differentiation test. Phys Ther 2020;100(1):192–200.
73. Domenech MA, Sizer PS, Dedrick GS, et al. The deep neck flexor endurance test: normative data scores in healthy adults. PM R 2011;3(2):105–10.

Vestibular Physical Therapy and Fall Risk Assessment

Wendy J. Carender, PT, MPT[a],*, Melissa Grzesiak, PT, DPT[a], Steven A. Telian, MD[b]

KEYWORDS

- Vestibular physical therapy • Vestibular rehabilitation • Dizziness • Balance
- Fall prevention

KEY POINTS

- The foundation of vestibular physical therapy includes a combination of 4 exercise modalities that target functional impairments to improve quality of life: gaze stabilization, habituation, balance/gait, and a walking program to build endurance.
- Emerging studies support initiating vestibular physical therapy early for individuals with peripheral or central causes of dizziness and imbalance.
- Clinicians should be familiar with vestibular test modalities and outcome measures that can document progress toward central compensation.
- Clinicians should screen for fall risk and provide appropriate recommendations and referrals to other specialists as indicated to reduce fall risk in individuals presenting with dizziness and balance impairments.

 Video content accompanies this article at http://www.oto.theclinics.com.

INTRODUCTION

Otolaryngologists and other clinicians are faced with the complexity of evaluating and treating patients with multiple forms of dizziness and imbalance. The astute clinician obtains a comprehensive history, considers comorbidities, performs a systematic clinical bedside examination, and reviews medical test results to formulate a differential diagnosis. Ultimately, the clinician guides the patient toward rational and effective treatment options, which may include medical management and/or surgical procedures.

[a] Department of Otolaryngology–Head & Neck Surgery, Michigan Medicine, University of Michigan, Michigan Balance Vestibular Testing and Rehabilitation, Med Inn Building, Room C166A, 1500 East Medical Center Drive, Ann Arbor, MI 48109-5816, USA; [b] Department of Otolaryngology–Head & Neck Surgery, University of Michigan, 1500 East Medical Center Drive, TC 1904L, Ann Arbor, MI 48109-5312, USA
* Corresponding author.
E-mail address: wcaren@med.umich.edu

Otolaryngol Clin N Am 54 (2021) 1015–1036
https://doi.org/10.1016/j.otc.2021.05.018
0030-6665/21/© 2021 Elsevier Inc. All rights reserved.

Vestibular physical therapy (VPT) is a specialized form of evidence-based therapy designed to alleviate symptoms related to vestibular disorders.[1,2] The primary presenting symptoms may include vertigo, dizziness, imbalance, gait instability, and/or falls. Clinical experience suggests that there are many secondary symptoms that add to significant discomfort and disability, such as deconditioning, cervical muscle tension, anxiety, reduced quality of life, fear of falling, and limitations imposed by fall or symptom-provoking avoidance behaviors.

THE ROLE OF VESTIBULAR PHYSICAL THERAPY

The primary goals of VPT are to decrease dizziness and visual symptoms, improve balance and gait stability, prevent falls, and increase activity level and conditioning. The overall objective is to facilitate return to daily activities, work, and recreation while improving quality of life. Important components of a VPT program include patient education regarding management of triggers/symptoms, minimizing use of vestibular suppressants, modifying lifestyle behaviors, and instruction in an individualized home exercise program (HEP).

VPT is beneficial for individuals with motion, visual or positional provoked dizziness, blurred vision with head movement, and postural instability, including slow and/or unsteady gait or more than 1 fall in the past 6 to 12 months. There is strong evidence to support VPT for individuals with acute or chronic uncompensated unilateral vestibular hypofunction (UVH) after injuries, such as ablative surgery, vestibular neuritis or labyrinthitis,[1] bilateral peripheral vestibular hypofunction (BVH),[3] and benign paroxysmal positional vertigo (BPPV).[4,5] VPT may improve symptoms in individuals with persistent postural-perceptual dizziness (PPPD or 3PD),[6,7] vestibular migraine,[8–12] cervicogenic dizziness,[13,14] and traumatic brain injury (TBI)/concussion[15–17]; however, additional studies are needed. **Table 1** provides more details. Clinical practice recommendations on the efficacy of VPT cannot be made for patients with neurologic disorders because of the lack of high-quality research and heterogeneity of treatment protocols.[18]

Patients with chronic imbalance related to later stages of Meniere's disease may benefit from balance retraining, but VPT is not recommended for individuals with early Meniere's who are experiencing frequent spontaneous spells of vertigo.[19] In general, patients with unstable or highly fluctuating episodic vestibular symptoms are not candidates for VPT. Contraindications for VPT include active cerebrospinal fluid leaks, traumatic perilymphatic fistula, or recent cervical fracture/instability (**Box 1**).

CENTRAL COMPENSATION

Following an acute disturbance of the peripheral vestibular system, the central vestibular system should compensate by adapting to the altered sensory input from the periphery. Vestibular exercises are aimed at promoting central compensation and improving functional abilities related to vestibular impairment or loss. Four different exercise categories have been identified as the foundation of evidence-based VPT programs: gaze stabilization, habituation, balance/gait, and endurance,[1] and are described in **Table 2**. Gaze stabilization (vestibulo-ocular reflex [VOR] adaptation and VOR substitution) exercises promote central adaptation with the goal of decreasing symptoms and improving gaze and postural stability.[1] Adaptation exercises encourage head movement while maintaining visual fixation on a target, which may be stationary (VOR × 1) or moving (VOR × 2).[1] A video demonstration and exercise handout of gaze stabilization VOR × 1 exercise can be viewed at: https://michmed.org/gkZZn. VOR substitution exercises (eye movements precede head movements) facilitate central preprogramming of eye movements to support gaze stability.

Table 1
Overview of conditions that improve with vestibular physical therapy

Diagnosis	Type of Exercise	Education	Plan of Care and Expected Outcomes
Acute unilateral vestibular hypofunction	• Gaze stabilization • Habituation • Balance training • Endurance	• Discontinue vestibular suppressants after the initial acute phase (days) • Movement facilitates recovery • Manage stress/anxiety	• Supervised VPT once per week for 2–3 wk combined with daily HEP • Expect return to all activities without dizziness or imbalance
Chronic unilateral vestibular hypofunction	• Gaze stabilization • Habituation • Balance training • Endurance	• Avoid vestibular suppressants • Movement facilitates recovery • Manage stress/anxiety	• Supervised VPT once per week for 4–6 wk combined with daily HEP • Older adults with balance deficits may require longer duration of VPT
Bilateral vestibular hypofunction	• Gaze stabilization • Sensory substitution • Balance training • Endurance	• Move eyes, then head to maintain stable vision • Caution on uneven surfaces and in dimly lit environments • Possible use of an assistive device • Avoid swimming alone: life vest for safety when boating • Driving safety	• Supervised VPT once per week for 8–12 wk combined with a daily HEP • Expect return to most activities with possible modifications (driving during daytime, safer occupation, use of assistive devices, and so forth)
Benign paroxysmal positional vertigo	• Particle repositioning maneuvers • Habituation • Balance training	• Educate patient how to determine involved ear • Subsequent self-management of BPPV relapses with PRMs	• Treatment is successful following 1 or 2 PRMs (79.4%–92.7%)[5] • Reassess within 1 mo to document resolution or persistence of symptoms
Meniere's disease producing chronic imbalance or uncompensated hypofunction	• Gaze stabilization • Habituation • Balance training • Endurance	• Low sodium diet • Diuretic compliance • Vestibular suppressant use restricted to acute episodes of vertigo	• Once episodic vertigo is effectively controlled, outcomes are expected to be consistent with those for individuals with UVH or BVH
Vestibular migraine	• Habituation • Balance training • Endurance	• Common migraine triggers, migraine diet, good sleep hygiene, adequate hydration, daily walking program	• Improvement in 5 studies, but control groups lacking.[64] HEP ranged from 5 d to 4 mo

(continued on next page)

Table 1
(continued)

Diagnosis	Type of Exercise	Education	Plan of Care and Expected Outcomes
Persistent postural-perceptual dizziness	• Gaze stabilization • Habituation • Visual desensitization • Balance training • Endurance	• Movement facilitates recovery • Exercises may provoke moderate dizziness • Good sleep hygiene, a healthy diet, and daily physical exercise • Stress/anxiety management	• VPT combined with CBT, SSRI/SNRI, and patient education • Supervised VPT once per week for at least 6 wk combined with a HEP
TBI/concussion	• Oculomotor (convergence) • Gaze stabilization • Habituation • Balance training • Endurance/exertion training If indicated: • PRMs • Cervical spine intervention	• Reduce risk of additional head injuries • After 24–48 h of rest, patients should engage in a progressive return to activities • Symptom-guided exercise progression: avoid more than a 3-point increase in headache, dizziness, or nausea during exercise or activity • Good sleep hygiene	• Most individuals do not have significant symptoms that last >1–3 mo' postinjury • Evidence supports cervical and vestibular therapy superior to rest and graded exertion for return to sport clearance[17] • Subjects who received cervical and VPT were 4 times more likely to be medically cleared for return to sport by 8 weeks[15]
Cervical vertigo	• Manual therapy/mobilizations • Cervical kinesthesia • Cervical ROM/strengthening • Vestibular exercises	• Good posture and ergonomics • Avoid forceful manipulation of the cervical vertebrae • Avoid exercises/activities that involve extreme head-on neck movements	• Diagnosis of exclusion because there are no clear diagnostic criteria • Limited studies to date that combine manual therapy and VPT or report on prognosis

Abbreviations: CBT, cognitive behavioral therapy; ROM, range of motion; SNRIs, serotonin norepinephrine reuptake inhibitors; SSRIs, selective serotonin reuptake inhibitors.

Box 1
Contraindications for vestibular physical therapy
Vestibular physical therapy is not indicated for the following: • Individuals with unstable or highly fluctuating symptoms • Individuals experiencing only spontaneous episodes of vertigo without motion provoked vertigo or imbalance Vestibular physical therapy is contraindicated for patients with the following: • Active cerebrospinal fluid leak • Traumatic perilymphatic fistula • Recent cervical fracture/instability

Table 2		
Overview of common vestibular exercises		
Type of Exercise	**Exercise Theory**	**Examples**
Gaze stabilization • VOR adaptation • VOR substitution	Improve gaze stability • Adaptation results from stimuli that produce error signals. The central nervous system reduces sensory mismatch by modifying the gain of the response • Substitution promotes central preprogramming of eye movements, including saccades	• VOR × 1 https://michmed.org/gkZZn • VOR × 2 • Eye-head movements between targets • Imaginary targets
Habituation	• Promotes desensitization by repeated exposure to a provocative stimulus • Therapist identifies specific movements that provoke the symptoms and develops an individualized exercise plan	• Horizontal/vertical head movements are commonly used • Gradually add visual conflict to the background
Balance/postural control • VSR substitution	• Static and dynamic balance exercises to improve postural control and decrease fall risk • VSR substitution improves postural control by promoting alternative strategies or increasing reliance on vision and proprioceptive feedback to substitute for impaired vestibular function • Sensory substitution/augmentation via vibrotactile feedback (trunk or tongue) to provide the user cues about body position in space	• Progression of static balance exercises altering base of support, visual input, proprioceptive input, adding a cognitive task • Dynamic balance exercises, including weight shift, walking with head movements
Endurance	Improve overall endurance and conditioning	Graded walking program

Abbreviation: VSR, vestibular spinal reflex.

Vestibular test results and the clinical examination using video goggles[20] are helpful in assessing compensation status or may explain the lack of compensation by identifying a pathologic process in the central nervous system. The specific test results that may be beneficial in making these key diagnostic distinctions are summarized in **Table 3**. Significant spontaneous, positional, or post–head shaking nystagmus on videonystagmography (VNG) or bedside video goggle examination provides evidence for failure of physiologic compensation in the VOR. Gaze stability can be assessed using the noninstrumented dynamic visual acuity (DVA) test.[21] A loss of 3 lines or greater correlates with clinically significant vestibular dysfunction. A persistent asymmetry in VOR responses at several rotational chair frequencies strongly suggests that the peripheral lesion is physiologically uncompensated.

Dynamic posturography can provide adjunctive functional information about the balance system in individuals with vestibular complaints despite essentially normal findings on VNG and rotational chair testing. Although there are limited studies that address the clinical utility at the individual level, dynamic posturography has been found to be a useful tool to understand the pathophysiological mechanism in patients with balance disorders at a group level.[22] Patients with an uncompensated vestibulopathy or poor ability to use vestibular inputs may demonstrate a vestibular dysfunction balance pattern, failing or "falling" on sensory organization test (SOT) condition 5 (eyes closed, sway referenced surface), and/or condition 6 (eyes open, sway referenced surface, sway referenced visual field). Balance training exercises should be provided for these patients.

OUTCOME MEASURES

Vestibular physical therapists rely on outcome measures to document and monitor functional progress and overall outcomes. The Vestibular Evidence Database to Guide Effectiveness task force has provided recommendations on outcome measures for individuals with vestibular hypofunction.[23] Subjective measures commonly used in practice include the Dizziness Handicap Inventory (DHI),[24] the Activities-Specific Balance Confidence Scale,[25] and more recently, the Vestibular Rehabilitation Benefit Questionnaire.[26] Measures related to postural control and gait include the SOT,[27] the modified Clinical Test of Sensory Interaction on Balance (mCTSIB),[28] the Mini BESTest,[29] the Dynamic Gait Index,[30] the Functional Gait Assessment,[31] and gait speed (10-m Walk Test).[32]

FACTORS THAT CONTRIBUTE TO OUTCOMES

Duration of VPT interventions and expected outcomes are outlined in **Table 1**. Age and gender have not been shown to affect VPT outcomes.[1] Comorbidities, including peripheral neuropathy,[33] anxiety,[34] migraine,[9,11] and long-term use of vestibular suppressants,[35] may limit outcomes and/or result in longer duration of care. Lack of physical activity, acquired visual disorders, impaired sleep, cognitive impairment, and fear of falling may also affect outcome.[36] Considerations for stopping VPT intervention are listed in **Box 2**. Telehealth may provide an avenue for patients who could benefit from ongoing care but have difficulty getting to a clinic. Therapist to physician correspondence and/or medical reassessment are indicated for patients who have prematurely plateaued, failed to compensate, or further regressed despite an adequate VPT trial (2–4 weeks), in attempt to determine potential reasons for lack of progress.

Table 3
Clinical decision making: vestibular tests and bedside exam results that assist in determining level of central compensation

Objective Findings	Unilateral Vestibular Dysfunction (UVH)	Indicative of an Uncompensated Vestibulopathy (UVH)	Compensated Vestibulopathy (UVH)	Unstable Labyrinthine Disease
Subjective symptoms	• Signature initial episode of violent vertigo lasting 6–72 h in duration • Nausea/emesis • Ongoing motion provoked dizziness • Postural instability • Blurred vision during head movement • Possible acute hearing loss	• Postural instability when walking in altered sensory conditions (head movements, dark, uneven ground) • Brief bouts of motion-provoked dizziness • Blurred vision with head movements	• Minimal to no postural instability • Minimal to no motion provoked dizziness • Clear vision with head movement	• Episodic spontaneous vertigo persisting; as severe as initial insult • Poor progress despite rehabilitation program
Vestibular tests				
Vestibular test results (ENG/VNG, rotary chair)	• Unilateral caloric weakness • Spontaneous or positional nystagmus despite normal oculomotor findings • Positive Dix-Hallpike or Roll test for BPPV • Abnormal rotational chair asymmetry	• Persistent spontaneous, gaze evoked, or positional nystagmus • Post-head shake nystagmus • Rotational chair asymmetry	• Resolution of nystagmus • Resolution of rotational chair asymmetry	• Persistent spontaneous, gaze evoked, or positional nystagmus • Post-head shake nystagmus • Rotational chair asymmetry
Posturography	SOT abnormalities on conditions 5 and/or 6	SOT abnormalities on conditions 5 and/or 6	Improved SOT (composite score performance)	May demonstrate SOT abnormalities on conditions 5 and/or 6
Clinical bedside exam				
Video-goggles (visual fixation removed)	• Spontaneous, gaze or post-head shake nystagmus • Positive Dix-Hallpike or Roll test for BPPV	Persistent spontaneous, gaze, positional, or post-head shake nystagmus	Resolution of nystagmus	Persistent spontaneous, gaze, positional or post-head shake nystagmus

(continued on next page)

Table 3
(continued)

Objective Findings	Unilateral Vestibular Dysfunction (UVH)	Indicative of an Uncompensated Vestibulopathy (UVH)	Compensated Vestibulopathy (UVH)	Unstable Labyrinthine Disease
Room light (with visual fixation)	• Positive head thrust test with refixation saccade • DVA $\geq$ 3-line difference	DVA $\geq$ 3-line difference	DVA < 3-line difference	DVA $\geq$ 3-line difference
Balance and gait	• Impaired mCTSIB • Gait instability when walking with altered sensory conditions (horizontal/vertical head movements, eyes closed, or uneven terrain)	• Impaired mCTSIB • Gait instability when walking with altered sensory conditions (horizontal/vertical head movements, eyes closed, or uneven terrain)	• Improved gait speed • Improved gait stability with head movements • Able to pass most/all mCTSIB conditions	• Impaired mCTSIB • Gait instability when walking with altered sensory conditions (horizontal/vertical head movements, eyes closed, or uneven terrain)

Box 2
Considerations for stopping vestibular physical therapy intervention

Potential reasons to end vestibular physical therapy intervention
- Resolution of symptoms
- Achievement of functional goals
- Improved balance, gait, and vestibular function (signs of compensation)
- Plateau in progress
- Patient preference
- Patient noncompliance
- Therapist/patient agreement
- Patient not improving despite adequate trial (2–4 weeks)

ANTICIPATED BENEFIT FROM VESTIBULAR REHABILITATION ON VARIOUS CONDITIONS

Acute Unilateral Vestibular Hypofunction

Based on level I evidence, clinicians should offer VPT to individuals with acute or sub-acute UVH with the overall goal of improving quality of life.[1] Recent evidence supports early initiation of VPT, within the first 2 weeks after onset, following acute vestibular neuritis.[37] Initiation of gaze stabilization exercises as early as postoperative day 3 following vestibular schwannoma resection is beneficial for reducing subjective dizziness.[38,39] Despite reported benefit in older studies, the use of methylprednisolone during the early acute period (20-mg tablets 3 times daily for 1 week tapered over another week) did not impact long-term outcomes in individuals with acute vestibular neuritis.[40] Studies support supervised physical therapy (PT) once per week for 2 to 3 weeks combined with a customized daily HEP consisting of gaze stabilization, habituation, and balance and conditioning exercises.[1] Improvement in balance occurs slower in older adults (60 years old and older) with UVH; thus, this population may benefit from additional vestibular therapy interventions.[41]

Postoperative Dizziness and Imbalance

Dizziness, vertigo, and imbalance have been documented following cochlear implantation (CI) possibly related to transient or permanent unilateral hypofunction, labyrinthitis, and/or BPPV.[42,43] VPT, including gaze stabilization, habituation exercises, balance retraining, and canalith repositioning maneuvers, as indicated, can assist in alleviating these symptoms.[44] Subjects greater than 60 years old are more likely to demonstrate decreased balance function and have an increased fall risk following CI; therefore, short-term VPT may be beneficial in the immediate postoperative period.[45]

Prolonged imbalance and residual motion sensitivity following posterior canal occlusion for intractable BPPV have been reported in the literature[46,47]; therefore, clinicians should consider referral to VPT either routinely or especially when these postsurgical symptoms are present. Balance measures (mCTSIB condition 4 and Dynamic Gait Index scores) were significantly impaired immediately following superior semicircular canal dehiscence (SSCD) repair, recovering by week 6.[48] Patients undergoing SSCD repair should undergo a postoperative fall risk assessment during the early postoperative recovery period. The clinician should also screen for postoperative motion-provoked dizziness, especially with head movements in the plane of the plugged canal.

Chronic Unilateral Vestibular Hypofunction

Evidence supports VPT for individuals with chronic (longer than 3 months) UVH with focus on gaze stabilization, habituation, and balance and endurance exercises combined with patient education in an HEP.[1] Supervised VPT has been found to be more effective than unsupervised intervention.[49] Individuals with chronic UVH who are experiencing ongoing dizziness and imbalance should participate in supervised VPT for 4 to 6 weeks combined with daily HEP.[1] Several different modes of treatment have been used, including virtual reality, tai chi, platform training, optokinetic stimuli, and vibrotactile feedback without a clear benefit of one mode over the other.

Bilateral Vestibular Hypofunction

Oscillopsia, unsteady gait, and impaired spatial memory are common sequelae related to bilateral vestibular hypofunction (BVH). Individuals with BVH often have difficulty performing work-related duties, driving, exercising, and participating in social and community activities. Similar to UVH, VPT for individuals with BVH should be initiated early in the setting of an acute onset, and longer periods of intervention may be required.[50]

Evidence supports the use of specific exercises (adaptation, substitution, balance, gait, and endurance)[51] to improve overall functional capacity, with therapeutic emphasis on the exercise principle of sensory substitution. The goal is to facilitate the use of proprioceptive and visual inputs to enhance postural control[52,53] and stabilize vision.[54] Other forms of technology-based sensory substitution options include vibrotactile feedback,[55,56] electrotactile tongue biofeedback,[57] and noisy galvanic stimulation.[58] These interventions have resulted in improved postural control for some individuals with BVH. Recently, clinical trials in humans using a vestibular prosthesis, which provides continuous, motion-modulated stimulation via electrodes in 3 semicircular canals, have demonstrated promise.[59] Subjects (n = 4) reported more stable vision and decreased postural unsteadiness and were able to return to driving within weeks of activating the device.

The ability to maintain stable vision can also occur via prefrontal planning, wherein the eye movements precede head rotation as head movement is anticipated.[54] These eye movements substitute for the deficient VOR, likely via central preprogramming and an efferent copy of the motor command.[54] In addition to adaptation (VOR $\times$ 1, VOR $\times$ 2) exercises, eye-head movements between 2 targets with emphasis on maintaining clear vision while performing horizontal and vertical eye-head movements are important for improving dynamic vision in this population.[54,60]

Benign Paroxysmal Positional Vertigo

Patients reporting brief episodes of vertigo/dizziness provoked by looking up, getting out of bed, rolling over in bed, quick head movements, and bending forward should undergo positional testing (Dix-Hallpike and Roll test) to rule out BPPV.[61] Some elderly individuals will not articulate these classic symptoms and should also be tested for this highly treatable condition. A large portion of patients (86%) with BPPV will experience interrupted daily activities or inability to work.[5] There is strong evidence to support successful performance of particle repositioning maneuvers (PRMs) by a clinician or by the patient at home when provided with proper instruction for effective treatment of posterior canal BPPV.[4,5] The short-term ($\geq$24 hours and <1 month) success rate for patients treated with PRMs by a clinician was found to be 67% to 95% compared with 10% to 38% resolution with a sham treatment.[4] In addition, clinician-performed PRMs combined with patient self-administered PRMs has been found to be more effective than the clinician administered PRMs alone.[4]

More recently, rarer apogeotropic variants of posterior canal[62] and horizontal canal[63] BPPV have been identified and successfully treated. Therefore, close observation of nystagmus patterns, using video goggles when available, is critical to accurate diagnosis, and more importantly, to efficient and effective treatment. An overview of commonly used PRMs can be found in the updated BPPV clinical practice guideline.[5] Postmaneuver restrictions have been deemed unnecessary.[5] Refer to article 6 for more information regarding BPPV.

Vestibular Migraine

Individuals with vestibular migraine may experience dizziness, motion sensitivity, visual vertigo, and imbalance, any of which would make them candidates for a trial of VPT. Although several studies reported improved functional outcome scores and subjective improvement of symptoms (DHI)[8–12] following a course of VPT (ranging from 5 days to 4 months with HEP), a further review of these studies[64] rated the evidence as inconclusive secondary to a lack of comparison to control groups. Habituation exercises were used in 4 of 5 studies in an attempt to decrease the heightened response to external stimuli.[8–11] Balance exercises were included in all 5 studies aimed at improving the organization and use of sensory information for postural control. Centrally acting medications did not appear to negate or enhance the benefit of VPT in 1 study,[11] but improved functional outcomes were noted in another study when the patient was taking antimigraine medication during VPT.[8]

Meniere's Disease

In current practice, VPT is not typically indicated in active Meniere's disease because of the spontaneous vertigo attacks with "normal" vestibular function between episodes. However, a session of therapy may reinforce important lifestyle modifications, improve activity confidence, and screen for potential fall risk. In a recent clinical practice guideline, Basura and colleagues[19] recommended that clinicians should offer VPT for patients with Meniere's disease with chronic imbalance. In addition, individuals with signs and symptoms of an uncompensated unilateral peripheral vestibular hypofunction following ablative medical (intratympanic gentamicin) or surgical (labyrinthectomy) procedures as well as those with bilateral vestibular loss from this disorder may benefit from VPT.[19] There are limited studies that have evaluated the type of exercises that may be beneficial in this population; however, there is strong supportive evidence for treatment of UVH and BVH focusing on gaze stabilization exercises and balance training.[1]

Persistent Postural-Perceptual Dizziness

Long-standing symptoms of dizziness, unsteadiness, and nonrotary vertigo may result in a clinical diagnosis of PPPD.[65] The precise cause of this chronic vestibular disorder is uncertain, but it manifests as waxing and waning nonspecific vestibular symptoms lasting greater than 3 months. Symptoms occur on most days, are exacerbated by upright posture, active or passive motion, and exposure to environments with moving or complex visual stimuli.[66]

Current treatment paradigms for PPPD include a combination of medication, cognitive behavioral therapy, vestibular rehabilitation, and patient education.[67–69] Selective serotonin reuptake inhibitors have been found to reduce symptoms in patients with chronic dizziness who completed 8 to 12 weeks of treatment.[70,71] Treatment with serotonin-norepinephrine reuptake inhibitors improves dizziness, headache, and anxiety in individuals with chronic subjective dizziness and vestibular migraine.[72] Cognitive behavioral therapy, especially if initiated within 8 months of symptom onset, has been shown to reduce dizziness, with improvements retained at 6 months.[73,74]

In a retrospective study, Thompson and colleagues[6] found that performance of a long-term (average 27.5 months) home-based habituation exercise program led to decreased motion and visually provoked dizziness. Improved functional, physical, and total DHI scores have been documented after 6 weeks of a customized HEP focused on progressively stimulating gaze and gait stabilization exercises.[7] More recently, 75% of individuals with PPPD who participated in 6 VPT sessions (once per week) combined with acceptance and commitment therapy, aimed at accepting versus controlling symptoms, demonstrated a significant decline in DHI scores at 6 months' posttreatment.[75] Staab[76] proposed that, in some cases, rather than promoting central compensation, VPT may have a positive effect through behavior modification. This behavior modification may include cognitive reframing to reduce fear and avoidance of movement, eliminate dependence on unnecessary assistive devices, and improve balance confidence.

Concussion/Traumatic Brain Injury

Dizziness following traumatic brain injury (TBI) may be peripheral or central in nature, with or without BPPV. Patients may present with a wide range of deficits and systems affected; thus, clinicians should conduct a comprehensive intake and examination.[17] VPT intervention should include a targeted approach and may include oculomotor training, gaze stabilization, balance training, motion and visual sensitivity training, PRMs, cervical treatment, and graduated exertion training.[77] Most individuals do not have significant symptoms lasting more than 1 to 3 months after concussion.[17] Early personalized VPT resulted in a shorter recovery period and was deemed safe and feasible in a randomized controlled trial comparing a group of adolescents with concussion and dizziness up to 14 days after injury to a control group.[16]

FALL RISK ASSESSMENT

Individuals with vestibular hypofunction commonly experience motion-provoked dizziness and imbalance with head movements, oscillopsia (visual blurring or bouncing of the environment), gait instability, and spatial disorientation, thereby increasing their risk for falling. A vestibular deficit was correlated with falls in 30% of individuals with UVH and 50% of individuals, ages 65 to 74, with BVH.[78] The recurrent fall rate in individuals with BVH has been found to be 30%.[79] Importantly, older adults with vestibular and balance impairments have a 5- to 8-fold increase in their risk of falling compared with age-matched healthy adults.[79,80]

Hearing loss has also been associated with higher fall risk, with 1 study finding a 1.4 hazard ratio for falling for every 10 dB of hearing loss.[81] Fear of falling can also contribute to falls. In 1 study, individuals with UVH and functional dizziness (chronic subjective dizziness) were significantly more concerned about falling compared with healthy participants.[79] Fear of falling develops in 20% to 40% of older adults who suffer a fall[82] and may lead to decreased activity, generalized weakness, and deconditioning, all of which further increase risk of falling.[83]

Clinicians should assess fall risk and fear of falling in individuals with dizziness and vestibular and balance disorders. The American Geriatrics Society/British Geriatrics Society Clinical Practice Guideline for prevention of falls in older persons recommends the use of 3 screening questions.[84] Patients are considered high risk if they affirm any of the following:

1. Two or more falls in the past year?
2. Presenting with an acute fall?
3. Difficulty with walking or balance?

When a patient screens positive for falls, the clinician should perform additional assessments that target 3 key risk factors: balance, medication, and home safety.[85]

Table 4
Fall risk balance and gait tests

Test	How to Administer	Interpretation of Findings	Test Assessment Forms Can Be Found:

Timed Up-and-Go (TUG)	Directions:
	• Patients can use a walking aid
	• Begin by having the patient sit back in a standard armchair and identify a line 3 m on the floor
	Instruct the patient: (always stand by patient for safety)
	• When I say "Go," I want you to:
	  1. Stand up from the chair
	  2. Walk to the line on the floor at your normal pace
	  3. Turn
	  4. Walk back to the chair at your normal pace
	  5. Sit down again
	• On the word "Go", begin timing
	• Stop timing after the patient sits back down
	• Record time
		An older adult who takes $\geq$12 s to complete the TUG is at risk for falling	https://www.cdc.gov/steadi/pdf/STEADI-Assessment-TUG-508.pdf

30-s chair stand test	Directions: • Begin by having the patient sit in a chair with a straight back without arm rests (seat 17 inches high) Instruct the patient: 1. Sit in the middle of the chair 2. Place your hands on the opposite shoulder crossed, at the wrists 3. Keep your feet flat on the floor	Below average scores: Age, y Men Women 60–64 <14 <12 65–69 <12 <11 70–74 <12 <10 75–79 <11 <10 80–84 <10 <9 85–89 <8 <8	https://www.cdc.gov/steadi/pdf/STEADI-Assessment-30sec-508.pdf

(continued on next page)

Table 4
(continued)

Test	How to Administer	Interpretation of Findings			Test Assessment Forms Can Be Found:
	4. Keep your back straight, and keep your arms against your chest 5. On "Go," rise to a full standing position, then sit back down again 6. Repeat this for 30 s • On the word "Go," begin timing • If the patient must use his/her arms to stand, stop the test. Record "0" for the number and score • Count the number of times the patient comes to a full standing position in 30 s • If the patient is over halfway to a standing position when 30 s have elapsed, count it as a stand • Record the number of times the patient stands in 30 s	90–94 Note: A below average score indicates a risk for falls.	<7	<4	
4-stage balance test	Instruct the patient: • "I'm going to show you 4 positions. Try to stand in each position for 10 s. You can hold your arms out, or move your body to help keep your balance, but don't move your feet" • For each position, I will say, "Ready, begin." Then, I will start timing. After 10 s, I will say, "Stop."	An older adult who cannot hold the tandem stance for at least 10 s is at increased risk of falling			https://www.cdc.gov/steadi/pdf/STEADI-Assessment-4Stage-508.pdf

1. Stand with your feet side by side
   Time: _____ seconds
2. Place the instep of 1 foot so it is touching the big toe of the other foot
   Time: _____ seconds
3. Tandem stand: Place 1 foot in front of the other, heel touching toe
   Time: _____ seconds
4. Stand on 1 foot
   Time: _____ seconds

Table 5	
Factors increasing fall risk	
Intrinsic Health Factors	**Environmental and Behavioral Factors**
• Dizziness	• Poor lighting
• Postural/orthostatic hypotension	• Throw rugs
• Pain	• Stairs without railing
• Impaired vision	• Shower/bath without grab bars
• Hearing loss	• Obstacles within walking path
• Peripheral neuropathy	• Complex unfamiliar environments
• Fear of falling	• Hard to reach objects
• Taking 4 or more medications	• Poor fitting or spongy footwear
• Leg weakness	• Rushing
• Moderate to severe cognitive impairment	• Distraction
• Low vitamin D levels	
• Depression, anxiety	
• Osteoporosis	

Three expeditious gait, strength, and balance tests (**Table 4**) are the Timed Up-and-Go, the 30-Second Chair Stand test, and the 4-Stage Balance test.[86] Clinicians should also be aware of common intrinsic or environmental factors that contribute to falls (**Table 5**).

Appropriate referrals should be made when a high fall risk is identified, including to a vestibular physical therapist for strengthening, balance, and gait training; an occupational therapist for a home safety evaluation; an audiologist for audiometry and a hearing aid trial; an optometrist for vision examination; and/or a neurologist for cognitive evaluation and sensory/proprioceptive testing. Referrals back to the primary care physician may be indicated for medication review, management of orthostatic hypotension, and further laboratory tests (vitamin B12 level, vitamin D level, complete blood count). Older adults, even with low fall risk, may benefit from a community exercise program that targets strengthening and balance, because this type of exercise is the single most effective intervention for reducing falls.[87]

SUMMARY

There is strong evidence to support VPT for individuals with acute or chronic uncompensated UVH and BVH and BPPV. Early VPT intervention may lessen the potential for the impairments to progress to secondary symptoms or a chronic condition, such as PPPD. Clinicians can use an individual's subjective symptom report, clinical bedside tests, and/or vestibular tests to assess a patient's compensation status and need for VPT. Individuals with vestibular disorders have higher fall rates and should be screened for balance impairments and fall risk. Clinicians should educate and encourage their patients to incorporate daily exercise, avoid long-term use of vestibular suppressants, and modify lifestyle behaviors to facilitate recovery.

CASE STUDY

See Video 1.

CLINICS CARE POINTS

- Clinicians should consider early referral to vestibular physical therapy to reduce the likelihood that vestibular impairments will result in a chronic condition associated with less favorable outcomes.

- There is strong evidence to support successful performance of particle repositioning maneuvers by a clinician or by the patient at home when provided with proper instruction for effective treatment of posterior canal benign paroxysmal positional vertigo.

- Clinicians should screen for fall risk and make appropriate recommendations and referrals to specialists to reduce fall risk in individuals with dizziness and balance impairments.

- Clinicians should educate and encourage their patients to incorporate daily exercise/movement, avoid long-term use of vestibular suppressants, and modify lifestyle behaviors to facilitate recovery from vestibular deficits.

DISCLOSURE

The authors have nothing to disclose.

SUPPLEMENTARY DATA

Supplementary data related to this article can be found online at https://doi.org/10.1016/j.otc.2021.05.018.

REFERENCES

1. Hall CD, Herdman SJ, Whitney SL, et al. Vestibular rehabilitation for peripheral vestibular hypofunction: an evidence-based clinical practice guideline: from the American Physical Therapy Association Neurology Section. J Neurol Phys Ther 2016;40(2):124–55.

2. American Academy of Otolaryngology—Head and Neck Surgery or Foundation (AAO-HNS/F) Boards of Directors. Position statement: vestibular rehabilitation. Available at: https://www.entnet.org/content/vestibular-rehabilitation. Revised October 13, 2020.

3. Herdman SJ, Hall CD, Maloney B, et al. Variables associated with outcome in patients with bilateral vestibular hypofunction: preliminary study. J Vestib Res 2015; 25(3–4):185–94.

4. Helminski JO, Zee DS, Janssen I, et al. Effectiveness of particle repositioning maneuvers in the treatment of benign paroxysmal positional vertigo: a systematic review. Phys Ther 2010;90(5):663–78.

5. Bhattacharyya N, Gubbels SP, Schwartz SR, et al. Clinical practice guideline: benign paroxysmal positional vertigo (update). Otolaryngol Head Neck Surg 2017;156(3_suppl):S1–47.

6. Thompson KJ, Goetting JC, Staab JP, et al. Retrospective review and telephone follow-up to evaluate a physical therapy protocol for treating persistent postural-perceptual dizziness: a pilot study. J Vestib Res 2015;25(02):97–103.

7. Nada EH, Ibraheem OA, Hassaan MR. Vestibular rehabilitation therapy outcomes in patients with persistent postural-perceptual dizziness. Ann Otology, Rhinology Laryngol 2019;128(4):323–9.

8. Whitney SL, Wrisley DM, Brown KE, et al. Physical therapy for migraine-related vestibulopathy and vestibular dysfunction with history of migraine. Laryngoscope 2000;110:1528–34.

9. Wrisley DM, Whitney SL, Furman JM. Vestibular rehabilitation outcomes in patients with a history of migraine. Otol Neurotol 2002;23:483–7.

10. Gottshall KR, Hoffer ME. Vestibular rehabilitation for migraine-associated dizziness. Int Tinnitus J 2005;11:81–4.

11. Vitkovic J, Winoto A, Rance G, et al. Vestibular rehabilitation outcomes in patients with and without vestibular migraine. J Neurol 2013;260:3039–48.

12. Sugaya N, Arai M, Goto F. Is the headache in patients with vestibular migraine attenuated by vestibular rehabilitation? Front Neurol 2017;8:124.

13. Wrisley DM, Sparto PJ, Whitney SL. Cervicogenic dizziness: a review of diagnosis and treatment. J Orthop Sports Phys Ther 2000;30(12):755–66.

14. Clendaniel RA, Landel R. Physical therapy management of cervicogenic dizziness. In: Herdman SJ, editor. Vestibular rehabilitation. 4th ed. Philadelphia: F.A. Davis Company; 2014. p. 590–609.

15. Schneider KJ, Meeuwisse WH, Nettel-Aguirre A, et al. Cervicovestibular rehabilitation in sport-related concussion: a randomized controlled trial. Br J Sports Med 2014;48:1294–8.

16. Reneker JC, Hassen A, Phillips RS, et al. Feasibility of early physical therapy for dizziness after a sports-related concussion: a randomized clinical trial. Scand J Med Sci Sports 2017;27:2009–18.

17. Quatman-Yates CC, Hunter-Giordano A, Shimamura KK, et al. Physical therapy evaluation and treatment after concussion/mild traumatic brain injury. J Orthop Sports Phys Ther 2020;50(4):CPG1–73.

18. Tramontano M, Russo V, Spitoni G, et al. The efficacy of vestibular rehabilitation in patients with neurological disorders: a systematic review. Arch Phys Med Rehabil 2020.

19. Basura GJ, Adams ME, Monfared A, et al. Clinical practice guideline: Ménière's disease. Otolaryngol Head Neck Surg 2020;162(2_suppl):S1–55.

20. Halmagyi GM, McGarvie LA, Strupp M. Nystagmus goggles: how to use them, what you find and what it means. Pract Neurol 2020;20:446–50.

21. Dannenbaum E, Paquet N, Chilingaryan G, et al. Clinical evaluation of dynamic visual acuity in subjects with unilateral vestibular hypofunction. Otol Neurotol 2009;30(3):368–72.

22. Visser JE, Carpenter MG, van der Kooij H, et al. The clinical utility of posturography. Clin Neurophysiol 2008;119(11):2424–36.

23. Vestibular evidence database to guide effectiveness. Available at: https://www.neuropt.org/practice-resources/neurology-section-outcome-measures-recommendations/vestibular-disorders. Accessed June 24, 2021.

24. Jacobson GP, Newman CW. The development of the dizziness handicap inventory. Arch Otolaryngol Head Neck Surg 1990;116(4):424–7.

25. Powell LE, Myers AM. The Activities-specific Balance Confidence (ABC) Scale. J Gerontol A Biol Sci Med Sci 1995;50A(1):M28–34.

26. Morris AE, Lutman ME, Yardley L. Measuring outcome from vestibular rehabilitation, part II: refinement and validation of a new self-report measure. Int J Audiol 2009;48(1):24–37.

27. Di Fabio RP. Sensitivity and specificity of platform posturography for identifying patients with vestibular dysfunction. Phys Ther 1995;75(4):290–305.

28. Shumway-Cook A, Horak FB. Assessing the influence of sensory interaction of balance. Suggestion from the field. Phys Ther 1986;66(10):1548–50.

29. Franchignoni F, Horak F, Godi M, et al. Using psychometric techniques to improve the balance evaluation systems test: the mini-BESTest. J Rehabil Med 2010;42(4):323–31.

30. Whitney SL, Hudak MK, Marchetti GF. The dynamic gait index related to self-reported fall history in individuals with vestibular dysfunction. J Vestib Res 2000;10(2):99–105.

31. Wrisley DM, Marchetti GF, Kuharsky DK, et al. Reliability, internal consistency, and validity of data obtained with the functional gait assessment. Phys Ther 2004;84(10):906–18.

32. Studenski S, Perera S, Patel K, et al. Gait speed and survival in older adults. JAMA 2011;305(1):50–8.

33. Aranda C, Meza A, Rodríguez R, et al. Diabetic polyneuropathy may increase the handicap related to vestibular disease. Arch Med Res 2009;40(3):180–5.

34. MacDowell SG, Wellons R, Bissell A, et al. The impact of symptoms of anxiety and depression on subjective and objective outcome measures in individuals with vestibular disorders. J Vestib Res 2018;27(5–6):295–303.

35. Shepard NT, Telian SA, Smith-Wheelock M. Habituation and balance retraining therapy. A retrospective review. Neurol Clin 1990;8(2):459–75.

36. Whitney SL, Sparto PJ, Furman JM. Vestibular rehabilitation and factors that can affect outcome. Semin Neurol 2020;40(1):165–72.

37. Lacour M, Laurent T, Alain T. Rehabilitation of dynamic visual acuity in patients with unilateral vestibular hypofunction: earlier is better. Eur Arch Otorhinolaryngol 2020;277(1):103–13.

38. Herdman SJ, Clendaniel RA, Mattox DE, et al. Vestibular adaptation exercises and recovery: acute stage after acoustic neuroma resection. Otolaryngol Head Neck Surg 1995;113(1):77–87.

39. Enticott JC, O'Leary SJ, Briggs RJ. Effects of vestibulo-ocular reflex exercises on vestibular compensation after vestibular schwannoma surgery. Otol Neurotol 2005;26(2):265–9.

40. Ismail EI, Morgan AE, Abdel Rahman AM. Corticosteroids versus vestibular rehabilitation in long-term outcomes in vestibular neuritis. J Vestib Res 2018;28(5–6):417–24.

41. Scheltinga A, Honegger F, Timmermans DP, et al. The effect of age on improvements in vestibulo-ocular reflexes and balance control after acute unilateral peripheral vestibular loss. Front Neurol 2016;7:18.

42. Rah YC, Park JH, Park JH, et al. Dizziness and vestibular function before and after cochlear implantation. Eur Arch Otorhinolaryngol 2016;273:3615–21.

43. Viccaro M, Mancini P, La Gamma R, et al. Positional vertigo and cochlear implantation. Otol Neurotol 2007;28(6):764–7.

44. Steenerson RL, Cronin GW, Gary LB. Vertigo after cochlear implantation. Otol Neurotol 2001;22(6):842–3.

45. Stevens MN, Baudhuin JE, Hullar TE, Washington University Cochlear Implant Study Group. Short-term risk of falling after cochlear implantation. Audiol Neurootol 2014;19(6):370–7.

46. Ahmed RM, Pohl DV, MacDougall HG, et al. Posterior semicircular canal occlusion for intractable benign positional vertigo: outcome in 55 ears in 53 patients operated upon over 20 years. J Laryngol Otol 2012;126(7):677–82.

47. Ramakrishna J, Goebel JA, Parnes LS. Efficacy and safety of bilateral posterior canal occlusion in patients with refractory benign paroxysmal positional vertigo: case report series. Otol Neurotol 2012;33(4):640–2.

48. Janky KL, Zuniga MG, Carey JP, et al. Balance dysfunction and recovery after surgery for superior canal dehiscence syndrome. Arch Otolaryngol Head Neck Surg 2012;138(8):723–30.

49. Smółka W, Smółka K, Markowski J, et al. The efficacy of vestibular rehabilitation in patients with chronic unilateral vestibular dysfunction. Int J Occup Med Environ Health 2020;33(3):273–82.

50. Ertugrul S, Emre Soylemez E. Investigation of the factors affecting the success of vestibular rehabilitation therapy in patients with idiopathic unilateral vestibular hypofunction and idiopathic bilateral vestibular hypofunction. ENT Updates 2019; 9(2):150–8.

51. Herdman SJ, Clendaniel RA. Physical therapy management of bilateral vestibular hypofunction and loss. In: Herdman SJ, editor. Clendaniel vestibular rehabilitation. Fourth Edition. Philedelphia, PA: F.A. Davis Co; 2014. p. 432–56.

52. Han BI, Song HS, Kim JS. Vestibular rehabilitation therapy: review of indications, mechanisms, and key exercises. J Clin Neurol 2011;7(04):184–96.

53. Porciuncula F, Johnson CC, Glickman LB. The effect of vestibular rehabilitation on adults with bilateral vestibular hypofunction: a systematic review. J Vestib Res 2012;22(5–6):283–98.

54. Herdman SJ, Schubert MC, Tusa RJ. Role of central preprogramming in dynamic visual acuity with vestibular loss. Arch Otolaryngol Head Neck Surg 2001;127: 1205–10.

55. Brugnera C, Bittar RS, Greters ME, et al. Effects of vibrotactile vestibular substitution on vestibular rehabilitation - preliminary study. Braz J Otorhinolaryngol 2015;81(6):616–21.

56. Kingma H, Felipe L, Gerards M-C, et al. Vibrotactile feedback improves balance and mobility in patients with severe bilateral vestibular loss. J Neurol 2019; 266(Suppl 1):19–26.

57. Barros CG, Bittar RS, Danilov Y. Effects of electrotactile vestibular substitution on rehabilitation of patients with bilateral vestibular loss. Neurosci Lett 2010;476(3): 123–6.

58. Wuehr M, Nusser E, Decker J, et al. Noisy vestibular stimulation improves dynamic walking stability in bilateral vestibulopathy. Neurology 2016;86(23): 2196–202.

59. Boutros PJ, Schoo DP, Rahman M, et al. Continuous vestibular implant stimulation partially restores eye-stabilizing reflexes. JCI Insight 2019;4(22):e12839.

60. Lehnen N, Kellerer S, Knorr AG, et al. Head-movement-emphasized rehabilitation in bilateral vestibulopathy. Front Neurol 2018;9:562.

61. Whitney SL, Marchetti GF, Morris LO. Usefulness of the dizziness handicap inventory in the screening for benign paroxysmal positional vertigo. Otol Neurotol 2005;26(5):1027–33.

62. Vannucchi P, Pecci R, Giannoni B, et al. Apogeotropic posterior semicircular canal benign paroxysmal positional vertigo: some clinical and therapeutic considerations. Audiol Res 2015;5(1):130.

63. Kim JS, Oh SY, Lee SH, et al. Randomized clinical trial for apogeotropic horizontal canal benign paroxysmal positional vertigo. Neurology 2012;78(3):159–66.

64. Alghadir AH, Anwer S. Effects of vestibular rehabilitation in the management of a vestibular migraine: a review. Front Neurol 2018;9:440.

65. Staab JP, Eckhardt-Henn A, Horii A, et al. Diagnostic criteria for persistent postural-perceptual dizziness (PPPD): consensus document of the Committee for the Classification of Vestibular Disorders of the Bárány Society. J Vestib Res 2017;27(4):191–208.

66. Staab JP. Persistent postural-perceptual dizziness. Semin Neurol 2020;40(1): 130–7.

67. Dieterich M, Staab JP. Functional dizziness: from phobic postural vertigo and chronic subjective dizziness to persistent postural-perceptual dizziness. Curr Opin Neurol 2017;30(1):107–13.

68. Trinidade A, Goebel JA. Persistent postural-perceptual dizziness-a systematic review of the literature for the balance specialist. Otol Neurotol 2018;39(10): 1291–303.

69. Axer H, Finn S, Wassermann A, et al. Multimodal treatment of persistent postural-perceptual dizziness. Brain Behav 2020;28:e01864.

70. Horii A, Mitani K, Kitahara T, et al. Paroxetine, a selective serotonin reuptake inhibitor, reduces depressive symptoms and subjective handicaps in patients with dizziness. Otol Neurotol 2004;25(04):536–43.

71. Horii A, Uno A, Kitahara T, et al. Effects of fluvoxamine on anxiety, depression, and subjective handicaps of chronic dizziness patients with or without neuro-otologic diseases. J Vestib Res 2007;17(01):1–8.

72. Horii A, Imai T, Kitahara T, et al. Psychiatric comorbidities and use of milnacipran in patients with chronic dizziness. J Vestib Res 2016;26(03):335–40.

73. Edelman S, Mahoney AE, Cremer PD. Cognitive behavior therapy for chronic subjective dizziness: a randomized, controlled trial. Am J Otolaryngol 2012; 33(04):395–401, 49.

74. Mahoney AE, Edelman S, Cremer PD. Cognitive behavior therapy for chronic subjective dizziness: longer-term gains and predictors of disability. Am J Otolaryngol 2013;34(02):115–20.

75. Kuwabara J, Kondo M, Kabaya K, et al. Acceptance and commitment therapy combined with vestibular rehabilitation for persistent postural-perceptual dizziness: a pilot study. Am J Otolaryngol 2020;41(6):102606.

76. Staab JP. Behavioral aspects of vestibular rehabilitation. NeuroRehabilitation 2011;29:179–83.

77. Morris L, Gottshall K. Physical therapy management of the patient with vestibular dysfunction from head trauma. In: Herdman SJ, editor. Clendaniel vestibular rehabilitation. Fourth Edition. Philedelphia, PA: F.A. Davis Co; 2014. p. 504–29.

78. Herdman SJ, Blatt P, Schubert MC, et al. Falls in patients with vestibular deficits. Am J Otol 2000;21(6):847–51.

79. Schlick C, Schniepp R, Loidl V, et al. Falls and fear of falling in vertigo and balance disorders: a controlled cross-sectional study. J Vestib Res 2016;25(5–6): 241–51.

80. Agrawal Y, Carey JP, Della Santina CC, et al. Disorders of balance and vestibular function in US adults. Arch Intern Med 2009;169:938–44.

81. Lin FR, Ferrucci L. Hearing loss and falls among older adults in the United States. Arch Intern Med 2012;172:369–71.

82. Scheffer AC, Schuurmans MJ, vanDijk N, et al. Fear of falling: measurement strategy, prevalence, risk factors and consequences among older persons. Age Aging 2008;37:19–24.

83. Friedman SM, Munoz B, West SK, et al. Falls and fear of falling: which comes first? A longitudinal prediction model suggests strategies for primary and secondary prevention. J Am Geriatr Soc 2002;50(8):1329–35.

84. Panel on Prevention of Falls in Older Persons. Summary of the Updated American Geriatrics Society/British Geriatrics Society clinical practice guideline for prevention of falls in older persons. J Am Geriatri Soc 2011;59: 148–57.

85. Stevens JA, Phelan EA. Development of STEADI: a fall prevention resource for health care providers. Health Promot Pract 2013;14:706–14.

86. STEADI tool kit. Available at: https://www.cdc.gov/steadi/materials.html. Accessed June 24, 2021.

87. Gillespie LD, Robertson MC, Gillespie WJ, et al. Interventions for preventing falls in older people living in the community. Cochrane Database Syst Rev 2012;9: CD007146.

Current and Emerging Medical Therapies for Dizziness

Mallory J. Raymond, MD[a], Esther X. Vivas, MD[b],*

KEYWORDS

- Pharmacotherapy • Dizziness • Central vertigo • Peripheral vertigo

KEY POINTS

- Pharmacotherapies for dizzy conditions are generally aimed at reducing dizziness, controlling the neurovegetative symptoms, or addressing its root cause.
- Pharmacotherapies for vertigo reduction and symptom management of acute peripheral and central vertigo include antihistamines, calcium channel blockers, and benzodiazepines.
- Evidence for oral prophylactic pharmacotherapies for Meniere's disease remains mixed, but betahistine and diuretics are reasonable first-line options.
- 4-Aminopyridine is the main pharmacologic agent shown to have benefit in patients with cerebellar dizziness and oculomotor disorders.
- Pharmacologic options for vestibular migraine, persistent postural perceptual dizziness, and mal de débarquement overlap and include selective serotonin reuptake inhibitors, serotonin-norepinephrine reuptake inhibitors, tricyclic antidepressants, and calcium channel blockers.

INTRODUCTION

Medical management of dizzy patients relies on a well-performed history and physical examination in order to determine the quality, type, site of origin of the dizziness, and associated symptoms. Pharmacotherapy is most commonly aimed at vertigo reduction and secondary symptom management but can also be directed at the origin of the pathologic process. Pharmacotherapy has roles in both acute and chronic dizziness, for abortive and prophylactic purposes, and for secondary neurovegetative symptoms. Many pharmacotherapies have widespread use across both central and

a Department of Otolaryngology–Head and Neck Surgery, Medical University of South Carolina, 135 Rutledge Avenue MSC 550, 11th Floor, Charleston, SC 29425, USA; b Department of Otolaryngology–Head and Neck Surgery, Emory University School of Medicine, 550 Peachtree Street Northeast, 11th Floor, Atlanta, GA 30308, USA
* Corresponding author.
E-mail address: evivas@emory.edu

Otolaryngol Clin N Am 54 (2021) 1037–1056
https://doi.org/10.1016/j.otc.2021.05.019
0030-6665/21/© 2021 Elsevier Inc. All rights reserved.

oto.theclinics.com

peripheral causes of dizziness because of the overlapping sites of action and the still largely unknown causes of many vertiginous conditions. This article reviews the major pharmacotherapy classes and the associated pharmacology that is available for the treatment of dizzy conditions, as well as the evidence behind medical therapies for specific disease entities.

NEUROPHARMACOLOGY OF THE VESTIBULAR PATHWAY
Inner Ear

Vestibular neuroepithelial hair cells synapse with afferent neurons and receive innervation from efferent neural projections. The main neurotransmitter of the afferent synapses is glutamate, and the main neurotransmitter of the efferent synapse is acetylcholine.[1] Glutamate released at afferent synapses interacts with excitatory amino acid receptors, such as N-methyl-D-aspartic acid (NMDA), which is responsible for basal discharge and tonic response to sustained stimuli.[2] Additional neurotransmission may occur through nitric oxide and opioid peptides.[3–5] In addition to sensory processing, vestibular hair cells also receive sympathetic and parasympathetic innervation. Pharmacologic agents aimed at the vestibular end-organ level target hair cells through ionic channel modulation or either afferent or efferent neuromodulation through neurotransmitters or receptor antagonists/agonists.[6]

Vestibular Nuclei

The Vestibular nuclei (VNs) contain a number of receptors and receive a complex network of projections from the vestibular nerve afferents, the visual pathway, and the proprioceptive pathway. Additional VN receptors include gamma-aminobutyric acid (GABA), glycine, histamine (H1, H2, and H3), serotonin (5HT1 and 5HT2), adrenergic, cholinergic, muscarinic, nicotinic, opioid, and glucocorticoid receptors.[7–10] Inhibitory GABAergic fibers from the cerebellum and contralateral VN activate GABA-A and GABA-B receptors. Histaminergic fibers originate from the tuberomammillary nucleus; serotonergic fibers originate from the raphe nuclei. Norepinephrine and dopamine modulate the reaction to vestibular stimuli centrally.[11] Given the multitude and diversity of synaptic connections and neurotransmitters, medications can target many processes, including input to the nuclei, the neuronal response, neuronal integration, excitability, and action potential discharge.[6]

Other Central Players

Stimulation of the chemoreceptor trigger zone within the area postrema of the brainstem induces vomiting and can be modulated with dopaminergic blockade.[12] The gastrointestinal tract plays a role in inducing vomiting as well through serotonergic (5HT3) pathways. Within the hypothalamus, histaminergic paths play a role in the vestibular-autonomic response to motion sickness.[13]

PHARMACOLOGIC CATEGORIES
Medications that Act on Neurotransmitter and Neuromodulator Receptors

Anticholinergics
Centrally acting anticholinergic medications, such as scopolamine and atropine, block muscarinic receptors, known to be present in the VN complex, and the vestibular afferent and efferent neurons.[6] Scopolamine is a nonselective competitive inhibitor of muscarinic acetylcholine receptors and has been most commonly used in a transdermal formulation for treatment of motion sickness.[6] Side effects include blurry vision, dry mouth, dilated pupils, urinary retention, and sedation. It is not

recommended that they be used for more than several days because of these side effects and potential for withdrawal. Scopolamine patches are used specifically for motion sickness.

Antihistamines

Histamine and histamine receptors have been found in the vestibular end organs and VN, and the ability of antihistamines to bind to these various sites accounts for their wide applicability. The most commonly prescribed medications are dimenhydrinate, diphenhydramine, meclizine, and promethazine. Although they are primarily H1 receptor antagonists, they also have anticholinergic activity, and all likely suppress vertigo and nausea equally. Side effects include hypersomnolence, dry mouth, and urinary retention.[14] Betahistine is a histamine analogue with antagonistic effects on H3 receptors and partial agonist effects on H1 and H2 receptors.[15,16] It is thought to reduce the incidence and severity of vertigo, nausea, and emesis through changes in inner ear blood flow.[17] Side effects are mild and may include headaches, nausea, feeling hot, eye irritation, palpitations, and upper gastrointestinal symptoms.[18,19] It should be avoided in patients with pheochromocytoma and used with caution for patients with peptic ulcer disease or asthma.[18,19]

Calcitonin gene–related peptide

Calcitonin gene–related peptide (CGRP) is a neuropeptide expressed in trigeminal neurons and is involved in pain perception. It is also a potent vasodilator and is postulated to play a major role in the pathogenesis of migraine. Anti-CGRP monoclonal antibodies have emerged as new and effective treatment options for chronic migraine and include galcanezumab, fremanezumab, eptinezumab, and erenumab. They are administered intravenously or subcutaneously on a monthly basis. Side effects include injection site reactions, upper respiratory symptoms, and constipation.[20] Further work is needed to assess their efficacy in vestibular migraine (VM).

Gamma-aminobutyric acid

Benzodiazepines are GABA receptor agonists and are effective at suppressing vertigo and vertigo-associated nausea.[21,22] Although a multitude of medications are available, the most commonly prescribed medications include diazepam, lorazepam, and clonazepam. There is no evidence for the superiority of one benzodiazepine over another and, similarly, for the superiority of the antivertiginous effects of benzodiazepines compared with antihistamines.[14] Adverse effects include habituation, sedation, memory impairment, and increased fall risk and consequent traumatic injury; they also carry a risk for drug dependence.[22] Benzodiazepines should be considered for patients with contraindications to anticholinergics or antihistamines.

Monoamines

Dopamine receptors have been found in the VN and end organs.[6] Dopamine antagonists have been used to treat acute peripheral vertigo or general vertigo.[6] Common agents include prochlorperazine and metoclopramide. Some dopamine receptor antagonists have antihistamine properties and, likewise, some antihistamines, such as promethazine, also possess antidopaminergic properties. Side effects include orthostatic hypotension, somnolence, parkinsonism, tardive dyskinesia, acute dystonia, endocrine abnormalities, and all of the anticholinergic adverse effects.[11]

Adrenergic activity in the VN is complex and is both excitatory and inhibitory, depending on the specific receptor. Inhibition of adrenergic reuptake through medications such as β-blockers and tricyclic antidepressants (TCAs) may be at play, with improvements found in patients with VM. β-Blockers in use include propranolol and metoprolol. TCAs include amitriptyline, a serotonin and norepinephrine reuptake inhibitor, and nortriptyline, which also has antihistamine and anticholinergic activity. Side effects of β-blockers include cold hands and feet, fatigue, weight gain, depression, and difficulty sleeping. Side effects of TCAs include dry mouth, slight blurring of vision, constipation, urinary retention, drowsiness, weight gain, sweating, and cardiac arrhythmias.

Spiral and vestibular ganglion cells express the serotonin receptors 5-HT1A, 5-HT1B, 5-HT1D, and 5-HT1F receptors.[23] Serotonergic innervation of the VN and the shared neural pathways and receptor expression of the vestibular ganglia, trigeminal ganglia, and spiral ganglia are thought to play a role in the associations of vestibular alterations, anxiety, and migraine.[24] Selective serotonin reuptake inhibitors (SSRIs), such as sertraline, and serotonin-norepinephrine reuptake inhibitors (SNRIs), such as venlafaxine and paroxetine, have been used for patients with VM or persistent postural perceptual dizziness (3PD). Side effects of SSRIs and SNRIs include indigestion, diarrhea, loss of appetite, insomnia and headaches, and sexual dysfunction.[25] Although rare, patients should be counseled about the possibility of serotonin syndrome, especially if on multiple medications that affect serotonin levels.

Medications that Act on Ion Channels

Calcium channel blockers
Calcium channels are responsible for neurotransmitter release at synaptic terminals at the level of the hair cells, afferent neurons, and VNs and are targets for the action of calcium channel blockers. The most common calcium channel blockers in use for vestibular disorders include nimodipine and verapamil, which inhibit the calcium current and neurotransmitter release in hair cells.[6] In Europe, cinnarizine and flunarizine have been used in the treatment of acute vertigo and VM. Aside from their peripheral calcium channel activity, they can block pressure-sensitive potassium channels and have additional antagonistic action on histamine and norepinephrine. Side effects include sedation, weight gain, extrapyramidal responses, and depression. In addition, gabapentin, originally thought to act at GABA receptors, also has calcium channel-blocking activity and has been used for the treatment of central vertigo.[26]

Sodium channel blockers
Voltage-gated sodium channels are expressed in the inner ear neuroepithelium and found within afferent neurons and the VNs.[6] Pharmacologic action on sodium channels leads to changes in excitability and discharge pattern of the afferent and VN neurons.[6] Although not recommended, transtympanic application of lidocaine, a sodium channel blocker, has resulted in vestibular symptom improvements.[6] Carbamazepine, an antiepileptic that stabilizes voltage-gated sodium channels, has been used for vestibular paroxysmia. Topiramate is another antiepileptic with multiple actions: blockade of voltage-gated sodium channels, enhancement of GABA neurotransmission, reduction of calcium currents from calcium channels, and inhibition of carbonic anhydrase.[27] The exact mechanism for its action in treatment of vestibular disorders is unknown, although it has been successfully used for VM. Side effects include paresthesia, fatigue, concentration difficulty, decreased appetite, and weight loss.[28] Lamotrigine and valproate are other antiepileptics that inhibit sodium channels and have also been used in treatment of VM. Side effects also include nausea, fatigue, and insomnia.

Potassium channel blockers
Potassium channels play a role in several pathologic processes, and many pharmacotherapies can act on these channels. However, their role in vestibular dysfunction has

been defined only by studies of the aminopyridines, voltage-gated potassium channel blockers. 4-Aminopyridine (4-AP) reduces slow-phase velocity of downbeat nystagmus, presumably by affecting the excitability and action potential of cerebellar Purkinje fibers.[6] 4-AP has also been used to treat episodic ataxia type 2 and upbeating nystagmus.[11] Side effects include abdominal discomfort and dizziness.

Antiinflammatory Medications

Glucocorticoid receptors have been found within the inner ear, leading to interest in the use of corticosteroids to modulate acute vestibulopathy. Corticosteroids, such as prednisone, methylprednisolone, and dexamethasone, have all been studied within the context of acute vestibulopathy and Meniere's disease (MD). Medication can be delivered orally, intravenously, or transtympanically. Side effects of systemic administration include glaucoma, insomnia, hyperglycemia, hypertension, muscle weakness, mood swings, stomach irritation, and bleeding.

Diuretics

Diuretics function primarily to alter sodium excretion by the kidneys but are thought to have additional effects on electrolyte balance of endolymph in the inner ear, leading to a reduction of endolymphatic volume.[14] Thiazide diuretics (hydrochlorothiazide, chlorthalidone, metolazone, indapamide) inhibit sodium and chloride reabsorption from the distal convoluted tubules of the kidney; loop diuretics (furosemide, bumetanide, ethacrynic acid) inhibit sodium reabsorption; potassium-sparing diuretics (triamterene, amiloride, spironolactone) inhibit the sodium-potassium exchange within the collecting ducts; carbonic anhydrase inhibitors (acetazolamide) increase excretion of sodium, potassium, bicarbonate, and water.[29] Combinations of thiazides and potassium-sparing agents, such as triamterene, are the most commonly prescribed diuretics for MD. Acetazolamide is considered a second-line agent and has also been used for episodic ataxia type 2. Thiazides can precipitate gout and are therefore contraindicated for patients with preexisting gout. In addition, potassium-sparing diuretics should not be used for patients with renal failure. General side effects include electrolyte imbalance, headache, thirst, and diarrhea. Acetazolamide can also cause distal extremity paresthesia.

TREATMENT BY CONDITION
Positional Vertigo

Benign paroxysmal positional vertigo

The gold standard of treatment of benign paroxysmal positional vertigo (BPPV) is canalith repositioning, and there is a limited role for pharmacotherapy. Vestibular suppressants in particular have been shown to be less efficacious than repositioning maneuvers in resolution and improvement of vertigo and, therefore, are not indicated for treatment of BPPV.[30,31] Vitamin D currently serves as the only pharmacotherapy target, because vitamin D deficiency has been associated with increased odds of BPPV occurrence and recurrence.[32–38] One explanation of this relationship is that vitamin D may play a role in the calcium metabolism of otoconia.[39] A 2020 meta-analysis of 5 trials (4 nonrandomized trials and 1 randomized controlled trial) of vitamin D supplementation in the setting of vitamin D deficiency and BPPV showed a significant prevention in recurrences compared with patients not receiving vitamin D supplementation.[40] However, dosages of vitamin D varied between the studies, ranging from low (800 IU vitamin D daily) to high (50,000 IU vitamin D3 weekly), so there is currently no gold standard for supplementation in the setting of BPPV. However, data from the most recent randomized trial suggest that patients with BPPV should be screened for vitamin D deficiency and, if found to be deficient, should be given vitamin D and calcium supplementation (800 IU vitamin D and 1000 mg calcium carbonate daily).[40,41]

Acute Peripheral and Central Vertigo

Pharmacotherapy for acute peripheral vertigo is initially aimed at neurovegetative symptom management (nausea, vomiting, palpitations, sweating, and anxiety) and secondarily at the cause of the vertigo and enhancing central adaptation.[42,43] There is no consensus on the first-line medication to be used for symptom reduction; however, several medications have been investigated, including antihistamines, calcium channel blockers, benzodiazepines, neuroleptics, and glucocorticoids.[44–48] Antihistamines have been the mainstay of treatment of acute peripheral vertigo because of their effect on the histaminergic signals from the VN to the vomiting center in the medulla and include meclizine, astemizole, and promethazine.[49,50] A major side effect of sedation has led investigators to compare betahistine with these H1 antagonists, and results suggest that betahistine may be as effective (or better) in controlling symptoms but without causing sedation.[51] Although H1 antagonists, such as promethazine, are effective in controlling vertigo, evidence suggests that ondansetron may be more effective at controlling the nausea and vomiting.[52] Historically, benzodiazepines, such as lorazepam and diazepam, were provided for symptom management of acute peripheral vertigo; however, promethazine may be more effective.[53,54] In addition, cinnarizine, a calcium channel blocker, has been used alone or in combination with antihistamines, such as dimenhydrinate or betahistine, to reduce symptoms, and evidence suggests that the medications used in combination are more effective in symptom reduction than when used as monotherapies.[55–57] The choice of initial medication remains primarily driven by physician comfort and preferences. However, prolonged use of any of the vestibular suppressants beyond the early and symptomatic stage is discouraged, because they may inhibit central compensation.[58]

Corticosteroids are aimed at the causative process of acute peripheral vertigo because of their antiinflammatory properties. There is mixed evidence regarding the symptomatic improvement after corticosteroid treatment; however, corticosteroids have been shown to improve the caloric recovery.[59–63] A 2011 Cochrane analysis found insufficient evidence to provide treatment recommendations for corticosteroids[64]; however, many investigators continue to argue for prompt (within 24 hours) treatment with them.[58,65] Additional agents that may enhance central vestibular compensation and recovery include N-acetyl-L-leucine and Ginkgo biloba extract EGb 761; however, further study is needed before making recommendations for their use.[66–69]

Vestibular paroxysmia

Vestibular paroxysmia is characterized by recurrent short-lived attacks of spontaneous spinning vertigo, relieved by carbamazepine or oxcarbazepine.[70] It is thought to be caused by neurovascular compression of the eighth nerve near the brainstem.[58] In 2 studies, low doses of these antiepileptic sodium channel blockers reduced the number of vertigo attacks.[71,72]

Meniere's Disease

Medical management of MD is aimed at reducing the severity and frequency of vertigo attacks and is considered complex because of the episodic and unpredictable nature of the disease as well as the limited understanding of its pathophysiology. Acute vertigo attacks are managed primarily with vestibular suppressants, similar to those discussed in relation to acute peripheral vertigo, including antihistamines, anticholinergics, and benzodiazepines. Although these medications are thought to be effective by both patients and providers, there is a lack of peer-reviewed evidence documenting their effectiveness. In addition, there is no evidence that suggests superiority of benzodiazepines compared with antihistamines or vice versa for vertigo control. In addition, anticholinergics are not commonly prescribed for vertigo control in MD because of their side effect profile.[14] Vestibular suppressants are not indicated for prophylactic use for MD.

Pharmacotherapy prophylaxis is typically recommended for patients who fail diet and lifestyle modifications, which include salt, caffeine, and alcohol intake restriction and stress reduction. Although several pathophysiologic mechanisms for MD have been proposed, diuretics and betahistine have been used to target the specific mechanisms of endolymphatic electrolyte imbalance and vestibular end-organ blood flow, respectively. A 2006 Cochrane systematic review identified 10 studies investigating the effectiveness of diuretics, but none met the inclusion criteria.[73] Despite this, some studies have shown an improvement in vertigo control with the use of diuretics, and the American Academy of Otolaryngology–Head and Neck Surgery (AAO-HNS) have designated diuretic use as an option to reduce symptoms or prevent vertigo attacks.[73,74] The study of betahistine has produced similarly mixed results in terms of vertigo control. Likely the best evidence to date from the BEMED trial (a double-blind randomized controlled trial [RCT] comparing placebo, low-dose betahistine [48 mg/d], and high-dose betahistine [144 mg/d]) does not show a difference in the number of vertigo attacks with betahistine treatment compared with placebo.[19] However, betahistine is considered an option for prophylactic management. Note that betahistine is not approved by the Food and Drug Administration (FDA) in the United States, and it can be difficult for patients to obtain. In addition, although oral steroids have historically been used for symptom management, only 1 pilot study has shown an overall improvement in vertigo.[75]

Intratympanic (IT) steroids are the next option to offer to patients with uncontrolled vertigo attacks. The mechanism of action is thought to be secondary to improvement in cochlear blood flow through antiinflammatory properties and cochlear ion and fluid homeostasis.[76–78] The AAO-HNS guidelines have designated IT steroids as an option, because both randomized controlled trials and systematic reviews have shown their efficacy compared with placebo.[79–82] Only 1 prospective, placebo-controlled trial of slow-release dexamethasone gel did not show a difference in rates of vertigo.[83] However, the 2 medications commonly used, methylprednisolone and dexamethasone, have different pharmacokinetics, and there is insufficient literature comparing their efficacy. Common dosages and administration frequency are listed in **Table 1**. Despite the lack of complete clarity on the use of IT steroids, they carry fewer side effects than oral steroids and are without the risk of hearing loss (compared with IT gentamicin). IT gentamicin should be offered to MD patients with symptoms uncontrolled by nonablative therapies. Several studies have shown improved symptom control with IT gentamicin compared with IT steroids (70%–87% vs 43%–90% of patients).[84–87] Reported rates of hearing loss vary, but, with low dosages and frequencies, the rate is considered low[14]; therefore, dosing is recommended on an as-needed basis.[88,89]

Chronic Central Vestibulopathies

Cerebellar dizziness and down beating nystagmus

Causes of chronic cerebellar dizziness include degenerative forms (cerebellar ataxia, multiple system atrophy, idiopathic downbeat nystagmus, and cerebellar ataxia with neuropathy and vestibular areflexia syndrome), hereditary forms (spinocerebellar ataxias and episodic ataxias), and acquired forms (autoimmune, toxin related, infectious).[90] Presentations of dizziness and vertigo can be recurrent or chronic. Therapy

Table 1
Current pharmacologic options for dizziness

Pharmacologic Categories	Medication Classes	Indications	Side Effects	Examples	Dosing Highlights[a]
Medications that act on neurotransmitter and neuromodulator receptors	Anticholinergics	Vestibular suppression Motion sickness Antiemetic	Blurry vision, dry mouth, dilated pupils, urinary retention and sedation	Scopolamine Atropine	Scopolamine 1 mg patch every 72 h
	Antihistamines	Vestibular suppression MD	Hypersomnolence, dry mouth, and urinary retention Headaches, nausea, feeling hot, eye irritation, palpitations, and upper gastrointestinal symptoms	Dimenhydrinate meclizine Promethazine Cinnarizine Betahistine	Meclizine 12.5–25 mg every 8 h Diphenhydramine 25–50 mg every 6 h Promethazine 12.5–25 mg every 4–6 h Betahistine 48 mg/d
	GABA (benzodiazepines)	Vestibular suppression MD Central nystagmus	Habituation, sedation, memory impairment, increased fall risk, dependence	Diazepam Lorazepam Clonazepam	Diazepam 2–10 mg every 8 h Lorazepam 1–2 mg every 8 h Clonazepam 0.5–1.0 mg every 8 h
	Dopamine agonists	Vestibular suppression Antiemetic	Orthostatic hypotension, somnolence, parkinsonism, tardive dyskinesia, acute dystonia, endocrinopathies, anticholinergic side effects	Prochlorperazine Metoclopramide	Prochlorperazine 5–10 mg every 6–8 h Metoclopramide 10 mg every 6 h
	Adrenergic antagonists or reuptake inhibitors	Vestibular suppression VM	Dry mouth, slight blurring of vision, constipation, urinary retention, drowsiness, weight gain, sweating, cardiac arrhythmias Cold hands and feet, fatigue, weight gain, depression,	TCAs • Nortriptyline • Amitriptyline β-Blockers • Metoprolol • Propranolol	Nortriptyline 25–75 mg/d Amitriptyline 10–50 mg/d Propranolol 80–240 mg/d Metoprolol 50–200 mg/d

	Indication	Side effects	Medications	Dosage
SSRIs/SNRIs	Vestibular suppression VM MD 3PD Mal de débarquement	and difficulty sleeping Indigestion, diarrhea, loss of appetite, insomnia, headaches, and sexual dysfunction	Sertraline Venlafaxine Paroxetine	Sertraline 25–150 mg/d Venlafaxine 37.5–75 mg/d Paroxetine 5–40 mg/d
Medications that act on ion channels				
Calcium channel blockers	Vestibular suppression VM MD	Sedation, weight gain, extrapyramidal responses and depression	Nimodipine Verapamil Gabapentin	Nimodipine 120 mg/d Verapamil 120–240 mg/d Gabapentin 300–900 mg/d
Sodium channel blockers	Vestibular paroxysmia VM	Paresthesia, fatigue, memory and concentration difficulty, decreased appetite, weight loss, nausea, insomnia	Topiramate Lamotrigine Valproate Carbamazepine Oxcarbazepine	Topiramate 25–50 mg/d Lamotrigine 25–100 mg/d Valproate 500–600 mg/d Carbamazepine 200–600 mg/d
Potassium channel blockers	Downbeat nystagmus Upbeat nystagmus Episodic ataxia type 2	Abdominal discomfort, dizziness	4-Aminopyridine	4-Aminopyridine 10–15 mg/d Fampridine 10–20 mg/d
Antiinflammatory medications				
Steroids	Acute vestibulopathy MD	Glaucoma, insomnia, hyperglycemia, hypertension, muscle weakness, mood swings, stomach irritation, or bleeding	Dexamethasone Prednisone Methylprednisolone	Oral or intravenous: Methylprednisolone 100 mg/d Prednisone 60 mg/d Transtympanic: Dexamethasone sodium phosphate 0.4–0.8 mL of 10 mg/mL Methylprednisolone sodium succinate 0.4–0.8 mg or 40 mg/mL

(continued on next page)

Table 1
(continued)

Pharmacologic Categories	Medication Classes	Indications	Side Effects	Examples	Dosing Highlights[a]
Diuretics	Thiazide, loop Potassium-sparing diuretics Carbonic anhydrase inhibitors	MD Episodic ataxia type 2 VM	Electrolyte imbalance, headache, thirst and diarrhea (generally)	Hydrochlorothiazide Furosemide Triamterene Acetazolamide	Triamterene/hydrochlorothiazide 37.5–25 mg/d Acetazolamide 250–500 mg/d
Vestibulotoxins	Gentamicin	MD	Hearing loss, tympanic membrane perforation	Gentamicin	Gentamicin, 0.75 mL of a 40-mg/mL gentamicin solution into the inner ear as needed

[a] Dosages provided are examples only and do not necessarily encompass the full dosage range and frequency for safety or effectiveness for all patients.

is multimodal and includes vestibular physical therapy for eye stabilization, posture and gait control, and pharmacotherapy.[91] Aminopyridines, chlorzoxazone, and N-acetyl-DL-leucine have had beneficial effects for patients with cerebellar dizziness and oculomotor disorders.[92,93] 4-AP was shown to reduce the intensity of downbeating nystagmus, alleviate symptoms of downbeating nystagmus, and improve visual acuity and motor performance in studies of patients with idiopathic downbeat nystagmus, cerebellar atrophy, and episodic ataxia type 2.[94–98] In a single, noncontrolled study, chlorzoxazone, a potassium channel agonist, led to improved postural stability for patients with downbeat nystagmus.[99] In addition, patients with cerebellar ataxia treated with N-acetyl-DL-leucine have shown improvements in ataxia scores, gait variability, and quality of life.[100,101]

Fixation nystagmus, upbeat nystagmus, central positioning nystagmus, and acquired pendular nystagmus

Other oculomotor disorders can be caused by lesions at several sites of the brainstem or cerebellum. Patients may complain of dizziness and oscillopsia. 4-AP has been used effectively in 2 case reports of upbeating nystagmus and central positional nystagmus.[26] Baclofen may be effective in managing upbeat or downbeat nystagmus as well as periodic alternating nystagmus.[102,103] It is thought to reduce nystagmus by inhibiting central vestibular pathways.[11] In addition, anticholinergic agents may be effective in reducing nystagmus intensity in acquired pendular nystagmus.[104] In addition, gabapentin was shown to reduce nystagmus and improve visual acuity for acquired pendular nystagmus.[105]

Vestibular Migraine

Pharmacotherapy management of VM (VM) includes both abortive and preventive medications; however, data regarding efficacy have been limited, in part because of the overlapping symptoms with MD, the concordance of VM with MD, and a lack of outcomes that define successful treatment. For this reason, many of the current treatments are derived from algorithms for the treatment of migraines. Initial prophylactic treatment revolves around dietary limitations (of caffeine, alcohol, artificial sweeteners, processed meats), stress reduction, sleep hygiene, and trigger avoidance. Supplementation of magnesium, vitamin B_2, and coenzyme Q may also be of initial benefit.[106]

Acute symptoms in VM can be managed similarly to acute peripheral vestibular disorders and treatments include antihistamine and anticholinergic vestibular suppressants, with a particular emphasis on controlling nausea. Promethazine is well suited for VM because of its potential antidopaminergic activity within the trigeminocervical complex; transdermal scopolamine can also be used, although infrequently, for patients with vertigo attacks lasting longer than 24 hours.[107] The triptan SSRIs (zolmitriptan and sumatriptan) have each been found effective in reducing vertigo, although the level of evidence is insufficient to make recommendations on their use.[108,109] In addition, intravenous methylprednisolone may be administered to patients with a prolonged severe vestibular attack.[110]

Indications for prophylactic medications for VM are derived from those for migraine and include recurring attacks that interfere with quality of life, 4 or more attacks per month, and failure of abortive medications.[111] Medications include benzodiazepines, β-blockers, calcium channel blockers, SSRIs, SNRIs, topiramate, and TCAs,[112] but there is insufficient evidence from RCTs to prove definitive efficacy in prevention of VM for many.[113] β-Blockers, such as propranolol, calcium channel blockers, such as verapamil, and antiepileptics, such as topiramate, have been successfully used for migraine prophylaxis.[114] Flunarizine, a calcium channel blocker, has been effective in reducing the severity and frequency of vertigo attacks, but it is not FDA approved.[115] Venlafaxine and propranolol have been effective in reducing vestibular symptoms, but venlafaxine also helped with depressive symptoms.[116] Cinnarizine is unavailable in the United States but has been shown to decrease both headache and vertigo frequency and severity.[117,118] In a retrospective study, lamotrigine reduced the frequency of vertigo but not of headache.[112] In addition, topiramate, well established as an effective choice for migraine prophylaxis, has also led to a reduction in vertigo frequency and severity.[28] A 2020 meta-analysis of pharmacotherapy studies for VM was unable to provide preferred treatment recommendations because of the heterogeneity and lack of standardized reporting outcomes from the included studies.[25] Therefore, clinicians should consider the side effect profile of each pharmacotherapy agent as well as patient comorbidities when choosing a regimen. An example algorithm for management of VM, presented by Liu and colleagues,[119] is: first-line treatment includes nortriptyline 20 to 50 mg at bedtime if the patient has insomnia issues, topiramate 50 to 100 mg daily for potential additive weight loss benefit, or venlafaxine 37.5 mg daily if there is underlying anxiety. Second-line treatment includes propranolol 80 mg 2 to 3 times daily or verapamil 120 mg daily or twice a day if the patient has hypertension. Verapamil is favored if there is a history of hemiplegic migraines.[119]

Botulinum toxin (Botox) injections are an additional option for patients with VM who have more than 15 headaches per month and are unresponsive to trials of 2 preventive medications from 2 different classes.[109] Botox injections are well supported in the literature for prevention of chronic migraine[120] and can be administered based on the PRE-EMPT (Phase 3 REsearch Evaluating Migraine Prophylaxis Therapy) trials.[121,122] Anti-CGRP monoclonal antibodies are emerging as effective options for management of chronic migraine as well, and they have potential use in VM.[123] A randomized, double-blinded, placebo-controlled trial comparing galcanezumab, a CGRP antagonist, with placebo for VM is currently in its recruitment phase.[124]

Persistent Postural Perceptual Dizziness

3PD is thought to be secondary to maladaptive strategies for balance control that develop after an acute episode of dizziness. Although treatment is aimed at fear modulation, activity avoidance, and reversing postural control and overcompensatory movement strategies through cognitive behavior therapy, vestibular rehabilitation, counseling and physiotherapy, medication has been used with variable success.[125] Specifically, SSRIs and SNRIs have been recommended for functional dizziness both with and without concordant psychiatric conditions.[126] Evidence comes from case control and retrospective studies and 1 RCT, investigating the response of patients with chronic subjective dizziness, psychogenic dizziness, and 3PD to sertraline, fluoxetine, paroxetine, citalopram, fluvoxamine, and venlafaxine.[127–132] Based on these studies, about half to two-thirds of patients can be expected to have a favorable response; therefore, clinicians should consider the addition of an SSRI or SNRI to a patient's treatment regimen, especially for those with significant comorbid depression and/or anxiety. When initiating medication, it is recommended to begin slowly and at lower doses in order to avoid bothersome side effects, which have the potential to lead to noncompliance. In addition, management of 3PD relies on readaptation strategies, and thus the use of vestibular suppressants should be avoided.

Mal de Débarquement

The pathophysiology of mal de débarquement syndrome is poorly understood but it is thought to share common pathways with migraine. It is not surprising, then, that prophylactic migraine therapies have been studied and found to have variable success. For example, benzodiazepines such as clonazepam and diazepam, as well as antidepressants, such as venlafaxine, have been found successful, but calcium channel blockers, such as verapamil, have not.[133-135] A 2017 prospective trial applied a migraine prophylaxis regimen of first-line therapies of nortriptyline, verapamil, or both and a second-line therapy of either acetazolamide or topiramate and found the regimen led to improved quality of life and symptom intensity.[136] Additional medications suggested to have benefit include SSRIs and TCAs.[137] Given the lack of understanding of the pathophysiologic mechanisms, migraine pharmacotherapy principles should be applied, and drug choice should be aimed at patient-specific factors.

SUMMARY

Medical therapies for dizziness are aimed at vertigo reduction, secondary symptom management, or the cause of the pathologic process. Acute peripheral vertigo pharmacotherapies include antihistamines, calcium channel blockers, and benzodiazepines, and their use must be balanced against the need for central compensation. Prophylactic pharmacotherapies vary between causes. For MD, betahistine and diuretics remain initial first-line oral options, whereas intratympanic steroids and intratympanic gentamicin are reserved for uncontrolled symptoms. For cerebellar dizziness and oculomotor disorders, 4-AP may provide benefit. For VM, 3PD, and mal de débarquement, treatment options overlap and include SSRIs, SNRIs, TCAs, and calcium channel blockers.

CLINICS CARE POINTS

- Pharmacotherapies for dizzy conditions are generally aimed at reducing dizziness, controlling the neurovegetative symptoms, or addressing its root cause.
- Pharmacotherapies for vertigo reduction and symptom management of acute peripheral and central vertigo include antihistamines, calcium channel blockers, and benzodiazepines.
- Evidence for oral prophylactic pharmacotherapies for MD remains mixed, but betahistine and diuretics are reasonable first-line options.
- 4-AP is the main pharmacologic agent shown to have benefit in patients with cerebellar dizziness and oculomotor disorders.
- Pharmacologic options for VM, 3PD, and mal de débarquement overlap and include SSRIs, SNRIs, TCAs, and calcium channel blockers.

DISCLOSURE

The authors have nothing to disclose.

REFERENCES

1. Soto E, Vega R. Neuropharmacology of vestibular system disorders. Curr Neuropharmacol 2010;8(1):26–40.
2. Soto E, Flores A, Eróstegui C, et al. Evidence for NMDA receptor in the afferent synaptic transmission of the vestibular system. Brain Res 1994;633(1–2): 289–96.
3. Hess A, Bloch W, Arnhold S, et al. Nitric oxide synthase in the vestibulocochlear system of mice. Brain Res 1998;813:97–102.

4. Hess A, Bloch W, Su JP, et al. Expression of inducible nitric oxide synthase in the vestibular system of hydropic guinea pigs. Neurosci Lett 1999;264:145–8.

5. Andrianov GN, Ryzhova IY. Opioid peptides as possible neuromodulators of the afferent synaptic transmission in the frog semicircular canal. Neuroscience 1999;93:801–6.

6. Soto E, Vega R, Seseña E. Neuropharmacological basis of vestibular system disorder treatment. J Vestib Res 2013;23(3):119–37.

7. Bergquist F, Dutia MB. Central histaminergic modulation of vestibular function - a review. Sheng Li Xue Bao 2006;58(4):293–304.

8. Halberstadt AL, Balaban CD. Selective anterograde tracing of the individual serotonergic and nonserotonergic components of the dorsal raphe nucleus projection to the vestibular nuclei. Neuroscience 2007;147(1):207–23.

9. Matsuoka I, Domino EF. Cholinergic mechanisms in the cat vestibular system. Neuropharmacology 1975;14(3):201–10.

10. Sulaiman MR, Dutia MB. Opioid inhibition of rat medial vestibular nucleus neurones in vitro and its dependence on age. Exp Brain Res 1998;122(2):196–202.

11. Colby C, Huang T. Medications used in treating acute and chronic vertigo and various vestibular disorders. In: Vertigo and disequilibrium a practical guide to diagnosis and management. New York: Thieme; 2017.

12. Rascol O, Hain TC, Brefel C, et al. Antivertigo medications and drug-induced vertigo. A pharmacological review. Drugs 1995;50(5):777–91.

13. Smith PF. Pharmacology of the vestibular system. Curr Opin Neurol 2000; 13(1):31–7.

14. Basura GJ, Adams ME, Monfared A, et al. Clinical practice guideline: Ménière's disease. Otolaryngol Head Neck Surg 2020;162(2_suppl):S1–55.

15. Arrang JM, Garbarg M, Quach TT, et al. Actions of betahistine at histamine receptors in the brain. Eur J Pharmacol 1985;111:73–84.

16. Wang JJ, Dutia MB. Effects of histamine and betahistine on rat medial vestibular nucleus neurones: possible mechanism of action of anti-histaminergic drugs in vertigo and motion sickness. Exp Brain Res 1995;105:18–24.

17. Martínez DM. The effect of Serc (betahistine hydrochloride) on the circulation of the inner ear in experimental animals. Acta Otolaryngol 1972;305:29–47.

18. Murdin L, Hussain K, Schilder AGM. Betahistine for symptoms of vertigo. Cochrane Database Syst Rev 2016;(6):CD010696.

19. Adrion C, Fischer CS, Wagner J, et al. Efficacy and safety of betahistine treatment in patients with Meniere's disease: primary results of a long term, multicentre, double blind, randomised, placebo controlled, dose defining trial (BEMED trial). BMJ 2016;352:h6816.

20. Szperka CL, VanderPluym J, Orr SL, et al. Recommendations on the use of Anti-CGRP monoclonal antibodies in children and adolescents. Headache 2018; 58(10):1658–69.

21. Brandt T, Zwergal A, Strupp M. Medical treatment of vestibular disorders. Expert Opin Pharmacother 2009;10(10):1537–48.

22. Lin E, Aligene K. Pharmacology of balance and dizziness. NeuroRehabilitation 2013;32(3):529–42.

23. Ahn SK, Balaban CD. Distribution of 5-HT1B and 5-HT1D receptors in the inner ear. Brain Res 2010;1346:92–101.

24. Balaban CD. Neural substrates linking balance control and anxiety. Physiol Behav 2002;77(4–5):469–75.

25. Byun YJ, Levy DA, Nguyen SA, et al. Treatment of vestibular migraine: a systematic review and meta-analysis. Laryngoscope 2021;131(1):186–94.

26. Zwergal A, Strupp M, Brandt T. Advances in pharmacotherapy of vestibular and ocular motor disorders. Expert Opin Pharmacother 2019;20(10):1267–76.
27. Mula M, Cavanna AE, Monaco F. Psychopharmacology of topiramate: from epilepsy to bipolar disorder. Neuropsychiatr Dis Treat 2006;2(4):475–88.
28. Gode S, Celebisoy N, Kirazli T, et al. Clinical assessment of topiramate therapy in patients with migrainous vertigo. Headache 2010;50(1):77–84.
29. Laurent S. Antihypertensive drugs. Pharmacol Res 2017;124:116–25.
30. Bhattacharyya N, Gubbels SP, Schwartz SR, et al. Clinical practice guideline: benign paroxysmal positional vertigo (update). Otolaryngol Head Neck Surg 2017;156:S1–47.
31. Sundararajan I, Rangachari V, Sumathi V, et al. Epley's manoeuvre versus Epley's manoeuvre plus labyrinthine sedative as management of benign paroxysmal positional vertigo: prospective, randomised study. J Laryngol Otol 2011;125:572–5.
32. Jeong SH, Kim JS, Shin JW, et al. Decreased serum vitamin D in idiopathic benign paroxysmal positional vertigo. J Neurol 2013;260(3):832–8.
33. Buki B, Ecker M, Junger H, et al. Vitamin D deficiency and benign paroxysmal positioning vertigo. Med Hypotheses 2013;80(2):201–4.
34. Talaat HS, Abuhadied G, Talaat AS, et al. Low bone mineral density and vitamin D deficiency in patients with benign positional paroxysmal vertigo. Eur Arch Otorhinolaryngol 2015;272(9):2249–53.
35. Rhim GI. Serum vitamin D and recurrent benign paroxysmal positional vertigo. Laryngoscope Investig Otolaryngol 2016;1(6):150–3.
36. Wu Y, Fan Z, Jin H, et al. Assessment of bone metabolism in male patients with benign paroxysmal positional vertigo. Front Neurol 2018;9:742.
37. Yang CJ, Kim Y, Lee HS, et al. Bone mineral density and serum 25-hydroxyvitamin D in patients with idiopathic benign paroxysmal positional vertigo. J Vestib Res 2018;27(5–6):287–94.
38. Han W, Fan Z, Zhou M, et al. Low 25-hydroxyvitamin D levels in postmenopausal female patients with benign paroxysmal positional vertigo. Acta Otolaryngol 2018;138(5):443–6.
39. Lundberg YW, Zhao X, Yamoah EN. Assembly of the otoconia complex to the macular sensory epithelium of the vestibule. Brain Res 2006;1091(1):47–57.
40. Jeong SH, Lee SU, Kim JS. Prevention of recurrent benign paroxysmal positional vertigo with vitamin D supplementation: a meta-analysis [published online ahead of print, 2020 Aug 7]. J Neurol 2020. https://doi.org/10.1007/s00415-020-09952-8.
41. Bigelow RT, Carey JP. Randomized controlled trial in support of vitamin D and calcium supplementation for BPPV. Neurology 2020;95(9):371–2.
42. Zatonski T, Temporale H, Holanowska J, et al. Current views on treatment of vertigo and dizziness. J Med Diagn Meth 2014;3:150.
43. Strupp M, Magnusson M. Acute unilateral vestibulopathy. Neurol Clin 2015;33:669–85.
44. Mira E, Guidetti G, Ghilardi L, et al. Betahistine dihydrochloride in the treatment of peripheral vestibular vertigo. Eur Arch Otorhinolaryngol 2003;260:73–7.
45. Marill KA, Walsh MJ, Nelson BK. Intravenous lorazepam versus dimenhydrinate for treatment of vertigo in the emergency department: a randomized clinical trial. Ann Emerg Med 2000;36:310–9.
46. Pianese CP, Hidalgo LO, Gonzalez RH, et al. New approaches to the management of peripheral vertigo: efficacy and safety of two calcium antagonists in a 12-week, multinational, double-blind study. Otol Neurotol 2002;23:357–63.

47. Irving C, Richman P, Kaiafas C, et al. Intramuscular droperidol versus intramuscular dimenhydrinate for the treatment of acute peripheral vertigo in the emergency department: a randomized clinical trial. Acad Emerg Med 2002;9:650–3.

48. Ariyasu L, Byl FM, Sprague MS, et al. The beneficial effect of methylprednisolone in acute vestibular vertigo. Arch Otolaryngol Head Neck Surg 1990;116:700–3.

49. Amini A, Heidari K, Kariman H, et al. Histamine antagonists for treatment of peripheral vertigo: a meta-analysis. J Int Adv Otol 2015;11(2):138–42.

50. Simons FE, Simons KJ. H1 antihistamines: current status and future directions. World Allergy Organ J 2008;1(9):145–55.

51. Motamed H, Moezzi M, Rooyfard AD, et al. A comparison of the effects and side effects of oral betahistine with injectable promethazine in the treatment of acute peripheral vertigo in emergency. J Clin Med Res 2017;9(12):994–7.

52. Saberi A, Pourshafie SH, Kazemnejad-Leili E, et al. Ondansetron or promethazine: which one is better for the treatment of acute peripheral vertigo? Am J Otolaryngol 2019;40(1):10–5.

53. Amini A, Heidari K, Asadollahi S, et al. Intravenous promethazine versus lorazepam for the treatment of peripheral vertigo in the emergency department: a double blind, randomized clinical trial of efficacy and safety. J Vestib Res 2014;24(1):39–47.

54. Shafipour L, Goli Khatir I, Shafipour V, et al. Intravenous promethazine versus diazepam for treatment of peripheral vertigo in emergency department. J Mazandaran Univ Med Sci 2017;27(149):88–98.

55. Scholtz AW, Steindl R, Burchardi N, et al. Comparison of the therapeutic efficacy of a fixed low-dose combination of cinnarizine and dimenhydrinate with betahistine in vestibular neuritis: a randomized, double-blind, non-inferiority study. Clin Drug Invest 2012;32:387–99.

56. Hahn A, Sejna I, Stefflova B, et al. A fixed combination of cinnarizine/dimenhydrinate for the treatment of patients with acute vertigo due to vestibular disorders: a randomized, reference-controlled clinical study. Clin Drug Invest 2008;28(2):89–99.

57. Asadi P, Zia Ziabari SM, Majdi A, et al. Cinnarizine/betahistine combination vs. the respective monotherapies in acute peripheral vertigo: a randomized triple-blind placebo-controlled trial. Eur J Clin Pharmacol 2019;75(11):1513–9.

58. Strupp M, Mandalà M, López-Escámez JA. Peripheral vestibular disorders: an update. Curr Opin Neurol 2019;32(1):165–73.

59. Strupp M, Zingler VC, Arbusow V, et al. Methylprednisolone, valacyclovir, or the combination for vestibular neuritis. N Engl J Med 2004;351:354–61, 18.

60. Batuecas-Caletrio A, Yanez-Gonzalez R, Sanchez-Blanco C, et al. Glucocorticoids improve acute dizziness symptoms following acute unilateral vestibulopathy. J Neurol 2015;262:2578–82.

61. Karlberg ML, Magnusson M. Treatment of acute vestibular neuronitis with glucocorticoids. Otol Neurotol 2011;32:1140–3.

62. Goudakos JK, Markou KD, Franco-Vidal V, et al. Corticosteroids in the treatment of vestibular neuritis: a systematic review and meta-analysis. Otol Neurotol 2010;31(2):183–9.

63. Ismail EI, Morgan AE, Abdel Rahman AM. Corticosteroids versus vestibular rehabilitation in long-term outcomes in vestibular neuritis. J Vestib Res 2019;28:417–24.

64. Fishman JM, Burgess C, Waddell A. Corticosteroids for the treatment of idiopathic acute vestibular dysfunction (vestibular neuritis). Cochrane Database Syst Rev 2011;(5):CD008607.

65. Sjorgen J, Magnusson M, Tjernstroem F, et al. Steroids for acute vestibular neuronitits – the earlier treatment, the better the outcome? Otol Neurotol 2019;40: 372–4.

66. Chabbert C. Principles of vestibular pharmacotherapy. Handb Clin Neurol 2016; 137:207–18.

67. Lindner M, Gosewisch A, Eilles E, et al. Ginkgo biloba extract EGb 761 improves vestibular compensation and modulates cerebral vestibular networks in the rat. Front Neurol 2019;10:147.

68. Tighilet B, Léonard J, Watabe I, et al. Betahistine treatment in a cat model of vestibular pathology: pharmacokinetic and pharmacodynamic approaches. Front Neurol 2018;9:431, eCollection 2018.

69. Hamann. Special ginkgo extract in cases of vertigo: a systematic review of randomised, double- blind, placebo controlled clinical examinations. HNO 2007;55: 258–63.

70. Strupp M, Lopez-Escamez JA, Kim JS, et al. Vestibular paroxysmia: diagnostic criteria. J Vestib Res 2016;26(5–6):409–15.

71. Hufner K, Barresi D, Glaser M, et al. Vestibular paroxysmia: diagnostic features and medical treatment. Neurology 2008;71(13):1006–14.

72. Bayer O, Brémová T, Strupp M, et al. A randomized double-blind, placebo-controlled, cross-over trial (Vestparoxy) of the treatment of vestibular paroxysmia with oxcarbazepine. J Neurol 2018;265(2):291–8.

73. Thirlwall AS, Kundu S. Diuretics for Ménière's disease or syndrome. Cochrane Database Syst Rev 2006;(3):CD003599.

74. Torok N. Old and new in Ménière disease. Laryngoscope 1977;87(11):1870–7.

75. Morales-Luckie E, Cornejo-Suarez A, Zaragoza-Contreras MA, et al. Oral administration of prednisone to control refractory vertigo in Ménière's disease: a pilot study. Otol Neurotol 2005;26(5):1022–6.

76. Shirwany NA, Seidman MD, Tang W. Effect of transtympanic injection of steroids on cochlear blood flow, auditory sensitivity, and histology in the guinea pig. Am J Otol 1998;19(2):230–5.

77. Pondugula S, Sanneman J, Wangemann P, et al. Glucocorticoids stimulate cation absorption by semicircular canal duct epithelium via epithelial sodium channel. Am J Physiol Ren Physiol 2004;286(6):F1127–35.

78. Otake H, Yamamoto H, Teranishi M, et al. Cochlear blood flow during occlusion and reperfusion of the anterior inferior cerebellar artery—effect of topical application of dexamethasone to the round window. Acta Otolaryngol 2009;129(2): 127–31.

79. Lavigne P, Lavigne F, Saliba I. Intratympanic corticosteroids injections: a systematic review of literature. Eur Arch Otorhinolaryngol 2016;273(9):2271–8.

80. Patel M. Intratympanic corticosteroids in Ménière's disease: a mini-review. J Otol 2017;12(3):117–24.

81. Paragache G, Panda NK, Ragunathan M, et al. Intratympanic dexamethasone application in Ménière's disease—is it superior to conventional therapy? Indian J Otolaryngol Head Neck Surg 2005;57(1):21–3.

82. Phillips JS, Westerberg B. Intratympanic steroids for Ménière's disease or syndrome. Cochrane Database Syst Rev 2011;(7):CD008514.

83. Lambert PR, Carey J, Mikulec AA, et al. Intratympanic sustained-exposure dexamethasone thermosensitive gel for symptoms of Ménière's disease: randomized phase 2b safety and efficacy trial. Otol Neurotol 2016;37(10):1669–76.

84. Casani AP, Piaggi P, Cerchiai N, et al. Intratympanic treatment of intractable unilateral Meniere disease: gentamicin or dexamethasone? A randomized controlled trial. Otolaryngol Head Neck Surg 2012;146(3):430–7.

85. ElBeltagy Y, Shafik A, Mahmoud A, et al. Intratympanic injection in Ménière's disease; symptomatic and audiovestibular; comparative, prospective randomized 1-year control study. Egypt J Otolaryngol 2012;28(3):171–83.

86. Patel M, Agarwal K, Arshad Q, et al. Intratympanic methylprednisolone versus gentamicin in patients with unilateral Ménière's disease: a randomised, double-blind, comparative effectiveness trial. Lancet 2016;388(10061):2753–62.

87. Sarafraz M, Saki N, Nikakhlagh S, et al. Comparison the efficacy of intratympanic injections of methylprednisolone and gentamicin to control vertigo in unilateral Ménière's disease. Biomed Pharmacol J 2015;8:705–9.

88. Bremer HG, van Rooy I, Pullens B, et al. Intratympanic gentamicin treatment for Ménière's disease: a randomized, double-blind, placebo-controlled trial on dose efficacy—results of a prematurely ended study. Trials 2014;15:328.

89. Chia SH, Gamst AC, Anderson JP, et al. Intratympanic gentamicin therapy for Ménière's disease: a meta-analysis. Otol Neurotol 2004;25(4):544–52.

90. Zwergal A, Feil K, Schniepp R, et al. Cerebellar dizziness and vertigo: etiologies, diagnostic assessment, and treatment. Semin Neurol 2020;40(1):87–96.

91. Stephen CD, Brizzi KT, Bouffard MA, et al. The comprehensive management of cerebellar ataxia in adults. Curr Treat Options Neurol 2019;21(03):9.

92. Strupp M, Teufel J, Zwergal A, et al. Aminopyridines for the treatment of neurologic disorders. Neurol Clin Pract 2017;7(01):65–76.

93. Kalla R, Strupp M. Aminopyridines and acetyl-DL-leucine: new therapies in cerebellar disorders. Curr Neuropharmacol 2019;17(01):7–13.

94. Schniepp R, Wuehr M, Neuhaeusser M, et al. 4-aminopyridine and cerebellar gait: a retrospective case series. J Neurol 2012;259(11):2491–3.

95. Strupp M, Schuler O, Krafczyk S, et al. Treatment of downbeat nystagmus with 3,4-diaminopyridine: a placebo-controlled study. Neurology 2003;61(02):165–70.

96. Kalla R, Spiegel R, Claassen J, et al. Comparison of 10-mg doses of 4-aminopyridine and 3,4-diaminopyridine for the treatment of downbeat nystagmus. J Neuroophthalmol 2011;31(04):320–5.

97. Claassen J, Spiegel R, Kalla R, et al. A randomised double-blind, cross-over trial of 4-aminopyridine for downbeat nystagmus– effects on slow phase eye velocity, postural stability, locomotion and symptoms. J Neurol Neurosurg Psychiatry 2013;84(12):1392–9.

98. Claassen J, Feil K, Bardins S, et al. Dalfampridine in patients with downbeat nystagmus–an observational study. J Neurol 2013;260(08):1992–6.

99. Feil K, Claaßen J, Bardins S, et al. Effect of chlorzoxazone in patients with downbeat nystagmus: a pilot trial. Neurology 2013 Sep 24;81(13):1152–8.

100. Strupp M, Teufel J, Habs M, et al. Effects of acetyl-DL-leucine in patients with cerebellar ataxia: a case series. J Neurol 2013;260(10):2556–61.

101. Schniepp R, Strupp M, Wuehr M, et al. Acetyl-DL-leucine improves gait variability in patients with cerebellar ataxia-a case series. Cerebellum Ataxias 2016;3:8.

102. Dieterich M, Straube A, Brandt T, et al. The effects of baclofen and cholinergic drugs on upbeat and downbeat nystagmus. J Neurol Neurosurg Psychiatry 1991;54:627–32.

103. Halmagyi GM, Rudge P, Gresty MA, et al. Treatment of periodic alternating nystagmus. Ann Neurol 1980;8:609–11.

104. Barton JJS, Huaman AG, Sharpe JA. Muscarinic antagonists in the treatment of acquired pendular and downbeat nystagmus: a double-blind, randomized trial of three intravenous drugs. Ann Neurol 1994;35:319–25.

105. Starck M, Albrecht H, Pöllmann W, et al. Acquired pendular nystagmus in multiple sclerosis: an examiner-blind cross-over treatment study of memantine and gabapentin. J Neurol 2010;257(3):322–7.

106. Gaul C, Diener HC, Danesch U, Migravent® Study Group. Improvement of migraine symptoms with a proprietary supplement containing riboflavin, magnesium and Q10: a randomized, placebo-controlled, double-blind, multicenter trial. J Headache Pain 2015;16:516.

107. Beh SC. Vestibular migraine: how to sort it out and what to do about it. J Neuroophthalmol 2019;39(2):208–19.

108. Neuhauser H, Radtke A, von Brevern M, et al. Zolmitriptan for treatment of migrainous vertigo: a placebo-controlled trial. Neurology 2003;60:882–3.

109. Bikhazi P, Jackson C, Ruckenstein MJ. Efficacy of antimigrainous therapy in the treatment of migraine associated dizziness. Am J Otol 1997;18:350–4.

110. Prakash S, Shah ND. Migrainous vertigo responsive to intravenous methylprednisolone: case reports. Headache 2009;49:1235–9.

111. Silberstein SD. Preventive migraine treatment. Continuum (Minneap Minn) 2015; 21(4 Headache):973–89.

112. Bisdorff AR. Management of vestibular migraine. Ther Adv Neurol Disord 2011; 4(3):183–91.

113. Maldonado Fernández M, Birdi JS, Irving GJ, et al. Pharmacological agents for the prevention of vestibular migraine. Cochrane Database Syst Rev 2015; 2015(6):CD010600.

114. Jackson JL, Cogbill E, Santana-Davila R, et al. A comparative effectiveness meta-analysis of drugs for the prophylaxis of migraine headache. PLoS One 2015;10:e0130733.

115. Lepcha A, Amalanathan S, Augustine AM, et al. Flunarizine in the prophylaxis of migrainous vertigo: a randomized controlled trial. Euro Arch Oto Rhino Laryngol 2014;271:2931–6.

116. Salviz M, Yuce T, Acar H, et al. Propranolol and venlafaxine for vestibular migraine prophylaxis: a randomized controlled trial. Laryngoscope 2016; 126(1):169–74.

117. Taghdiri F, Togha M, Jahromi SR, et al. Cinnarizine for the prophylaxis of migraine associated vertigo: a retrospective study. Spring 2014;3:231.

118. Teggi R, Colombo B, Gatti O, et al. Fixed combination of cinnarizine and dimenhydrinate in the prophylactic therapy of vestibular migraine: an observational study. Neurol Sci 2015;36(10):1869–73.

119. Liu YF, Macias D, Donaldson L, et al. Pharmacotherapy failure and progression to botulinum toxin injection in vestibular migraine. J Laryngol Otol 2020;134(7): 586–91.

120. Herd CP, Tomlinson CL, Rick C, et al. Cochrane systematic review and meta-analysis of botulinum toxin for the prevention of migraine. BMJ Open 2019;9: e027953.

121. Aurora SK, Dodick DW, Turkel CC, et al. OnabotulinumtoxinA for treatment of chronic migraine: results from the double-blind, randomized, placebo-controlled phase of the PREEMPT 1 trial. Cephalalgia 2010;30(7):793–803.

122. Diener HC, Dodick DW, Aurora SK, et al. OnabotulinumtoxinA for treatment of chronic migraine: results from the double-blind, randomized, placebo-controlled phase of the PREEMPT 2 trial. Cephalalgia 2010;30(7):804–14.

123. Agostoni EC, Barbanti P, Calabresi P, et al. Current and emerging evidence-based treatment options in chronic migraine: a narrative review. J Headache Pain 2019;20(1):92.

124. Sharon. Galcanezumab for Vestibular Migraine (NCT04417361). Available at: https://clinicaltrials.gov/ct2/show/NCT04417361. Accessed January 15, 2021.

125. Popkirov S, Stone J, Holle-Lee D. Treatment of Persistent Postural-Perceptual Dizziness (PPPD) and Related Disorders. Curr Treat Options Neurol 2018; 20(12):50.

126. Staab JP. Chronic subjective dizziness. Continuum (Minneap Minn) 2012;18(5): 1118–24.

127. Staab JP, Ruckenstein MJ, Solomon D, et al. Serotonin reuptake inhibitors for dizziness with psychiatric symptoms. Arch Otolaryngol Head Neck Surg 2002; 128(5):554–60.

128. Staab JP, Ruckenstein MJ, Amsterdam JD. A prospective trial of sertraline for chronic subjective dizziness. Laryngoscope 2004;114(9):1637–41.

129. Staab JP, Ruckenstein MJ. Chronic dizziness and anxiety: effect of course of illness on treatment outcome. Arch Otolaryngolheadneck Surg 2005;131(8): 675–9.

130. Horii A, Uno A, Kitahara T, et al. Effects of fluvoxamine on anxiety, depression, and subjective handicaps of chronic dizziness patients with or without neuro-otologic diseases. J Vestib Res 2007;17(1):1–8.

131. Staab JP. Clinical clues to a dizzying headache. J Vestib Res 2011;21(6): 331–40.

132. Staab JP, Eggers SD, Neff BA, et al. Vestibular migraine and persistent postural perceptual dizziness: results of a double-blind, parallel group, pharmacological dissection trial using verapamil and sertraline. Cephalgia 2015;35:65.

133. Hain T, Hanna P, Rheinberger M. Mal de debarquement. Arch Otolaryngol Head Neck Surg 1999;125:615–20.

134. Van Ombergen A, Van Rompaey V, Maes LK, et al. Mal de debarquement syndrome: a systematic review. J Neurol 2016;263:843–54.

135. Beh SC, Chiang HS, Sanderson C. The Interconnections of mal de Débarquement syndrome and vestibular migraine. Laryngoscope 2020;131(5):E1653–61.

136. Ghavami Y, Haidar YM, Ziai KN, et al. Management of mal de debarquement syndrome as vestibular migraines. Laryngoscope 2017;127(7):1670–5.

137. Canceri JM, Brown R, Watson SR, et al. Examination of current treatments and symptom management strategies used by patients with mal de debarquement syndrome. Front Neurol 2018;9:943.

Allergy, Immunotherapy, and Alternative Treatments for Dizziness

M. Jennifer Derebery, MD[a],*, Laura Christopher, MD[b]

KEYWORDS

- Dizziness • Allergy • Immunotherapy • Meniere disease
- Autoimmune inner ear disease

KEY POINTS

- Allergic reactions may result in central symptoms of dizziness.
- Most pharmacotherapies used to treat allergic rhinitis have limited benefit in treating those individuals with allergically induced or related dizziness.
- Allergy treatment using immunotherapy and elimination diet in patients with Meniere disease and allergy may improve their Meniere symptoms, including dizziness.
- Treatment of autoimmune inner ear disease may lead to improvements in dizzy symptoms and hearing stabilization.

INTRODUCTION

That dizziness might be a symptom of underlying allergy was first published in reference to Meniere disease (MD) in 1923.[1,2] Early articles were based on observations that patients with diagnosed allergy sometimes suffered seasonal exacerbation of their MD symptoms or in conjunction with other classic allergic rhinitis symptoms. Descriptions of allergic dizziness include chronic imbalance with or without accompanying brain fog, MD, vestibular migraines, and autoimmune inner ear disease (AIED). Vestibular migraine is covered elsewhere in this issue; the focus here is the role of allergy in chronic dizziness of MD and AIED.

PATHOPHYSIOLOGY

On allergic stimulation, tissue-bound mast cells and their counterpart, circulating basophils, release mediators within minutes (immediate-phase reaction) with a later phase some 2 to 4 hours later. Histamine, the primary immediate phase mediator, causes capillary dilatation and increased permeability to white blood cells, which

[a] House Ear Clinic and Institute, 2100 West Third Street, Los Angeles, CA 90057, USA; [b] Jackson Ear Clinic, 290 East Layfair Drive, Flowood, MS 39232, USA
* Corresponding author.
E-mail address: jderebery@houseclinic.com

Otolaryngol Clin N Am 54 (2021) 1057–1068
https://doi.org/10.1016/j.otc.2021.05.020
0030-6665/21/© 2021 Elsevier Inc. All rights reserved.

target and attack foreign bodies in the affected tissue. The late-phase reaction involves release of mediators and inflammatory cells including leukotrienes, tumor necrosis factor-α (TNF-α) prostaglandins, kinins, platelet-activating factor, cytokines, and chemokines. Increasingly, late-phase reactions are believed to be more important in the chronic symptoms of allergy and possibly in MD.

As foreign antigens bind to mucosal IgE-sensitized mast cells, several responses occur. Immediate-phase histamine-induced sensorineural stimulation leads to the familiar peripheral symptoms of allergy, including sneezing, nasal congestion, pruritis, bronchoconstriction, gastric acid secretion, and rhinorrhea.

Histamine additionally produces central effects. Histamine neurons are found in the tuberomammillary nuclei of the posterior hypothalamus, with extension into the cortex and medial forebrain bundle. Non–mast cell histamine is released in the brain, acting as a neurotransmitter with an increase in wakefulness/sleep prevention and a potent stimulant of cochlear blood flow.

The particular central or peripheral symptoms of allergy depend on which of four histamine receptor subtypes are bound. The organ of Corti, spiral ganglion, vestibular ganglion, vestibular sensory epithelium, and endolymphatic sac (ES) cells all show an immunofluorescent reaction to H_1, H_2, H_3, and H_4 receptors. Additionally, HRH_1 is found in the epithelial lining of the ES, and HRH_3 exclusively in the subepithelial capillary network.[3]

At the molecular level, and in animal models, the ES has been found capable of antigen recognition and processing for initiation of an immune response, including an allergic type I hypersensitivity reaction.[4–6] The pathogenesis of MD is unknown; however, one theory is that fluid disruption causes a hydropic distention of the ES.[7] The ES, responsible for a major part of the inner ear transepithelial ion transport, exhibits molecular mechanisms similar to the kidney collecting duct epithelia. Dysfunction of this transepithelial ion transport has been hypothesized as the reason that endolymphatic hydrops occurs in MD.

THERAPEUTIC OPTIONS

The most common options used to treat the symptoms of allergy include: avoidance of known or suspected allergens; antihistamines; injectable, intranasal, or oral steroids; leukotriene receptor antagonists; and allergy immunotherapy for desensitization (**Box 1**). Excepting first-generation antihistamines and oral or intratympanic (IT)

Box 1
Medications used to treat allergy-related dizziness

- First-generation antihistamines
  - Dimenhydrinate
  - Meclizine
  - Diphenhydramine
  - Promethazine
  - Cinnarizine

- Steroids
  - Oral
  - Intratympanic

- Leukotriene receptor antagonists (montelukast)

- Immunotherapy

steroids, the medications used to treat allergic rhinitis have little benefit in the treatment of allergically related dizziness and vertigo.

Most patients with any form of dizziness of labyrinthine or central origin are treated with some form of medication targeted toward allergy. The primary treatments of acute and chronic dizziness are vestibular suppressants, primarily benzodiazepams, anticholinergic agents, and antihistamines.

Because of ease of access, over-the-counter availability, and cost, the most commonly used vestibular suppressants are first-generation antihistamines, developed to treat the peripheral symptoms of allergy. These include dimenhydrinate (25–50 mg every 6 hours), meclizine (12.5–25 mg every 8 hours), or diphenhydramine (25–50 mg every 6 hours).

The exact mechanism of how antihistamines suppress vestibular symptoms is unknown. First-generation antihistamines cross the blood-brain and blood-labyrinthine barriers and bind to several neurotransmitter receptors, including histamine and muscarinic acetylcholine receptors, reducing the central allergic symptom of dizziness produced by H_1 binding.[8] Their ability to bind to these sites likely accounts for suppression of vertigo and nausea. All first-generation antihistamines also have anticholinergic activity; some argue that their antivertiginous property is caused by central anticholinergic actions, not H_1 effects.

The routine use of first-generation antihistamines for the peripheral symptoms of H_1 binding is limited, secondary to undesirable central side effects of sedation, urinary retention, and weight gain. They have been supplanted for this purpose by second-generation antihistamines, such as fexofenadine, cetirizine, and loratadine, which do not cross the blood-brain or blood-labyrinthine barriers. Although second-generation antihistamines are more useful clinically for the peripheral symptoms of allergy, they are ineffective for central symptoms, including dizziness.

Antihistamines as a class are notorious for the development of tolerance to their beneficial effect, making them of limited benefit in patients whose dizziness may be related to months-long pollen or mold antigens, or routinely for food-induced allergic dizziness secondary to chronic ingestion of undiagnosed dietary allergens. Vestibular suppressants, including first-generation antihistamines, should be used only to suppress acute vertiginous events. Their chronic use is undesirable, possibly suppressing central adaptation/compensation to vestibular loss and perpetuating symptoms of chronic imbalance.

Steroids, although non–Food and Drug Administration approved for vertigo, are often used orally or by IT injection for acute exacerbations of vertigo and/or hearing loss in MD and AIED. The action of steroids on the inner ear remains speculative, but may involve anti-inflammatory effects, immunosuppression, and/or ion homeostasis on the multiple glucocorticoid receptors in the vestibular and cochlear systems.[9] Oral steroids are often used as "rescue medications" for acute-onset hearing loss and fluctuation, or an exacerbation of underlying MD, and other symptoms including but not limited to chronic rhinosinusitis, food allergy–induced urticaria or angioedema, and asthma. Although nonotologic symptoms of allergy often improve with a short-term steroid burst, we find that the typical short-term treatment with low-dose steroids or a Medrol Dose Pak is less effective for vertigo control than a higher dose regimen of 1 mg/kg for a minimum of 5 days, tapered over a minimum of 5 days.

Although effective immunosuppressants, chronic oral steroid use is not recommended for treatment of peripheral or central symptoms of allergy. Their known side effects include hyperglycemia, osteoporosis, cataracts glaucoma, weight gain, steroid-induced psychosis, and potentially Cushing syndrome or adrenal insufficiency. Because of these limitations, steroids used for the labyrinthine exacerbations of dizziness or hearing loss are often given IT. The limitations of long-term or frequent use of IT steroids as a rescue treatment include the risk of a permanent perforation of the tympanic membrane; discomfort; reduced efficacy secondary to anatomic abnormalities, such as scarring over the round window; and general reluctance of most patients to have multiple injections through the tympanic membrane.

Intranasal steroids are commonly used in allergic rhinitis. The systemic bioavailability of most intranasal steroids is small, as low as 0.01%, and of limited benefit in the treatment of allergically induced vertigo.

The role of immunotherapy for treatment of dizziness is discussed later.

MENIERE DISEASE
Pathophysiology

Theories relating allergy to MD that center on inflammation within the ES have been described.[10] These include: (1) the ES's fenestrated blood supply allows potential antigen entry, mast cell degranulation, and inflammation; (2) circulating immune complexes entering ES circulation and the stria vascularis cause inflammation, increased permeability, and fluid balance disruption; and (3) occurrence of a viral antigen-allergic interaction. Virally induced histamine release can exacerbate allergic symptoms by damaging epithelial surfaces and trigger T-cell migration to the ES.[11] Another potential mediator involved in hydropic changes are leukotrienes. Takeda and colleagues[12] have shown that allergically sensitized guinea pigs develop endolymphatic hydrops when exposed to their relevant allergen. The timing of this development suggests a likely late-phase reaction. Pretreatment of the animals with a leukotriene receptor antagonist blocked the development of endolymphatic hydrops in the treated group, but not the control animals.[12] A double-blind, placebo-controlled pilot clinical trial is underway at our institution to assess possible effects of a leukotriene receptor antagonist (montelukast) on patients with MD who have diagnosed allergies.

We find that for significant central effects of allergy, including chronic dizziness and the vertigo associated with MD in patients who also have allergy, targeted allergic treatment using immunotherapy for confirmed inhalant allergies and elimination diets for food allergies gives effective and immunologically sound results.[13,14]

Evaluation

We have previously described how to select which patients with MD should undergo diagnostic testing for allergy.[15] Indicators are shown in **Box 2**.

Testing modalities include prick testing, intradermal, intradermal titration, intradermal dilutional provocative food testing, and in vitro. Given different opinions regarding

---

Box 2
Indications for allergy diagnostic testing

- A suggestive history, including a seasonal relationship of symptoms
- Presence of other symptoms suggesting allergy, such as rhinitis
- Bilateral symptoms in patients with MD
- Strong family history of allergy
- History of childhood allergy even if outgrown
- Production of MD symptoms shortly after exposure to a food or inhaled antigen

the relative sensitivity versus specificity of various tests, the reader is encouraged to perform her/his own review of the subject. The patient should be tested with inhalants and food antigens. We find that reactivity of patients with suspected inhalant allergic triggers to their MD symptoms is often low, in the range of 1/500 wt/vol of antigen. Because prick testing exhibits more specificity but less sensitivity than intradermal testing, we prefer the superiority of intradermal tests to diagnose more moderate allergic skin reactions, although abnormal electrocochleography changes have been reported from before to after prick testing in patients with MD.[16] Similar electrocochleography changes have been noted in MD patients with provocative food testing, nasal provocation with inhalant antigens, and prick testing.[17]

The reader is advised that the purpose of allergy testing is to objectively establish whether a patient is allergic to a particular allergen, not to infer that the amount of antigen producing a positive skin test directly relates to the severity of symptom production.

Derebery and Berliner[13] evaluated the effect of specific allergy immunotherapy and food elimination of suspected food allergens on 113 patients with allergy with MD. Those treated by desensitization and diet showed a significant improvement after treatment, in allergic rhinitis and Meniere symptoms. Patient ratings of frequency, severity, and interference with daily activities of their Meniere symptoms improved after allergy treatment, compared with ratings from the control group of untreated patients. Results indicated that patients with MD can show improvement in tinnitus and vertigo when receiving specific allergy therapy. Because this study used retrospective recall, a second prospective study was performed with 68 patients completing a questionnaire before allergy treatment and at an average of 23 months after treatment.[14] Severity of vertigo, tinnitus, and unsteadiness improved significantly, as did frequency of vertigo, frequency and interference of unsteadiness, and ratings on the American Academy of Otolaryngology–Head and Neck Surgery disability scale. Statistical analyses strongly suggested that improvements were independent of natural history and other medical treatment of MD received during the immunotherapy period.

A weakness of these and other studies is the lack of control groups receiving saline injections or given diets eliminating foods negative on testing. Patients with MD are understandably reluctant to commit to months of possible placebo injections.

AUTOIMMUNE INNER EAR DISEASE
Pathophysiology

AIED is defined as an organ-specific immunologic attack of the inner ear. The specific pathologic mechanism by which AIED causes symptoms is unknown. Temporal bones of patients with AIED show evidence of endolymphatic hydrops and immunoreactivity in the ES and duct, suggesting that these sites may be involved in the cause.[18]

Bilateral MD or delayed endolymphatic hydrops is by definition a form of AIED, but many patients first diagnosed with unilateral MD are not recognized as having AIED after the contralateral ear becomes affected, resulting in missing potential beneficial treatment options. Audiovestibular symptoms may also be present in a variety of systemic autoimmune diseases.[19] However, recent literature suggests that AIED is organ-specific, because only 15% to 30% of patients with AIED have other known autoimmune conditions. AIED should remain on the differential for dizzy patients without an autoimmune history, although concurrent autoimmune disease may increase suspicion of AIED. Knowledge regarding diagnosis and treatment of AIED is beneficial during the work-up of a dizzy patient.

Evaluation

Although classically described as progressive hearing loss responsive to corticosteroids, the reader is reminded that response to steroids regarding improved symptoms does not make an entity by default, autoimmune. It instead suggests there is an inflammatory component to the symptom, but not necessarily via an autoimmune response. The diagnosis of AIED may at times be difficult because it must be made clinically using pattern and timing of hearing loss, with no confirmatory diagnostic tests. It presents with rapidly progressive and ultimately bilateral sensorineural hearing loss (SNHL), accompanied by vestibular symptoms in 50% of patients, which may be the presenting symptom.[20] Factors used in the diagnosis are listed in **Box 3**.[21]

The search for an antigen-specific laboratory test revealed that sera from patients with AIED, MD, and sudden deafness reacted strongly with several inner ear antigens or proteins, the strongest being a 68-kDa protein.[22] The role of this protein, termed heat shock protein 70, is unknown, and is not specific for an AIED diagnosis.

AIED was initially described in European literature, with symptoms of bilateral profound deafness in addition to vestibulopathy.[23–25] **Box 4** is a more current list of clinical symptoms suggestive of AIED, as described by Harris.[25]

TREATMENT

AIED was initially described in European literature as inevitably ending in the symptoms of bilateral profound deafness in addition to vestibulopathy.[23–25] Although not the first to describe the entity, McCabe's work was notable in attempting to find interventional treatment to prevent the severe outcome. McCabe's initial treatment of AIED was high-dose steroid and cyclophosphamide.[24,25] Since his initial results, cyclophosphamide fell out of favor, whereas high-dose steroids remain the gold standard treatment. Prednisone (60 mg per day) is recommended for 1 month, with varying slow-tapering regimens. Hearing improvement may decline as steroids are tapered, and steroids are often continued at the lowest dose required to maintain stable hearing and balance. Additionally, IT steroids may be used as an adjunctive treatment option.

The negative side effect profile of long-term steroid use has been well-described, leading to a search for alternatives. The following steroid-sparing treatment options have been proposed for AIED and MD, the latter of which is believed to be a form of AIED if it does progress to bilaterality (**Box 5**).

The reader is directed to a more comprehensive discussion of some of these therapies next.

Box 3
Clinical symptoms suggestive of AIED

- Otherwise unexplained history
- Timing: loss occurs over weeks to months or bilateral sudden SNHL
- Presence of other known autoimmune disease, condition (15%–30% of patients)
- Response to corticosteroids
- Abnormal nonspecific immunologic laboratory test results (eg, ESR [erythrocyte sedimentation rate], ANA [anti-nuclear antibody])
- Antigen-specific laboratory tests

Box 4
Clinical symptoms suggestive of AIED

- Rapidly progressive bilateral SNHL
  - Bilateral sudden SNHL
- Rapidly progressive bilateral SNHL with systemic autoimmune disease
- Immune-mediated MD
- Bilateral MD
- Delayed contralateral endolymphatic hydrops
- Rapidly progressive bilateral SNHL with inflammatory disease
- Immune-mediated SNHL with discrete organ system disease (Cogan syndrome, Wegener granulomatosis, relapsing polychondritis)
- Nonimmune rapidly progressive SNHL (oxycodone, paraneoplastic syndrome)

Chemotherapeutic Agents

Studies have shown improved hearing and balance in patients with AIED and MD with methotrexate, with vertigo improvement rates ranging from 53% to 69%.[26–28] However, a large randomized, double-blind, placebo-controlled trial of methotrexate in AIED demonstrated no effectiveness in maintaining hearing improvement, and it has since not been recommended for treatment.[29] A recent retrospective review of a small number of patients did show improvement in vertigo in AIED patients treated with methotrexate.[30]

Box 5
Possible steroid-sparing treatments for AIED

- Methotrexate
- Azathioprine
- Etanercept
- Plasmapheresis
- Intravenous γ-globulin
- TNF-α blockers
- Hydroxychloroquine
- Allergy immunotherapy
- Other biologic agents
- Betahistine
- Diuretics
- Diet (low sodium, food allergy elimination diet)
- Migraine management, including dietary restrictions
- Antivirals
- Alternative treatments

Plasmapheresis

Plasmapheresis was proposed as a treatment option for AIED because of its well-documented benefits in other autoimmune diseases. Although some patients experience improved or stable hearing, there is no reported effect on balance.[31,32]

Biologics

Categories of biologics that have been tried as treatment of AIED include:

- TNF-α blockers (adalimumab, certolizumab, etanercept, golimumab, and infliximab)
- Monoclonal antibodies (rituximab)
- Interleukin-1 antagonist (anakinra)

Five TNF-α blockers approved by the Food and Drug Administration for systemic autoimmune disease, include infliximab, adalimumab, certolizumab, etanercept, and golimumab. A weekly IT injection of infliximab for 4 weeks showed some evidence for hearing stabilization.[33] IT golimumab in long-term steroid-dependent AIED patients allowed either significant decrease or discontinuation of steroid with stable hearing.[34]

Additional biologic agents studied for AIED treatment include rituximab and anakinra. A small open-label pilot study of intravenous infusion of rituximab in patients with AIED found that five of seven patients were able to maintain or improve hearing to that of steroid treatment levels after weaning from the steroids.[35]

A retrospective review of patients with AIED found that although hearing did not improve with the TNF-α blockers rituximab and adalimumab, some patients did experience improvement in vertigo, tinnitus, and fullness.[36]

Anakinra is an injectable interleukin-1 antagonist used in rheumatoid arthritis. It has been suggested that interleukin-1β is abnormally regulated in patients with steroid-resistant AIED.[37] A small clinical trial of anakinra in patients with steroid-unresponsive AIED found evidence of hearing improvement and reduced plasma levels of interleukin-1β, but no reported effect on dizziness.[38]

Most research on biologics in AIED focuses on hearing improvement and stability, seeking to prevent bilateral profound hearing loss. Many of these biologic agents show improvement in other audiovestibular symptoms including vertigo without substantial hearing improvement.[26,30,36]

For patients with AIED who have become steroid dependent, early referral to rheumatology is useful, because these patients will likely benefit from biologic medications in the future. Additional situations in which referral is appropriate include patients with rapidly progressive hearing loss, symptoms in an only-hearing ear, or systemic autoimmune diseases.

Alternative Treatments for Dizziness/Vertigo in Meniere Disease and Autoimmune Inner Ear Disease

Antivirals

Antivirals have been proposed as a treatment option in MD because of the potential relationship between herpes simplex virus–induced basophil degranulation and MD. A temporal bone study found viral particles in vestibular ganglion cells of MD patients, supporting a potential viral cause.[39] A prospective study showed hearing and balance improvement in 12 of 31 patients with MD treated with either acyclovir or famciclovir.[40] However, a randomized, double-blinded, placebo-controlled trial involving famciclovir showed reduced hearing fluctuations without significant effect on vertigo or dizziness.[41]

Homeopathic/alternatives

Many alternative or homeopathic treatments for dizziness associated with MD have been described, including salicylicum acidum, salicylicum natrum, nux vomica, Chenopodium, and Vertigoheel.[41] Herbal medications, including ginkgo biloba and ginger, are more commonly cited as alternative therapies for MD. Other alternative treatments recommended include: kava, lysine, manganese, vinpocetine, valerian, chamomile tea, garlic oil, and nystatin.[42,43] However, herbal and homeopathic treatments for MD have no large randomized controlled trials showing improvements; may have unwanted side effects; and interact with other medications, including anticoagulants.[42]

Tai chi, massage, meditation, acupuncture, and psychotherapy have been suggested to improve symptoms of MD, citing benefits in balance and stress reduction. Although these interventions may reduce patient anxiety and are not likely harmful, no evidence exists to support improvement of dizziness or MD symptoms in peer-reviewed literature.

SUMMARY

Allergic reactions may result in central symptoms of dizziness, including nonspecific chronic imbalance, MD, and AIED. Excepting first-generation antihistamines and short-term steroids, most pharmacotherapies used to treat allergic rhinitis have limited benefit in treating individuals with allergically induced or related dizziness. Allergy immunotherapy and/or an elimination diet for diagnosed food allergies have been found to be effective treatments. Individuals diagnosed with AIED, including bilateral MD, who have poor control of dizziness or vertigo, may require high-dose, long-term steroid treatment, immunotherapy, biologics, or immunomodulators for symptom control. Newer biologic agents require further research to determine their role in treatment. Homeopathic treatment, although not shown efficacious for treatment of vertigo or dizziness, may result in lessened patient anxiety.

MD has as a defining characteristic, the symptom of vertigo, and frequently includes dizziness and/or imbalance. AIED may present with vestibular symptoms in addition to hearing loss. Therefore, these diagnoses and delayed endolymphatic hydrops and systemic autoimmune conditions should be considered in the evaluation of a dizzy patient with associated hearing loss.

CLINICS CARE POINTS

- Allergic reactions may result in central symptoms of dizziness, including nonspecific chronic imbalance, Meniere disease, and AIED.

- Most pharmacotherapies used to treat allergic rhinitis have limited benefit in treating those individuals with allergically induced or related dizziness.

- Allergy immunotherapy and/or an elimination diet for diagnosed food allergies can be effective in reducing symptoms of dizziness in patients with test-confirmed allergy.

- Allergy testing establishes objectively whether a patient is allergic to a particular allergen. Do not infer that the strength of antigen producing a positive skin test directly relates to the severity of symptoms produced.

- Vestibular suppressants should be used only for acute vertiginous events. Chronic use can suppress central adaptation/compensation to vestibular loss, perpetuating symptoms of chronic imbalance.

- Treatment of AIED may lead to improvements in dizzy symptoms and hearing stabilization.

DISCLOSURES

The authors have received a grant from the House Ear Institute and the CURES foundation for a clinical trial of the use of montelukast in patients with allergy who also have been diagnosed with Meniere disease.

REFERENCES

1. Duke WW. Menière's syndrome caused by allergy. JAMA 1923;81:2179–82.
2. Espenshade TA, Browman KE, Bitner RS, et al. The histamine H_3 receptor: an attractive target for the treatment of cognitive disorders. Br J Pharma 2008;154: 1166–81.
3. Møller MN, Kirkeby S, Vikeså J. Expression of histamine receptors in the human endolymphatic sac: the molecular rationale for betahistine use in Menieres disease. Eur Arch Otorhinolaryngol 2016;273:1705–10.
4. Møller MN, Kirkeby S, Cayé-Thomasen P. Innate immune defense in the inner ear: mucines are expressed by the human endolymphatic sac. J Anat 2017;230: 297–302.
5. Møller MN, Kirkeby S, Vikesa J. Gene expression demonstrates an immunological capacity of the human endolymphatic sac. Laryngoscope 2015;125:E269–75.
6. Yan Z, Wang JB, Gong SS, et al. Cell proliferation in the endolymphatic sac in situ after the rat Waldeyer ring equivalent immunostimulation. Laryngoscope 2003; 113:1609–14.
7. Paparella MM, Djalilian HR. Etiology, pathophysiology of symptoms, and pathogenesis of Meniere's disease. Otolaryngol Clin N Am 2002;35:529–45.
8. Hain TC, Yacovino D. Pharmacologic treatment of persons with dizziness. Neurol Clin 2005;23:831–53.
9. Hamid M, Trune D. Issues, indications, and controversies regarding intratympanic steroid perfusion. Curr Opin Otolaryngol Head Neck Surg 2008;16:434–40.
10. Derebery MJ, Berliner KI. Allergy and its relation to Menière's disease. Otolaryngol Clin North Am 2010;43:1047–58.
11. Savastano M, Giacomelli L, Marioni G. Non-specific immunological determinations in Menière's disease: any role in clinical practice? Eur Arch Otorhinolaryngol 2007;264:15–9.
12. Takeda T, Takeda S, Egami N, et al. Type 1 allergy-induced endolymphatic hydrops and the suppressive effect of leukotriene receptor antagonist. Otol Neurotol 2012;33:886–90.
13. Derebery MJ, Berliner KI. Prevalence of allergy in Mèniére's disease. Otolaryngol Head Neck Surg 2000;123:69–75.
14. Derebery MJ, Berliner KI. Allergic management in Mèniére's disease: a prospective study. Presented at the American Academy of Otolaryngic Allergy Annual Meeting. Orlando (FL); September 19, 2003.
15. Derebery MJ. Allergic and immunologic features of Ménière's disease. Otolaryngol Clin N Am 2011;44:655–66.
16. Topuz B, Ogmen G, Ardiç FN, et al. Provocation of endolymphatic hydrops with a prick test in Meniere's disease. Adv Ther 2007;24:819–25.
17. Gibbs SR, Mabry RL, Roland PS, et al. Electrocochleographic changes after intranasal allergen challenge: a possible diagnostic tool in patients with Meniere's disease. Otolaryngol Head Neck Surg 1999;121:283–4.
18. Altermatt HJ, Gebbers JO, Müller C, et al. Human endolymphatic sac: evidence for a role in inner ear immune defense. ORL J Otorhinolaryngol Relat Spec 1990; 52:143–8.

19. Bovo R, Aimoni C, Martini A. Immune-mediated inner ear disease. Acta Otolaryngol 2006;126:1012–21.
20. Girasoli L, Cazzador D, Padoan R, et al. Update on vertigo in autoimmune disorders, from diagnosis to treatment. J Immunol Res 2018;2018:5072582.
21. Ghossaini SN, et al. Laryngoscope 2013;123:2840–4.
22. Boulassel MR, Deggouj N, Tomasi JP, et al. Inner ear autoantibodies and their targets in patients with autoimmune inner ear diseases. Acta Otolaryngol 2001;121: 28–34.
23. Lehnhardt E. Sudden hearing disorders occurring simultaneously or successively on both sides (German). Z Laryngol Rhinol Otol 1958;37:1–16.
24. McCabe BF. Autoimmune sensorineural hearing loss. Ann Otol Rhinol Laryngol 1979;88:585–9.
25. Harris J, et al. Otolaryngol Head Neck Surg 2002;396–407.
26. Sismanis A, Wise CM, Johnson GD. Methotrexate management of immune-mediated cochleovestibular disorders. Otolaryngol Head Neck Surg 1997;116: 146–52.
27. Matteson EL, Fabry DA, Facer GW, et al. Open trial of methotrexate as treatment for autoimmune hearing loss. Arthritis Rheum 2001;45:146–50.
28. Salley LH Jr, Grimm M, Sismanis A, et al. Methotrexate in the management of immune mediated cochleovesitibular disorders: clinical experience with 53 patients. J Rheumatol 2001;28:1037–40.
29. Harris JP, Weisman MH, Derebery JM, et al. Treatment of corticosteroid-responsive autoimmune inner ear disease with methotrexate: a randomized controlled trial. JAMA 2003;290:1875–83.
30. García-Berrocal JR, Ibáñez A, Rodríguez A, et al. Alternatives to systemic steroid therapy for refractory immune-mediated inner ear disease: a physiopathologic approach. Eur Arch Otorhinolaryngol 2006;263:977–82.
31. Luetje CM. Theoretical and practical implications for plasmapheresis in autoimmune inner ear disease. Laryngoscope 1989;99:1137–46.
32. Luetje CM, Berliner KI. Plasmapheresis in autoimmune inner ear disease: long-term follow-up. Am J Otol 1997;18:572–6.
33. Van Wijk F, Staecker H, Keithley E, et al. Local perfusion of the tumor necrosis factor alpha blocker infliximab to the inner ear improves autoimmune neurosensory hearing loss. Audiol Neurootol 2006;11:357–65.
34. Derebery MJ, Fisher LM, Voelker CC, et al. An open label study to evaluate the safety and efficacy of intratympanic golimumab therapy in patients with autoimmune inner ear disease. Otol Neurotol 2014;35:1515–21.
35. Cohen S, Roland P, Shoup A, et al. A pilot study of rituximab in immune-mediated inner ear disease. Audiol Neurootol 2011;16:214–21.
36. Matsuoka AJ, Harris JP. Autoimmune inner ear disease: a retrospective review of forty-seven patients. Audiol Neurootol 2013;18:228–39.
37. Pathak S, Goldofsky E, Vivas EX, et al. IL-1β is overexpressed and aberrantly regulated in corticosteroid nonresponders with autoimmune inner ear disease. J Immunol 2011;186:1870–9.
38. Vambutas A, Lesser M, Mullooly V, et al. Early efficacy trial of anakinra in corticosteroid-resistant autoimmune inner ear disease. J Clin Invest 2014;124: 4115–22.
39. Gacek RR. Ménière's disease is a viral neuropathy. ORL J Otorhinolaryngol Relat Spec 2009;71:78–86.
40. Gacek RR. Recovery of hearing in Meniere's disease after antiviral treatment. Am J Otolaryngol 2015;36:315–23.

41. Derebery MJ, Fisher LM, Iqbal Z. Randomized double-blinded, placebo-controlled trial of famciclovir for reduction of Meniere's disease symptoms. Otolaryngol Head Neck Surg 2004;131:877–84.

42. Sen P, Papesch M. Is there any evidence for complementary and alternative therapy in Menieres disease. Internet J Otorhinolaryngol 2004;4:1–6.

43. Available at: https://www.dizziness-and-balance.com/disorders/menieres/treatment/men_alt.html

New Frontiers in Managing the Dizzy Patient

Desi P. Schoo, MD, Bryan K. Ward, MD*

KEYWORDS

- Vestibular • Dizziness • Labyrinth • Perception • MRI • CT • Inner ear

KEY POINTS

- A common language for vestibular disorders and the symptoms they cause is being developed by the International Classification of Vestibular Disorders and will streamline communication, diagnosis, and progress in the understanding of vestibular disease.
- Virtual evaluation and management of patients with dizziness will continue, with new technology to remotely monitor eye movements. Ambulatory event monitoring of nystagmus will help clinicians diagnose patients with episodic dizziness.
- Similar to pure tone audiometry, perceptual threshold testing for vestibular sensation will become integrated into clinical practice at tertiary centers.
- Improved spatial resolution for both computed tomography and MRI will identify new vestibular disorders and help to understand better the pathophysiology of existing ones.
- Vestibular implants will enter clinical practice as a treatment of patients with bilateral vestibulopathy.

In the last 2 decades, a great progress has been seen in the understanding of the clinical management of patients presenting with dizziness or vertigo. The lifetime prevalence of dizziness has been estimated to be around 30%, with approximately 3% of adults experiencing dizziness in any year. True vertigo occurs much less often (21% and 1.4%, respectively). In the United States, dizziness accounts for 4 million visits to emergency departments per year.[1–3] Dizziness symptoms or signs are more prevalent with increasing age, have been found to increase the risk of falls,[4] and are associated with cognitive impairment,[5] 2 of the most debilitating and expensive health care conditions in society. These data emphasize the important public health aspects of vestibular disorders and the urgent need for better diagnosis and management. Despite progress, much remains poorly understood about vestibular pathophysiology and its management. The aim of this narrative review is to highlight key developments and research in vestibular disorders that are likely to be adopted in clinical practice in the next 20 years.

Department of Otolaryngology–Head and Neck Surgery, Johns Hopkins University School of Medicine, 601 North Caroline Street, Baltimore, MD 21287, USA
* Corresponding author.
E-mail address: bward15@jh.edu

Otolaryngol Clin N Am 54 (2021) 1069–1080
https://doi.org/10.1016/j.otc.2021.06.003
0030-6665/21/© 2021 Elsevier Inc. All rights reserved.

A COMMON LANGUAGE FOR DIZZINESS AND ASSOCIATED DISORDERS

The use of language is a fundamental problem for vestibular disorders. Most vestibular disorders do not have a clinical test capable of establishing a diagnosis. Instead, when deciding on a diagnosis, clinicians rely primarily on the symptoms that a patient reports. Terms such as "dizziness" or "vertigo" can have different meanings to patients and providers. Because vertigo occurs only when the vestibular system is not functioning properly, patients struggle to describe their new experiences, even as an adult. This challenge is magnified when clinicians define terms differently or when some common terms such as vertigo do not translate well across languages. Furthermore, research studies use different diagnostic terms to describe patient symptoms or diagnoses, some of which are specific to regions or medical centers.

The Bárány society, an international organization of neurologists, otolaryngologists, engineers, scientists, and rehabilitation specialists, has established the International Classification for Vestibular Disorders (ICVD) that aims to provide standard definitions of symptoms and signs of vestibular disorders and diagnostic criteria.[6] Already, diagnostic criteria have been updated for Ménière disease,[7] vestibular migraine,[8] bilateral vestibulopathy,[9] vestibular paroxysmia,[10] benign paroxysmal positional vertigo,[11] and mal de debarquement syndrome.[12] Diagnoses that have had different criteria depending on the academic medical center such as persistent postural perceptual dizziness (PPPD) have been combined under a single diagnostic term.[13] Some conditions such as presbyvestibulopathy,[14] a labyrinth analog to presbycusis in the cochlea, and orthostatic dizziness[15] are now established diagnoses. As the diagnostic and statistical manual for psychiatric disorders, the ICVD organizes a common language for physicians and specialists, allowing them to communicate better about patients and to establish rigorous definitions for making progress in research.

New diagnostic criteria are being published for vestibular migraine of childhood and superior semicircular canal dehiscence syndrome, with others such as motion sickness, acute unilateral vestibulopathy, perilymphatic fistula, and labyrinthine concussion under development. The published definitions will be updated regularly as the understanding of these disorders and their pathophysiology improves. Clear diagnostic criteria have also led to understanding that dizziness disorders are often not seen in isolation.[16] The ICVD diagnostic criteria are an essential foundation and will become even more integrated in the care of patients with dizziness.

REMOTELY MANAGING THE DIZZY PATIENT

Clinicians have rapidly adopted telehealth, driven by the infectious risk of severe acute respiratory syndrome coronavirus 2 (SARS-CoV-2) and by measures to relax regulations and support reimbursement for virtual clinical encounters.[17] For several years before SARS-CoV-2, the use of telehealth by otolaryngologists has increased.[18] Emergency providers and neurologists have worked together to provide virtual evaluations of dizzy patients in the emergency setting,[19,20] promising improved resource utilization.[21] During the SARS-CoV-2 pandemic, as many clinical medicine visits shifted to remote encounters, telehealth algorithms were developed and applied to outpatient visits for patients with dizziness.[22–24] Despite technical challenges related to software and network connectivity, patients and providers are satisfied with virtual visits, suggesting telehealth after SARS-CoV-2 is likely to continue at greater frequency than before the pandemic.[25]

Virtual visits are well suited to diagnoses such as vestibular disorders that are primarily based on patient symptoms and assessments of eye movements. However, we will need to develop algorithms to better triage patients for in-person visits.

Patients with chronic dizziness symptoms consistent with vestibular migraine or PPPD for instance may be appropriate for a telemedicine visit before in-person evaluation. Some patients with new, persistent dizziness, however, are having a stroke and require urgent in-person assessment. Improved access to physicians via telemedicine may lead to patients with an acute vestibular syndrome seeing an otolaryngologist before an emergency medicine provider. Virtual evaluations of an acutely dizzy patient require video adequate for assessing eye movements,[26] an examination important for separating central from peripheral pathology.[19,27] Fortunately, this examination is readily accessible in a virtual visit, and standards for remote assessments of a dizzy patient are being developed.[23,26] Management may be possible as well, with evidence that vestibular rehabilitation is effective via telehealth.[28] Although there are technical challenges to telehealth and virtual assessment of eye movements, these can be overcome with current technology.[24]

EVENT MONITORING FOR DIZZINESS EPISODES

Many patients with vestibular disorders do not experience episodes of vertigo or nystagmus when seen in the office. Patients may be encouraged to keep a diary of their episodes; however, these provide limited information to the clinician aside from the duration and presence of an episode of dizziness. In other fields in which patients have paroxysmal symptoms such as cardiac electrophysiology or epilepsy, event monitors record physiologic data during an event, sometimes transmitting these data remotely for interpretation. A similar approach has been applied to patients with dizziness,[29] in which patients were provided goggles that were donned during episodes to record nystagmus. The eye movements were later processed and interpreted.

Event monitoring in episodic dizziness has diagnostic value and can be used with commercially available technology. Wearable technology such as electronic watches and heart rate monitors are diagnosing cardiac arrhythmias.[30] There has been similar interest in using widely available smartphone technology for eye movement analysis for vestibular diagnoses.[31] Eye movement tracking using optical head-mounted displays is under development for commercial use. Similar to current partnerships with companies producing this technology for cardiac event monitoring, researchers could minimize barriers to development by collaborating with commercial developers.

QUANTIFYING VESTIBULAR PERCEPTION

Patients with vestibular disorders perceive dizziness or vertigo, yet there are no tests of vestibular perceptual thresholds used in the clinic. Tests of subjective visual vertical or horizontal are the closest to a currently available perceptual test. Patients align a bar with the assumed gravity vector or horizon. Although not widely used in clinical practice, the tests are shown to have promise for assessing otoconial organ function. Inexpensive versions have been developed.[32] The commonly performed vestibular assessments (rotary chair, caloric testing, video head impulse testing, and vestibular evoked myogenic potentials [VEMPs]) are physiologic tests that measure performance of reflex pathways from the vestibular organs. Although these tests have advanced the ability to diagnose patients with dizziness, reflex pathway testing correlates poorly with vestibular symptoms.[33,34] This disconnect, in addition to the appeal of developing tests of perceptual limits as those used in audiometry, has led to renewed interest in perceptual testing of the vestibular system.

During perceptual threshold testing for the vestibular system, patients are seated in a chair. Low-velocity, low-acceleration motions are delivered via a motorized moving platform, sled, or rotary chair(**Fig. 1**).[35–38] When the patient perceives motion, they signal the direction of movement. The semicircular canals and otoconial end organs can be tested using movements that are rotations (in the X "tilt-roll," Y "pitch," or Z "yaw" axes) or translations (in the X "surge," Y "heave," or Z "bob" planes). To the extent possible, patients are isolated from external visual, auditory, and somatosensory stimulation. The minimal perceptual threshold is found using the staircase method. Similar to assessing pure tone thresholds, at first the stimulus intensity is easily detected and then is decreased until the motion is imperceptible, at which point the intensity is increased again until a correct response is achieved, on which it reverses again. Current testing protocols are time consuming, taking up to 100 trials to find the perceptual threshold for each motion vector, thus limiting its clinical application.[39] A testing protocol using a 12-motion forced choice paradigm has recently been proposed as more suitable for clinical testing.[40]

Threshold testing can add perceptual information about vestibular performance that is direction and frequency specific. Higher thresholds have been observed in patients with bilateral vestibulopathy[41] and Ménière disease,[42] whereas patients with vestibular migraine have lower thresholds.[43] Importantly, thresholds seem stable when repeated, suggesting they can be followed over time.[44] Similar to vestibulo-ocular reflex and VEMP responses, perceptual responses seem to decrease with age starting in the fifth decade.[39] Clinical testing procedures are needed that balance thoroughness with the time constraints of a clinical encounter. Studies are also needed on a wider variety of vestibular disorders and the response of testing to treatment. Although perceptual thresholds might intuitively correlate with patient symptoms and risk of falls, this needs to be demonstrated. If perceptual threshold tests correlate with symptoms, they are likely to become more common in tertiary clinical centers in coming years.

SEEING PATHOLOGY OF THE INNER EAR WITH IMAGING

The labyrinth has been difficult to image because it is deep within the skull, tiny, and surrounded by a mixture of materials of different densities. Computed tomography (CT) provides vivid contrast between otic capsule bone and fluid or soft tissue structures, whereas MRI discriminates better among soft tissues of differing proton densities (ie, water density) and has potential for imaging the membranous labyrinth. CT and MRI will continue to be complementary techniques in the management of patients with dizziness. There have been new technological developments in both CT and MRI that are aiding the diagnosis of patients with dizziness and are likely to see greater adoption in clinical practice.

Flat-panel CT scanners use a cone-shaped beam of X rays and a sensor arranged in a flat panel. These scanners are widely used in dental offices and are being used to image the inner ear, with spatial resolution exceeding that of conventional helical temporal bone CT scanners (**Fig. 2**).[45] For the diagnosis of thin versus dehiscent bone over the superior semicircular canal, images from flat-panel scans correlate better with intraoperative findings.[46] These scanners are also useful for improving CT image quality of inner ear implants.[47,48] As flat-panel CT scanners become more widely used by otolaryngologists and neurologists, we will learn more about disorders affecting the bony labyrinth. Any bony dehiscence of the otic capsule likely contributes to symptoms of a third mobile window.[49] Patients with a dehiscence of other parts of the inner ear such as the posterior semicircular canal and cochlea, as well as patients with a presumed inner ear dehiscence, but without evidence of a dehiscence on conventional CT,[50] have been reported. CT images with higher spatial resolution will help

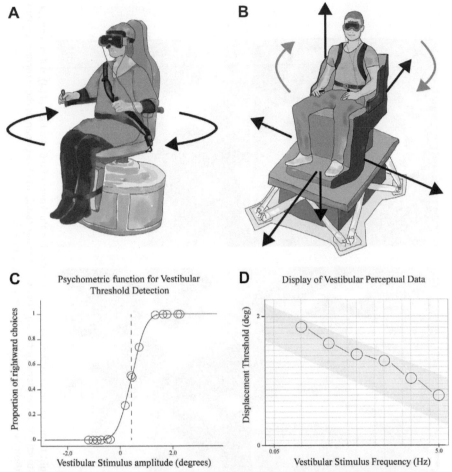

Fig. 1. Perceptual threshold testing. (*A*) Conventional rotary chairs could be adapted for threshold testing but with limited degrees of freedom. (*B*) A 6-degrees-of-freedom motion platform allows stimuli in any direction of translation or rotation. (*C*) Participants indicate the perceived direction of rotation for each stimulus, and psychometric functions are fitted to determine a perceptual threshold. (*D*) Thresholds can be measured for a variety of stimulus frequencies and plotted as a function of stimulus magnitude (amplitude, velocity, or acceleration), similar to pure tone audiometry.

clarify these disorders and whether patients with other dehiscences in otic capsule bone present differently than those with superior semicircular canal dehiscence syndrome.

MRI of the inner ear has advanced with the combination of 3 T clinical scanners, improved gradient technology, and new pulse sequences. Gadolinium-based contrast agents (GBCA) have been found to be taken up in the perilymphatic space, and not the endolymphatic space,[51,52] with a delay of approximately 4 hours following intravenous administration of GBCA[53] or 24 hours following transtympanic injection.[54] The differential uptake of gadolinium in the perilymph allows image contrast with the endolymph space, permitting assessments of the volume of endolymph, and this has been helpful in studies of Ménière disease, in which dilation of the endolymph space (ie,

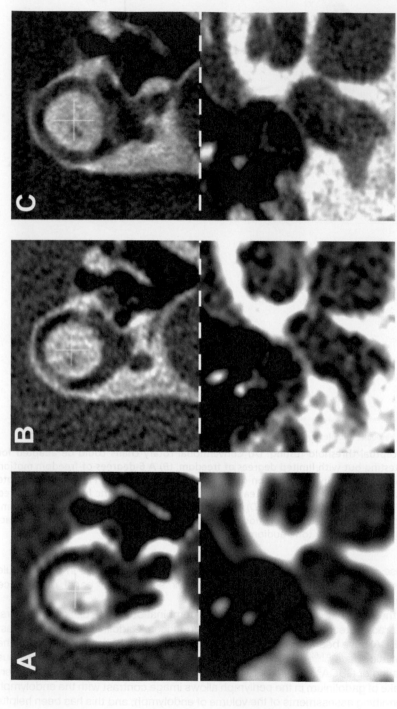

Fig. 2. Examples of high-resolution CT imaging of the right temporal bone in the same patient with slice thickness of 0.6 mm helical (*A*), 0.4 mm helical (*B*), and 0.1 mm flat panel (*C*). Upper panels show reconstructions in the plane of the superior semicircular canal, and lower panels show reconstructions in the plane of the stapes. In these images the only pathology is a dehiscence over the tegmen tympani.

endolymphatic hydrops) is common.[55] Thus far, the ability to see endolymphatic hydrops in vivo has revealed an association between the severity of endolymphatic hydrops and sensorineural hearing loss in patients with Ménière disease.[56] In patients with various disease states, some have observed enhancement earlier than expected or with greater signal intensity, leading to speculation that these observations reflect a leakiness of the blood-labyrinth barrier.[57] If GBCA were a marker of permeability of the blood-labyrinth barrier, these studies could improve understanding of inner ear pathophysiology. Improved gradient technology and higher strength static magnetic fields are likely to further increase spatial resolution, potentially allowing the diagnosis of several inner ear disorders that have been theoretic or identifiable only in postmortem specimens.

With increasing magnetic field strength, there is increased signal available for generating images with MRI, and there is interest in imaging the inner ear at 7 T.[58] Dizziness and vertigo are also common symptoms when people are exposed to strong MRI machines.[59] Without visual fixation, all healthy humans tested thus far have nystagmus in strong MRI machines and the sensation of dizziness and velocity of nystagmus scales with increasing magnetic field strength.[60] The strong static magnetic field of an MRI machine interacts with the natural ionic currents entering the hair cells of the utricle, causing a force in the endolymph (ie, a Lorentz force). This force displaces the cupulae of the superior and lateral semicircular canals, causing a sensation of vertigo and a persistent nystagmus the entire time someone is in a strong MRI machine.[61] As stronger MRI machines become more widely available, this strange effect on the inner ear will need to be mitigated. This mechanism may be a useful way to stimulate the inner ear, and there is evidence that the brain is learning to adapt to the stimulus while in the MRI,[62] suggesting a role for this effect in vestibular rehabilitation.

RESTORING VESTIBULAR SENSATION WITH A VESTIBULAR IMPLANT

Important advancements have been made in the development and implementation of vestibular implants (VI). Four research groups are currently conducting human clinical trials studying the effects of electrical vestibular stimulation on vestibular reflexes and balance function in patients with bilateral vestibulopathy.[63–67] These devices sense head motion and deliver electrical stimulation via electrodes placed surgically in the ampullae of the semicircular canals. Different device designs have been used, including unmodified cochlear implants, combined vestibulo-cochlear implants, and dedicated vestibular implants. The targeted end-organ, implantation techniques, and inclusion criteria have varied across studies. The outcomes from these early studies are promising, with important findings including the relative safety of implantation compared with other surgeries of the inner ear, the ability to drive electrically evoked vestibular responses (motion perception, vestibulo-ocular reflexes, vestibulo-cervical reflexes, and vestibulo-spinal reflexes), improvements in assessments of balance and gait, and patient tolerance of device use both in an acute and chronic setting.[63–66]

Although the existing collective experience supports great potential for this technology to provide relief to patients suffering from vestibular dysfunction, more work is needed to establish VI as a treatment. Recently, groups developing a VI published a joint statement about criteria for patient selection in future trials.[68] The investigators recommended a stricter requirement for determining candidacy than the definition of bilateral vestibulopathy proposed by the ICVD,[9] emphasizing the importance of defining severity of vestibular loss similar to assessments of auditory function. Similarly, electrophysiologic tests of the vestibular periphery would be helpful, and some evidence supports a vestibular microphonic similar to the cochlear microphonic that could be developed into an electrophysiological test.[69] As vestibular implants become incorporated into clinical practice, centers will need to develop resources to support implantation, electrode mapping, and vestibular rehabilitation.

SUMMARY

Although this review necessarily excludes unexpected developments, its aim is to highlight areas of current research that are likely to affect the diagnosis and management of the dizzy patient. Several diagnostic approaches are under development with immediate clinical applicability, as well as a technology in vestibular implants that is likely to transform the way otolaryngologists approach patients with dizziness.

CLINICS CARE POINTS

- Most diagnoses of vestibular disorders are based on symptoms. Clinical consensus diagnostic criteria have been developed by the International Classification of Vestibular Disorders and are currently available for most vestibular disorders.

- When evaluating a patient for acute vestibular syndrome via telemedicine, clinicians should be aware that patients presenting with a first episode of spinning vertigo, risk factors for vascular disease or advanced patient age are at increased risk of stroke and require evaluation in an emergency department.

- High resolution CT scans of the temporal bone have variable slice thickness. For small structures like the superior semicircular canal, scans with larger slice thickness can lead to partial volume averaging, leading to the appearance of an anatomic dehiscence when one may not be present.

DISCLOSURE

BW was supported by clinician-scientist awards from the American Otological Society and Johns Hopkins University School of Medicine, as well as K23DC018302.

REFERENCES

1. Newman-Toker DE, Hsieh Y-H, Camargo CA Jr, et al. Spectrum of dizziness visits to US emergency departments: cross-sectional analysis from a nationally representative sample. Mayo Clin Proc 2008;83(7):765–75.
2. Neuhauser HK, Radtke A, von Brevern M, et al. Burden of dizziness and vertigo in the community. Arch Intern Med 2008;168(19):2118–24.
3. Murdin L, Schilder AGM. Epidemiology of balance symptoms and disorders in the community: a systematic review. Otol Neurotol 2015;36(3):387–92.
4. Agrawal Y, Carey JP, Della Santina CC, et al. Disorders of balance and vestibular function in US adults: data from the National Health and Nutrition Examination Survey, 2001-2004. Arch Intern Med 2009;169(10):938–44.
5. Agrawal Y, Smith PF, Rosenberg PB. Vestibular impairment, cognitive decline and Alzheimer's disease: balancing the evidence. Aging Ment Health 2020;24(5): 705–8.
6. Bisdorff A, Von Brevern M, Lempert T, et al. Classification of vestibular symptoms: towards an international classification of vestibular disorders. J Vestib Res 2009; 19(1–2):1–13.

7. Lopez-Escamez JA, Carey J, Chung W-H, et al. Diagnostic criteria for Menière's disease. J Vestib Res 2015;25(1):1–7.
8. Lempert T, Olesen J, Furman J, et al. Vestibular migraine: diagnostic criteria. J Vestib Res 2012;22(4):167–72.
9. Strupp M, Kim JS, Murofushi T, et al. Bilateral vestibulopathy: Diagnostic criteria Consensus document of the Classification Committee of the Barany Society. J Vestib Res 2017;27(4):177–89.
10. Strupp M, Lopez-Escamez JA, Kim J-S, et al. Vestibular paroxysmia: Diagnostic criteria. J Vestib Res 2016;26(5–6):409–15.
11. Von Brevern M, Bertholon P, Brandt T, et al. Benign paroxysmal positional vertigo: diagnostic criteria. J Vestib Res 2015;25(3,4):105–17.
12. Cha Y-H, Baloh RW, Cho C, et al. Mal de débarquement syndrome diagnostic criteria: Consensus document of the Classification Committee of the Bárány Society. J Vestib Res 2020;30(5):285–93.
13. Staab JP, Eckhardt-Henn A, Horii A, et al. Diagnostic criteria for persistent postural-perceptual dizziness (PPPD): Consensus document of the committee for the classification of Vestibular Disorders of the Bárány Society. J Vestib Res 2017;27(4):191–208.
14. Agrawal Y, Van de Berg R, Wuyts F, et al. Presbyvestibulopathy: Diagnostic criteria Consensus document of the classification committee of the Bárány Society. J Vestib Res 2019;29(4):161–70.
15. Kim HA, Bisdorff A, Bronstein AM, et al. Hemodynamic orthostatic dizziness/vertigo: Diagnostic criteria. J Vestib Res 2019;29(2–3):45–56.
16. Zhu RT, Van Rompaey V, Ward BK, et al. The Interrelations Between Different Causes of Dizziness: A Conceptual Framework for Understanding Vestibular Disorders. Ann Otol Rhinol Laryngol 2019;128(9):869–78.
17. Keesara S, Jonas A, Schulman K. Covid-19 and Health Care's Digital Revolution. N Engl J Med 2020;382(23):e82.
18. Miller LE, Rathi VK, Kozin ED, et al. Telemedicine Services Provided to Medicare Beneficiaries by Otolaryngologists Between 2010 and 2018. JAMA Otolaryngol Head Neck Surg 2020;146(9):816–21.
19. Gold D, Tourkevich R, Shemesh A, et al. A Novel Tele-Dizzy Consultation Program in the Emergency Department Using Portable Video-Oculography to Improve Peripheral Vestibular and Stroke Diagnosis (S28.002). Neurology 2019;92(15 Supplement). Available at: https://n.neurology.org/content/92/15_Supplement/S28.002.abstract.
20. Müller-Barna P, Hubert ND, Bergner C, et al. TeleVertigo: Diagnosing Stroke in Acute Dizziness: A Telemedicine-Supported Approach. Stroke 2019;50(11):3293–8.
21. Newman-Toker DE, Saber Tehrani AS, Mantokoudis G, et al. Quantitative video-oculography to help diagnose stroke in acute vertigo and dizziness: toward an ECG for the eyes. Stroke 2013;44(4):1158–61.
22. Chari DA, Wu MJ, Crowson MG, et al. Telemedicine Algorithm for the Management of Dizzy Patients. Otolaryngol Head Neck Surg 2020;163(5):857–9.
23. Bertholon P, Thai-Van H, Bouccara D, et al. Guidelines of the French Society of Otorhinolaryngology (SFORL) for teleconsultation in patients with vertigo during the COVID-19 pandemic. Eur Ann Otorhinolaryngol Head Neck Dis 2020. https://doi.org/10.1016/j.anorl.2020.11.011.
24. Green KE, Pogson JM, Otero-Millan J, et al. Opinion and Special Articles: Remote Evaluation of Acute Vertigo: Strategies and Technological Considerations. Neurology 2021;96(1):34–8.

25. Ning AY, Cabrera CI, D'Anza B. Telemedicine in Otolaryngology: A Systematic Review of Image Quality, Diagnostic Concordance, and Patient and Provider Satisfaction. Ann Otol Rhinol Laryngol 2021;130(2):195–204.

26. Shaikh AG, Bronstein A, Carmona S, et al. Consensus on Virtual Management of Vestibular Disorders: Urgent Versus Expedited Care. Cerebellum 2020. https://doi.org/10.1007/s12311-020-01178-8.

27. Mantokoudis G, Gold DR, Newman-Toker DE. Video-Oculography in the Emergency Department: An "ECG" for the Eyes in the Acute Vestibular Syndrome. In: Shaikh A, Ghasia F, editors. Advances in translational neuroscience of eye movement disorders. Springer International Publishing; 2019. p. 283–307.

28. van Vugt VA, van der Wouden JC, Essery R, et al. Internet based vestibular rehabilitation with and without physiotherapy support for adults aged 50 and older with a chronic vestibular syndrome in general practice: three armed randomised controlled trial. BMJ 2019;367.

29. Young AS, Lechner C, Bradshaw AP, et al. Capturing acute vertigo: A vestibular event monitor. Neurology 2019;92(24):e2743–53.

30. Ip JE. Wearable Devices for Cardiac Rhythm Diagnosis and Management. JAMA 2019;321(4):337–8.

31. Parker TM, Farrell N, Otero-Millan J, et al. Proof of Concept for an "eyePhone" App to Measure Video Head Impulses. Digit Biomark 2021;5(1):1–8.

32. Celis-Aguilar E, Castro-Urquizo A, Mariscal-Castro J. Evaluation and interpretation of the bucket test in healthy individuals. Acta Otolaryngol 2018;138(5):458–62.

33. Patel M, Arshad Q, Roberts RE, et al. Chronic Symptoms After Vestibular Neuritis and the High-Velocity Vestibulo-Ocular Reflex. Otol Neurotol 2016;37(2):179–84.

34. Yip CW, Strupp M. The Dizziness Handicap Inventory does not correlate with vestibular function tests: a prospective study. J Neurol 2018;265(5):1210–8.

35. Grabherr L, Nicoucar K, Mast FW, et al. Vestibular thresholds for yaw rotation about an earth-vertical axis as a function of frequency. Exp Brain Res 2008;186(4):677–81.

36. Janssen M, Lauvenberg M, van der Ven W, et al. Perception Threshold for Tilt. Otol Neurotol 2011;32(5):818.

37. Chaudhuri SE, Merfeld DM. Signal detection theory and vestibular perception: III. Estimating unbiased fit parameters for psychometric functions. Exp Brain Res 2013;225(1):133–46.

38. Cousins S, Kaski D, Cutfield N, et al. Vestibular perception following acute unilateral vestibular lesions. PLoS One 2013;8(5):e61862.

39. Bermúdez Rey MC, Clark TK, Wang W, et al. Vestibular Perceptual Thresholds Increase above the Age of 40. Front Neurol 2016;7:162.

40. Dupuits B, Pleshkov M, Lucieer F, et al. A New and Faster Test to Assess Vestibular Perception. Front Neurol 2019;10:707.

41. Priesol AJ, Valko Y, Merfeld DM, et al. Motion Perception in Patients with Idiopathic Bilateral Vestibular Hypofunction. Otolaryngol Head Neck Surg 2014;150(6):1040–2.

42. Bremova T, Caushaj A, Ertl M, et al. Comparison of linear motion perception thresholds in vestibular migraine and Menière's disease. Eur Arch Otorhinolaryngol 2016;273(10):2931–9.

43. King S, Priesol AJ, Davidi SE, et al. Self-motion perception is sensitized in vestibular migraine: pathophysiologic and clinical implications. Sci Rep 2019;9(1):14323.

44. Lee TL, Shayman CS, Oh Y, et al. Reliability of Vestibular Perceptual Threshold Testing About the Yaw Axis. Ear Hear 2020;41(6):1772–4.

45. Piergallini L, Scola E, Tuscano B, et al. Flat-panel CT versus 128-slice CT in temporal bone imaging: Assessment of image quality and radiation dose. Eur J Radiol 2018;106:106–13.

46. Tunkel A, Carey JP, Pearl M. Flat Panel Computed Tomography in the Diagnosis of Superior Semicircular Canal Dehiscence Syndrome. Otol Neurotol 2019;40(2): 213–7.

47. Jiam NT, Jiradejvong P, Pearl MS, et al. The Effect of Round Window vs Cochleostomy Surgical Approaches on Cochlear Implant Electrode Position: A Flat-Panel Computed Tomography Study. JAMA Otolaryngol Head Neck Surg 2016; 142(9):873–80.

48. Hedjoudje A, Schoo DP, Ward BK, et al. Vestibular Implant Imaging. AJNR Am J Neuroradiol 2021;42(2):370–6.

49. Merchant SN, Rosowski JJ. Conductive hearing loss caused by third-window lesions of the inner ear. Otol Neurotol 2008;29(3):282–9.

50. Wackym PA, Wood SJ, Siker DA, et al. Otic capsule dehiscence syndrome: Superior semicircular canal dehiscence syndrome with no radiographically visible dehiscence. Ear Nose Throat J 2015;94(8):E8–24.

51. Counter SA, Bjelke B, Borg E, et al. Magnetic resonance imaging of the membranous labyrinth during in vivo gadolinium (Gd-DTPA-BMA) uptake in the normal and lesioned cochlea. Neuroreport 2000;11(18):3979–83.

52. Zou J, Zhang W, Poe D, et al. Differential passage of gadolinium through the mouse inner ear barriers evaluated with 4.7T MRI. Hearing Res 2010;259(1–2): 36–43.

53. Naganawa S, Komada T, Fukatsu H, et al. Observation of contrast enhancement in the cochlear fluid space of healthy subjects using a 3D-FLAIR sequence at 3 Tesla. Eur Radiol 2006;16(3):733–7.

54. Nakashima T, Naganawa S, Sugiura M, et al. Visualization of endolymphatic hydrops in patients with Meniere's disease. Laryngoscope 2007;117(3):415–20.

55. Rauch SD, Merchant SN, Thedinger BA. Meniere's syndrome and endolymphatic hydrops: double-blind temporal bone study. Ann Otol Rhinol Laryngol 1989; 98(11):873–83.

56. Zhang W, Hui L, Zhang B, et al. The Correlation Between Endolymphatic Hydrops and Clinical Features of Meniere Disease. Laryngoscope 2021;131(1):E144–50.

57. Song CI, Pogson JM, Andresen NS, et al. MRI with Gadolinium as a Measure of Blood-Labyrinth Barrier Integrity in Patients with Inner Ear Symptoms: A Scoping Review. Front Neurol 2021;12:746.

58. van Egmond SL, Visser F, Pameijer FA, et al. Ex vivo and in vivo imaging of the inner ear at 7 Tesla MRI. Otol Neurotol 2014;35(4):725–9.

59. Hansson B, Markenroth Bloch K, Owman T, et al. Subjectively reported effects experienced in an actively shielded 7T MRI: A large-scale study: Subjective effects in 7T MRI; Large-scale. J Magn Reson Imaging 2020;52(4):1265–76.

60. Roberts DC, Marcelli V, Gillen JS, et al. MRI magnetic field stimulates rotational sensors of the brain. Curr Biol 2011;21(19):1635–40.

61. Ward BK, Roberts DC, Otero-Millan J, et al. A decade of magnetic vestibular stimulation: from serendipity to physics to the clinic. J Neurophysiol 2019;121(6): 2013–9.

62. Jareonsettasin P, Otero-Millan J, Ward BK, et al. Multiple Time Courses of Vestibular Set-Point Adaptation Revealed by Sustained Magnetic Field Stimulation of the Labyrinth. Curr Biol 2016;26(10):1359–66.

63. Guinand N, van de Berg R, Cavuscens S, et al. Vestibular Implants: 8 Years of Experience with Electrical Stimulation of the Vestibular Nerve in 11 Patients with Bilateral Vestibular Loss. ORL J Otorhinolaryngol Relat Spec 2015;77(4): 227–40.

64. Boutros PJ, Schoo DP, Rahman M, et al. Continuous vestibular implant stimulation partially restores eye-stabilizing reflexes. JCI Insight 2019;4(22). https://doi.org/10.1172/jci.insight.128397.

65. Ramos Macias A, Ramos de Miguel A, Rodriguez Montesdeoca I, et al. Chronic Electrical Stimulation of the Otolith Organ: Preliminary Results in Humans with Bilateral Vestibulopathy and Sensorineural Hearing Loss. Audiol Neurootol 2020;25(1–2):79–90.

66. Rubinstein JT, Ling L, Nowack A, et al. Results From a Second-Generation Vestibular Implant in Human Subjects: Diagnosis May Impact Electrical Sensitivity of Vestibular Afferents. Otol Neurotol 2020;41(1):68–77.

67. Fornos AP, van de Berg R, Armand S, et al. Cervical myogenic potentials and controlled postural responses elicited by a prototype vestibular implant. J Neurol 2019;266(Suppl 1):33–41.

68. van de Berg R, Ramos A, van Rompaey V, et al. The vestibular implant: Opinion statement on implantation criteria for research. J Vestib Res 2020;30(3):213–23.

69. Pastras CJ, Curthoys IS, Brown DJ. In vivo recording of the vestibular microphonic in mammals. Hear Res 2017;354:38–47.

1. Publication Title	2. Publication Number	3. Filing Date
OTOLARYNGOLOGIC CLINICS OF NORTH AMERICA	466 – 550	9/18/2021

4. Issue Frequency	5. Number of Issues Published Annually	6. Annual Subscription Price
FEB, APR, JUN, AUG, OCT, DEC	6	$437.00

7. Complete Mailing Address of Known Office of Publication (Not printer) (Street, city, county, state, and ZIP+4®)

ELSEVIER INC.
230 Park Avenue, Suite 800
New York, NY 10169

Contact Person
Malathi Samayan

Telephone (Include area code)
91-44-4299-4507

8. Complete Mailing Address of Headquarters or General Business Office of Publisher (Not printer)

ELSEVIER INC.
230 Park Avenue, Suite 800
New York, NY 10169

9. Full Names and Complete Mailing Addresses of Publisher, Editor, and Managing Editor (Do not leave blank)

Publisher (Name and complete mailing address)

DOLORES MELONI, ELSEVIER INC.
1600 JOHN F KENNEDY BLVD. SUITE 1800
PHILADELPHIA, PA 19103-2899

Editor (Name and complete mailing address)

Stacy Eastman, ELSEVIER INC.
1600 JOHN F KENNEDY BLVD. SUITE 1800
PHILADELPHIA, PA 19103-2899

Managing Editor (Name and complete mailing address)

PATRICK MANLEY, ELSEVIER INC.
1600 JOHN F KENNEDY BLVD. SUITE 1800
PHILADELPHIA, PA 19103-2899

10. Owner (Do not leave blank. If the publication is owned by a corporation, give the name and address of the corporation immediately followed by the names and addresses of all stockholders owning or holding 1 percent or more of the total amount of stock. If not owned by a corporation, give the names and addresses of the individual owners. If owned by a partnership or other unincorporated firm, give its name and address as well as those of each individual owner. If the publication is published by a nonprofit organization, give its name and address.)

Full Name	Complete Mailing Address
WHOLLY OWNED SUBSIDIARY OF REED/ELSEVIER, US HOLDINGS	1600 JOHN F KENNEDY BLVD. SUITE 1800 PHILADELPHIA, PA 19103-2899

11. Known Bondholders, Mortgagees, and Other Security Holders Owning or Holding 1 Percent or More of Total Amount of Bonds, Mortgages, or Other Securities. If none, check box ► ☐ None

Full Name	Complete Mailing Address
N/A	

12. Tax Status (For completion by nonprofit organizations authorized to mail at nonprofit rates) (Check one)
The purpose, function, and nonprofit status of this organization and the exempt status for federal income tax purposes:
☒ Has Not Changed During Preceding 12 Months
☐ Has Changed During Preceding 12 Months (Publisher must submit explanation of change with this statement)

PS Form **3526**, July 2014 [Page 1 of 4 (see instructions page 4)] PSN: 7530-01-000-9831 PRIVACY NOTICE: See our privacy policy on www.usps.com.

13. Publication Title		14. Issue Date for Circulation Data Below
OTOLARYNGOLOGIC CLINICS OF NORTH AMERICA		JUNE 2021

15. Extent and Nature of Circulation			Average No. Copies Each Issue During Preceding 12 Months	No. Copies of Single Issue Published Nearest to Filing Date
a. Total Number of Copies (Net press run)			287	230
b. Paid Circulation (By Mail and Outside the Mail)	(1)	Mailed Outside-County Paid Subscriptions Stated on PS Form 3541 (Include paid distribution above nominal rate, advertiser's proof copies, and exchange copies)	144	113
	(2)	Mailed In-County Paid Subscriptions Stated on PS Form 3541 (Include paid distribution above nominal rate, advertiser's proof copies, and exchange copies)	0	0
	(3)	Paid Distribution Outside the Mails Including Sales Through Dealers and Carriers, Street Vendors, Counter Sales, and Other Paid Distribution Outside USPS®	101	69
	(4)	Paid Distribution by Other Classes of Mail Through the USPS (e.g. First-Class Mail®)	0	0
c. Total Paid Distribution (Sum of 15b (1), (2), (3), and (4))		►	245	182
d. Free or Nominal Rate Distribution (By Mail and Outside the Mail)	(1)	Free or Nominal Rate Outside-County Copies included on PS Form 3541	22	28
	(2)	Free or Nominal Rate In-County Copies Included on PS Form 3541	0	0
	(3)	Free or Nominal Rate Copies Mailed at Other Classes Through the USPS (e.g. First-Class Mail)	0	0
	(4)	Free or Nominal Rate Distribution Outside the Mail (Carriers or other means)	0	0
e. Total Free or Nominal Rate Distribution (Sum of 15d (1), (2), (3) and (4))		►	22	28
f. Total Distribution (Sum of 15c and 15e)		►	267	210
g. Copies not Distributed (See Instructions to Publishers #4 (page 43))		►	20	20
h. Total (Sum of 15f and g)		►	287	230
i. Percent Paid (15c divided by 15f times 100)		►	91.76%	86.66%

* If you are claiming electronic copies, go to line 16 on page 3. If you are not claiming electronic copies, skip to line 17 on page 3.

PS Form **3526**, July 2014 (Page 2 of 4)

16. Electronic Copy Circulation	Average No. Copies Each Issue During Preceding 12 Months	No. Copies of Single Issue Published Nearest to Filing Date
a. Paid Electronic Copies	►	
b. Total Paid Print Copies (Line 15c) + Paid Electronic Copies (Line 16a)	►	
c. Total Print Distribution (Line 15f) + Paid Electronic Copies (Line 16a)	►	
d. Percent Paid (Both Print & Electronic Copies) (16b divided by 16c × 100)	►	

☒ I certify that 50% of all my distributed copies (electronic and print) are paid above a nominal price.

17. Publication of Statement of Ownership

☒ If the publication is a general publication, publication of this statement is required. Will be printed in the October 2021 issue of this publication.   ☐ Publication not required.

18. Signature and Title of Editor, Publisher, Business Manager, or Owner

Malathi Samayan - Distribution Controller   *Malathi Samayan*   Date 9/18/2021

I certify that all information furnished on this form is true and complete. I understand that anyone who furnishes false or misleading information on this form or who omits material or information requested on the form may be subject to criminal sanctions (including fines and imprisonment) and/or civil sanctions (including civil penalties).

PS Form **3526**, July 2014 (Page 3 of 4)   PRIVACY NOTICE: See our privacy policy on www.usps.com

Moving?

Make sure your subscription moves with you!

To notify us of your new address, find your **Clinics Account Number** (located on your mailing label above your name), and contact customer service at:

Email: journalscustomerservice-usa@elsevier.com

800-654-2452 (subscribers in the U.S. & Canada)
314-447-8871 (subscribers outside of the U.S. & Canada)

Fax number: 314-447-8029

Elsevier Health Sciences Division
Subscription Customer Service
3251 Riverport Lane
Maryland Heights, MO 63043

ELSEVIER

Moving?

**Make sure your subscription
moves with you!**

To notify us of your new address, find your Clinics Account **Number** (located on your mailing label above your name), and contact customer service at:

Email: journalscustomerservice-usa@elsevier.com

800-654-2452 (subscribers in the U.S. & Canada)
314-447-8871 (subscribers outside of the U.S. & Canada)

Fax number: 314-447-8029

**Elsevier Health Sciences Division
Subscription Customer Service
3251 Riverport Lane
Maryland Heights, MO 63043**

*To ensure uninterrupted delivery of your subscription, please notify us at least 4 weeks in advance of move.

Printed and bound by CPI Group (UK) Ltd, Croydon, CR0 4YY

03/10/2024

01040307-0002